T0263287

The Liver and Renal Disease

Editor

DAVID BERNSTEIN

CLINICS IN LIVER DISEASE

www.liver.theclinics.com

Consulting Editor
NORMAN GITLIN

May 2022 • Volume 26 • Number 2

ELSEVIER

1600 John F. Kennedy Boulevard • Suite 1800 • Philadelphia, Pennsylvania, 19103-2899

http://www.theclinics.com

CLINICS IN LIVER DISEASE Volume 26, Number 2
May 2022 ISSN 1089-3261, ISBN-13: 978-0-323-89758-7

Editor: Kerry Holland
Developmental Editor: Ann Gielou M. Posedio

© **2022 Elsevier Inc. All rights reserved.**

This periodical and the individual contributions contained in it are protected under copyright by Elsevier, and the following terms and conditions apply to their use:

Photocopying

Single photocopies of single articles may be made for personal use as allowed by national copyright laws. Permission of the Publisher and payment of a fee is required for all other photocopying, including multiple or systematic copying, copying for advertising or promotional purposes, resale, and all forms of document delivery. Special rates are available for educational institutions that wish to make photocopies for non-profit educational classroom use. For information on how to seek permission visit www.elsevier.com/permissions or call: (+44) 1865 843830 (UK)/ (+1) 215 239 3804 (USA).

Derivative Works

Subscribers may reproduce tables of contents or prepare lists of articles including abstracts for internal circulation within their institutions. Permission of the Publisher is required for resale or distribution outside the institution. Permission of the Publisher is required for all other derivative works, including compilations and translations (please consult www.elsevier.com/permissions).

Electronic Storage or Usage

Permission of the Publisher is required to store or use electronically any material contained in this periodical, including any article or part of an article (please consult www.elsevier.com/permissions). Except as outlined above, no part of this publication may be reproduced, stored in a retrieval system or transmitted in any form or by any means, electronic, mechanical, photocopying, recording or otherwise, without prior written permission of the Publisher.

Notice

No responsibility is assumed by the Publisher for any injury and/or damage to persons or property as a matter of products liability, negligence or otherwise, or from any use or operation of any methods, products, instructions or ideas contained in the material herein. Because of rapid advances in the medical sciences, in particular, independent verification of diagnoses and drug dosages should be made.

Although all advertising material is expected to conform to ethical (medical) standards, inclusion in this publication does not constitute a guarantee or endorsement of the quality or value of such product or of the claims made of it by its manufacturer.

Clinics in Liver Disease (ISSN 1089-3261) is published quarterly by Elsevier Inc., 360 Park Avenue South, New York, NY 10010-1710. Months of issue are February, May, August, and November. Business and Editorial Offices: 1600 John F. Kennedy Blvd., Ste. 1800, Philadelphia, PA 19103-2899. Customer Service Office: 3251 Riverport Lane, Maryland Heights, MO 63043. Periodicals postage paid at New York, NY and additional mailing offices. Subscription prices are $329.00 per year (U.S. individuals), $100.00 per year (U.S. student/resident), $782.00 per year (U.S. institutions), $421.00 per year (international individuals), $200.00 per year (international student/resident), $813.00 per year (international instituitions), $382.00 per year (Canadian individuals), $100.00 per year (Canadian student/resident), and $813.00 per year (Canadian institutions). Foreign air speed delivery is included in all *Clinics* subscription prices. All prices are subject to change without notice. **POSTMASTER:** Send address changes to *Clinics in Liver Disease*, Elsevier Health Sciences Division, Subscription Customer Service, 3251 Riverport Lane, Maryland Heights, MO 63043. **Customer Service: Telephone: 1-800-654-2452 (U.S. and Canada); 314-447-8871 (outside U.S. and Canada). Fax: 314-447-8029. E-mail: journalscustomer service-usa@elsevier.com (for print support); journalsonlinesupport-usa@elsevier.com (for online support).**

Reprints. For copies of 100 or more of articles in this publication, please contact the Commercial Reprints Department, Elsevier Inc., 360 Park Avenue South, New York, NY 10010-1710. Tel.: 212-633-3874; Fax: 212-633-3820; E-mail: reprints@elsevier.com.

Clinics in Liver Disease is covered in *MEDLINE/PubMed (Index Medicus)*, Science Citation Index Expanded, Journal Citation Reports/Science Edition, and Current Contents/Clinical Medicine.

Contributors

CONSULTING EDITOR

NORMAN GITLIN, MD, FRCP (LONDON), FRCPE (EDINBURGH), FAASLD, FACP, FACG
Head of Hepatology, Southern California Liver Centers, San Clemente, California, USA

EDITOR

DAVID BERNSTEIN, MD, FAASLD, MACG, FACP, AGAF
Head, Liver Sub-Specialty Service Line, Vice Chair of Medicine for Clinical Trials, Chief, Division of Hepatology and Sandra Atlas Bass Center for Liver Diseases, Northwell Health, Professor of Medicine and Educational Sciences, Donald and Barbara Zucker School of Medicine at Hofstra/Northwell, Manhasset, New York, USA

AUTHORS

MEDHA AIRY, MD, MPH
Assistant Professor of Medicine, Selzman Kidney Institute, Baylor College of Medicine, Houston, Texas, USA

ZOHAIB BAGHA, MD
Hofstra University at Northwell Health, Manhasset, New York, USA

SEBASTIANO BUCCHERI, MD
Department of Internal Medicine, Donald and Barbara Zucker School of Medicine at Hofstra/Northwell, Northwell Health, Manhasset, New York, USA

ANDRES F. CARRION, MD
Division of Digestive Health and Liver Diseases, Department of Medicine, University of Miami Miller School of Medicine, Miami, Florida, USA

VINCENT CASINGAL, MD
Chief, Transplant Surgery, Atrium Health Wake Forest Baptist, Atrium Health-Carolinas Medical Center, Charlotte, North Carolina, USA

PRAMODH CHANUMOLU, MD
Fellow, Division of Nephrology, Department of Medicine, Icahn School of Medicine, New York, New York, USA

TIMEA CSAK, MD, PhD
Assistant Professor, Sandra Atlas Bass Center for Liver Diseases, Donald and Barbara Zucker School of Medicine at Hofstra/Northwell, Northwell Health, Manhasset, New York, USA

BEN L. DA, MD
Department of Internal Medicine, Division of Hepatology, Sandra Atlas Bass Center for Liver Diseases, North Shore University Hospital, Assistant Professor of Medicine, Donald and Barbara Zucker School of Medicine at Hofstra/Northwell, Northwell Health, Manhasset, New York, USA

PRIYA DESHPANDE, MD
Assistant Professor, Division of Nephrology, Department of Medicine, Icahn School of Medicine, New York, New York, USA

DOUGLAS DIETERICH, MD
Professor, Division of Liver Disease, Department of Medicine, Icahn School of Medicine, New York, New York, USA

ELLIOT I. GRODSTEIN, MD, FACS
Fellowship Director, Transplant Surgery Fellowship, Assistant Professor of Surgery, Donald and Barbara Zucker School of Medicine at Hofstra/Northwell, Northwell Health, Manhasset, New York, USA

RAJIV HEDA, MD
Department of Internal Medicine, Tulane University School of Medicine, New Orleans, Louisiana, USA

ALEXANDER J. KOVALIC, MD
Department of Internal Medicine, Division of Gastroenterology and Hepatology, Donald and Barbara Zucker School of Medicine at Hofstra/Northwell, Northwell Health, Hempstead, New York, USA

KARTHIK KOVVURU MD, FASN
Assistant Professor of Medicine, Department of Nephrology, Ochsner Health, New Orleans, Louisiana, USA; The University of Queensland/Ochsner Clinical School, Brisbane, Queensland, Australia

CHRISTIAN KUNTZEN, MD
Hofstra University at Northwell Health, Manhasset, New York, USA

DANIEL LIA, MD, MS
Northwell Northshore-LIJ Residency

PAUL MARTIN, MD
Division of Digestive Health and Liver Diseases, Department of Medicine, University of Miami Miller School of Medicine, Miami, Florida, USA

RAMON O. MINJARES, MD
Department of Internal Medicine, University of Miami Miller School of Medicine, Miami, Florida, USA

GAYATRI NAIR, MD
Assistant Professor of Medicine, Division of Kidney Disease and Hypertension, Donald and Barbara Zucker School of Medicine at Hofstra/Northwell, Hempstead, New York, USA

VINAY NAIR, DO
Associate Professor of Medicine and Surgery, Division of Kidney Disease and Hypertension, Donald and Barbara Zucker School of Medicine at Hofstra/Northwell, Hempstead, New York, USA

MAZEN NOUREDDIN, MD, MHSc
Department of Medicine, Karsh Division of Gastroenterology and Hepatology, Director, Cedars-Sinai Fatty Liver Program, Division of Digestive and Liver Diseases, Department of Medicine, Cedars-Sinai Medical Center, Comprehensive Transplant Center, Los Angeles, California, USA

REBECCA ROEDIGER, MD
Assistant Professor, Division of Liver Disease, Department of Medicine, Icahn School of Medicine, New York, New York, USA

HELBERT RONDON-BERRIOS, MD, MS
Associate Professor, Department of Medicine, Renal-Electrolyte Division, University of Pittsburgh School of Medicine, Pittsburgh, Pennsylvania, USA

MARK W. RUSSO, MD, MPH
Professor of Medicine, Chief, Division of Hepatology, Atrium Health Wake Forest Baptist, Atrium Health-Carolinas Medical Center, Charlotte, North Carolina, USA

SANJAYA K. SATAPATHY, MBBS, MD, DM, MS, FACG, AGAF, FASGE, FAASLD
Department of Internal Medicine, Division of Gastroenterology and Hepatology, Donald and Barbara Zucker School of Medicine at Hofstra/Northwell, Northwell Health, Hempstead, New York, USA; Medical Director, Liver Transplantation, Division of Hepatology, Sandra Atlas Bass Center for Liver Diseases, Professor of Medicine, Barbara and Zucker School of Medicine at Hofstra/Northwell, Northwell Health, Manhasset, New York, USA

PURVA SHARMA, MD
Assistant Professor of Medicine, Division of Kidney Disease and Hypertension, Director, The Glomerular Disease Center at Northwell Health, Donald and Barbara Zucker School of Medicine at Hofstra/Northwell, Great Neck, New York, USA

EMILY TRUONG, MD
Department of Medicine, Cedars-Sinai Medical Center, Los Angeles, California, USA

JUAN CARLOS Q. VELEZ MD, FASN
Professor of Medicine, Department of Nephrology, Ochsner Health, New Orleans, Louisiana, USA; Professor, The University of Queensland/Ochsner Clinical School, Brisbane, Queensland, Australia

Contents

Hyponatremia is the most common electrolyte disorder encountered in clinical practice, and it is a common complication of cirrhosis reflecting an increase in nonosmotic secretion of arginine vasopressin as a result of of the circulatory dysfunction that is characteristic of advanced liver disease. Hyponatremia in cirrhosis has been associated with poor clinical outcomes including increased risk of morbidity and mortality, poor quality of life, and heightened health care utilization. Despite this, the treatment of hyponatremia in cirrhosis remains challenging as conventional therapies such as fluid restriction are frequently ineffective. In this review, we discuss the epidemiology, clinical outcomes, pathogenesis, etiology, evaluation, and management of hyponatremia in cirrhosis.

Hepatorenal syndrome (HRS) is defined as a functional renal failure without major histologic changes in individuals with severe liver disease and it is associated with a high mortality rate. Renal hypoperfusion due to marked vasoconstriction as a result of complex circulatory dysfunction has been suggested to be the cornerstone of HRS. Splanchnic and peripheral arterial vasodilation and cirrhotic cardiomyopathy result in effective arterial hypovolemia and compensatory activation of vasoconstrictor mechanisms. The efficacy of current therapeutic strategies targeting this circulatory dysfunction is limited. Increasing evidence suggests a substantial role of systemic inflammation in HRS via either vascular or direct renal effects. Here we summarize the current understanding of HRS pathophysiology.

Hepatorenal syndrome (HRS) is a hemodynamically driven process mediated by renal dysregulation and inflammatory response. Albumin, antibiotics, and β-blockers are among therapies that have been studied in HRS prevention. There are no Food and Drug Administration–approved treatments for HRS although multiple liver societies have recommended terlipressin as first-line pharmacotherapy. Renal replacement therapy is the primary modality used to bridge to definitive therapy with orthotopic liver transplant or simultaneous liver-kidney transplant. Advances in our understanding of HRS pathophysiology and emerging therapeutic modalities are needed to change outcomes for this vulnerable population.

complemented with paracentesis. Peritoneal dialysis has not been widely used, but recent literature shows promising outcomes barring for publication bias. Albumin dialysis could be a lifesaving procedure for a carefully selected subgroup of patients with liver failure.

Rajiv Heda, Alexander J. Kovalic, and Sanjaya K. Satapathy

Renal function is intricately tied to Model for End-Stage Liver Disease score and overall prognosis among patients with cirrhosis. The estimation of glomerular filtration rate (GFR) and etiology of renal impairment are even more magnified among cirrhotic patients in the period surrounding liver transplantation. Novel biomarkers including cystatin C and urinary neutrophil gelatinase-associated lipocalin have been demonstrated to more accurately assess renal dysfunction and aid in the diagnosis of competing etiologies. Accurately identifying the severity and chronicity of renal dysfunction among transplant candidates is an imperative component with respect to stratifying patients toward simultaneous liver-kidney transplantation versus liver transplantation alone.

Mark W. Russo and Vincent Casingal

The number of patients presenting with cirrhosis with kidney injury and the potential need for SLKT is increasing. In 2017, standardized criteria were implemented to identify candidates for SLKT as well as criteria for prioritizing LTA recipients for kidney transplant if they developed kidney failure, which is referred to as the 'safety net rule.' Goal of the safety net rule is to provide a pathway that provides increased priority to LTA recipients with renal failure who may have previously undergone SLKT. This article reviews the pros and cons of the safety net rule for liver transplant recipients who develop ESRD.

Daniel Lia and Elliot I. Grodstein

The number of liver transplant candidates with concomitant renal disease has been steadily rising since the implementation of MELD-based allocation in 2002. Consequently, the number of simultaneous liver-kidney (SLK) transplants being performed each year has also increased. However, the establishment of well-defined criteria for when to choose SLK over liver transplant alone has lagged behind. The lack of clear guidelines has worsened an already large shortage of transplantable kidneys. This article further explores the rationale for and outlines the implementation of the SLK allocation policy.

The use of hepatitis C virus (HCV) -positive organs in HCV-negative recipients with posttransplant antiviral treatment has increasingly been studied since the introduction of new direct-acting antivirals. This article reviews existing experience in liver and kidney transplant. Fifteen studies with 218 HCV D+/R− liver transplants, with 182 from viremic donors, show a sustained viral response for 12 weeks (SVR12) rate of 99.5%. Nine studies involving 204 HCV donor-positive recipient-negative kidney transplant recipients had an SVR12 rate of 99.5%. Complications are infrequent. Preemptive treatment in kidney transplant of for only 4 weeks or even 4 days showed surprising success rates.

End-stage kidney disease (ESKD) after liver transplantation is associated with high morbidity and mortality. This increase in mortality can be offset by performing a kidney transplant at the time of the liver transplant in select cases. Accordingly, Margreiter and colleague; s performed the first simultaneous liver–kidney (SLK) transplant in 1983. The number of SLK transplants has increased by more than 300% since then. In 1990%, 1.7% of all liver transplants in the United States were SLK transplants which increased to 9.9% by 2016. This steep increase was likely due to the implementation of the model of end-stage liver disease (MELD) scoring system in 2002, which is heavily weighted by serum creatinine.

Improved survival after liver transplantation has led to an aging cohort of recipients at risk of renal dysfunction. The etiology of renal dysfunction is typically multifactorial; calcineurin inhibitors nephrotoxicity, pretransplant renal dysfunction, and perioperative acute kidney injury are important risk factors. Metabolic complications such as hypertension, diabetes mellitus, and metabolic-associated fatty liver disease also contribute to the development of renal disease. Most LT recipients will eventually develop some degree of renal dysfunction. Criteria to select candidates for simultaneous liver and kidney transplantation have been established. Both delayed introduction of CNIs and renal-sparing immunosuppressive regimens may reduce progression of renal dysfunction.

CLINICS IN LIVER DISEASE

SERIES OF RELATED INTEREST

Gastroenterology Clinics of North America
https://www.gastro.theclinics.com

THE CLINICS ARE AVAILABLE ONLINE!
Access your subscription at:
www.theclinics.com

CLINICS IN LIVER DISEASE

Preface

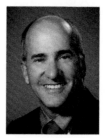

David Bernstein, MD, FAASLD, MACG, FACP, AGAF
Editor

The relationship between the kidney and the liver in disease is important for clinicians to recognize and understand. Liver disease, both mild and especially cirrhosis of any cause, can lead to the development of kidney disease. Chronic hepatitis B and C can lead to the development of significant glomerular disease. The presence of portal hypertension and ascites can lead to vasoconstriction of the renal vessels, causing hepatorenal syndrome, which can rapidly lead to renal failure and the need for renal replacement therapy. Formerly termed hepatorenal syndrome 1 and 2, this condition has recently been reclassified as hepatorenal–acute kidney injury and hepatorenal syndrome–chronic kidney disease. The pathophysiology, diagnosis, and management strategies, including new therapies, of both forms of the hepatorenal syndrome are discussed.

Nowhere is the special relationship between the kidney and the liver more prominent than in the consideration of kidney, liver, and combined liver-kidney transplantation. The advent of highly effective direct-acting antiviral therapies for the treatment of chronic hepatitis C has allowed the treatment of patients with chronic kidney disease stages 4 and 5. In addition, the effectiveness of these direct-acting antiviral therapies has allowed for the use of hepatitis C–positive organs in hepatitis C–negative recipients. The availability of these organs has significantly shortened kidney transplant waiting times for many patients. This important topic is elaborated on in this issue.

Kidney disease occurs in liver disease patients awaiting liver transplantation and may also develop de novo following liver transplantation. This issue discusses the management of kidney disease in patients awaiting liver transplantation and also discusses the indications for simultaneous liver-kidney transplantation. The causes and management of kidney disease that develops after liver transplantation are also covered.

This issue of *Clinics in Liver Disease* should be a useful reference for practitioners caring for patients with liver disease who develop kidney disorders. I would like to thank Dr Norman Gitlin for offering me the opportunity to serve as the editor for this

Clin Liver Dis 26 (2022) xiii–xiv
https://doi.org/10.1016/j.cld.2022.02.001
1089-3261/22/© 2022 Published by Elsevier Inc.

liver.theclinics.com

issue. I would also like to thank Kerry Holland and her staff for their tireless assistance in preparing the articles for publication.

David Bernstein, MD, FAASLD, MACG, FACP, AGAF
Chief, Division of Hepatology and Sandra Atlas Bass Center for Liver Diseases,
Northwell Health, Zucker School of Medicine at Hofstra/Northwell, 400 Community
Drive, Manhasset, NY 11030, USA

E-mail address:
dav31475@gmail.com

Hyponatremia in Cirrhosis

Helbert Rondon-Berrios, MD, MS[a],*, Juan Carlos Q. Velez, MD[b,c]

KEYWORDS

- Hyponatremia • Cirrhosis • Liver transplantation • Ascites • Albumin
- Arginine vasopressin • Osmotic demyelination syndrome
- Central pontine myelinolysis

KEY POINTS

- Hyponatremia is the most common electrolyte abnormality in cirrhosis, and it is associated with ominous outcomes.
- The most common type of hyponatremia in cirrhosis is mediated by an arginine vasopressin-dependent mechanism of water retention.
- Treatment of hyponatremia of cirrhosis should start with conservative measures including fluid restriction (FR), correction of hypokalemia, and discontinuation of diuretics.

INTRODUCTION

Hyponatremia, arbitrarily defined as a serum sodium concentration (SNa) of less than 130 mmol/L, is the most common electrolyte disorder and a well-known complication of cirrhosis.[1] Hyponatremia in cirrhosis is a predictor of poor outcomes, and its treatment remains challenging. In this review, we summarize the current understanding of the epidemiology, clinical outcomes, pathogenesis, etiology, evaluation, and management of hyponatremia in cirrhosis.

Epidemiology and Clinical Outcomes

The prevalence of hyponatremia in cirrhosis varies depending on the definition used and the population studied, ranging between 20% and 60%.[2–5] Hyponatremia is more likely to be present in more advanced stages of cirrhosis. As a result, the incidence of hyponatremia among patients hospitalized with decompensated cirrhosis is much higher than what is observed in the outpatient setting. Hyponatremia has been found in 15%–20% and 30%–40% of those with Child-Pugh class B and class C, respectively.[2,3] Similarly, hyponatremia is strongly associated with severity of liver disease (odds ratio for Model for End-Stage Liver Disease [MELD] >16 = 7.84).[5]

[a] Department of Medicine, Renal-Electrolyte Division, University of Pittsburgh School of Medicine, 3550 Terrace Street, A915 Scaife Hall, Pittsburgh, PA 15261, USA; [b] Department of Nephrology, Ochsner Health, 1514 Jefferson Highway, Clinic Tower 5th, Floor, Room 5E328, New Orleans, LA 70121, USA; [c] Ochsner Clinical School/The University of Queensland, Brisbane, Queensland, Australia
* Corresponding author.
E-mail address: rondonberriosh@upmc.edu
Twitter: @NephroMD (H.R.-B.); @VelezNephHepato (J.C.Q.V.)

Clin Liver Dis 26 (2022) 149–164
https://doi.org/10.1016/j.cld.2022.01.001
1089-3261/22/© 2022 Elsevier Inc. All rights reserved.

Furthermore, among those affected with hepatorenal syndrome type 1 (HRS-1), an ominous form of acute kidney injury in advanced cirrhosis, hyponatremia is virtually universal and may be used as a clue to point toward HRS-1 diagnosis.[6]

Hyponatremia in cirrhosis has been associated with important clinical outcomes including increased mortality and increase risk of cirrhotic complications as well as reduced quality of life and increased health care burden (**Fig. 1**).

Mortality

It has long been recognized that hyponatremia in cirrhosis is a predictor of mortality.[7] An analysis of a registry of 6796 patients awaiting liver transplant estimated a 5% increase in the risk of death (HR = 1.05; 95% CI: 1.03–1.08; $P < .001$) per unit decrease in SNa for SNa levels between 125 and 140 mmol/L.[8] In 2002, allocation for deceased donor livers in the United States changed to a "sickest first" policy, with priority based on a MELD score.[9] Several single-center retrospective studies have shown that the addition of SNa to MELD score (MELD-Na) significantly increases the accuracy to predict mortality.[10] It is estimated that the use of MELD-Na scores could have averted 7% of deaths in patients awaiting liver transplant.[8] These findings led to the United Network for Organ Sharing to incorporate SNa in the calculation of the MELD score for organ allocation in 2016.[11]

Cirrhosis Complications

Hyponatremia has been implicated in the pathogenesis of hepatic encephalopathy (HE). A study of 997 patients demonstrated a higher frequency of HE episodes within a 4-week period with decreasing baseline SNa levels (HE in 15%, 24%, and 38% in patients with baseline SNa >135, 131–135, and ≤130 mmol/L, respectively).[2] In

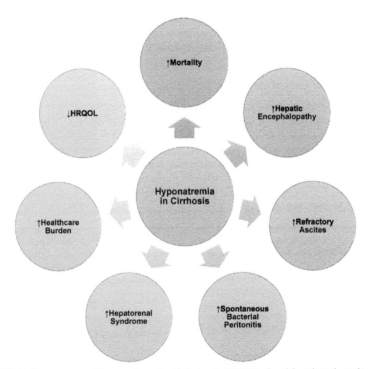

Fig. 1. Clinical outcomes of hyponatremia of cirrhosis. HRQOL, health-related quality of life.

another study of 61 patients with cirrhosis, hyponatremia was found to be an independent predictor of overt HE (OR = 10.5, 95% CI: 5.44–20.30, P < .001).[12] The relationship between hyponatremia and HE could be explained by brain adaptation to hyponatremia. Reduction in plasma tonicity causes water movement into brain cells, specifically astrocytes, which adapt to acute swelling by releasing solutes to the extracellular space. Initially, electrolytes (potassium and chloride ions) are lost, but further cell volume reduction is achieved by the loss of organic osmolytes such as glutamate, glutamine, and myo-inositol (MI).[13]

HE similarly reflects the manifestations of a low-grade cerebral edema without clinically overt increase in intracranial pressure.[14] Ammonia is exclusively metabolized in astrocytes by glutamine synthase, which converts ammonia and glutamate into glutamine. It has been hypothesized that glutamine contributes to the pathogenesis of HE, at least in part, by acting as an osmolyte causing water translocation and astrocyte swelling.[15] Consistent with this, proton magnetic resonance spectroscopy has noted a reduction of MI signal in the brain of cirrhotic patients confirming an osmotic adaptation.[16] Under conditions of low-grade cerebral edema associated with HE where MI stores for counteraction of cell swelling are largely depleted, hyponatremia may act as a second osmotic hit resulting in overt HE.[12]

Hyponatremia has been associated with refractory ascites with higher incidences observed at more severe degrees of hyponatremia.[2] In a retrospective study of 188 hospitalized patients with cirrhosis, patients with hyponatremia had a significant risk of developing ascites (OR = 2.708, 95% CI: 1.034–7.092, P = .043).[3] In addition, hyponatremia has been linked to greater ascitic fluid accumulation, greater likelihood of undergoing paracentesis, greater requirement for large volume paracentesis, and shorter time interval between paracentesis[2] and decreased sensitivity to diuretics.[17] Hyponatremia is also an important predictor for spontaneous bacterial peritonitis (SBP).[2,3]

HRS-1 is more common in patients with hyponatremia and ascites (OR = 3.45, 95% CI: 2.04–5.82 for patients with SNa of 130 mmol/L or lower).[2] A prospective study of 234 cirrhotic patients with ascites followed more than 5 years demonstrated that SNa of 133 mmol/L or lower was strongly predictive of HRS-1.[18]

In addition, hyponatremia may also have an impact on health-related quality of life and health care burden in patients with cirrhosis.[19,20]

Post Liver Transplant Outcomes

Early European studies demonstrated an association between pre-liver transplant (pre-LT) hyponatremia and increased post-liver transplant (post-LT) mortality and complications.[4,21] A single-center retrospective study of 241 patients with cirrhosis in Spain showed that patients with pre-LT hyponatremia had a higher post-LT 90-day mortality than patients with pre-LT normonatremia after adjusting for cofounders (84% vs 95%, respectively, P < .05).[4] In addition, patients with pre-LT hyponatremia had a greater risk of postoperative complications. In a multicenter study based on a registry of 5152 liver transplant recipients from the United Kingdom and Ireland, patients with pre-LT hyponatremia had a greater adjusted risk of post-LT 90-day mortality than pre-LT normonatremic patients (HR = 1.55, 95% CI: 1.18–2.04; P < .002).[21] However, cofounders could have affected the findings of the above studies.[22] More recent and larger studies have not confirmed these initial findings.[23]

PATHOGENESIS

The development of portal hypertension is the cornerstone of the pathogenesis of hyponatremia in individuals with cirrhosis. Increase in hydraulic pressure in the hepatic sinusoids resulting from liver fibrosis translates into increases in portal vein pressure. This phenomenon results in the development of ascites.[24] As a consequence of the increased intrahepatic sinusoidal pressure, vasodilators are released, specifically nitric oxide and prostaglandins.[25] These vasodilators exert their effects in peripheral vascular beds. Thus, splanchnic arterial vasodilatation ensues leading to pooling of blood, decrease in systemic vascular resistance, and compensatory increase in cardiac output, that is, hyperdynamic circulation. Early on, this adaptation maintains systemic arterial blood pressure. However, at advanced stages, this adaptive mechanism becomes insufficient, and the mean arterial pressure starts to decrease. This cascade of events leads to a reduction in effective arterial blood volume (EABV).[26] Baroreceptors localized in the carotid sinus, aortic arch, and other areas sense the decrease in EABV and activate the Sympathetic Nervous System (SNS). The renin-angiotensin-aldosterone system (RAAS) is also activated by two related mechanisms: (1) β-adrenergic receptor stimulation originated by the activated SNS leads to renin release; (2) decrease in EABV leads to decrease in kidney perfusion, decrease in glomerular filtration rate (GFR), decrease in the delivery of filtered chloride to the macula densa, activation of prostaglandins, and renin release. Renin is responsible for the cleavage of angiotensinogen into angiotensin I which is further converted into angiotensin II. In turn, the activation of the SNS and RAAS induces an increase in sodium and water retention in the kidney (**Fig. 2**).

Independently of the activation of the SNS and the RAAS, baroreceptor stimulation by low EABV signals to the hypothalamus via afferent sympathetic nerves to induce nonosmotic synthesis and release of Arginine Vasopressin (AVP).[27] The net result of avid reabsorption of water mediated by AVP is hyponatremia.

Although the hyponatremia of cirrhosis is primarily dilutional, there are data suggesting it might also be a function of potassium deficiency.[28] Edelman empirically showed that the SNa is determined by the ratio between total body exchangeable sodium and potassium and total body water[29] with changes in potassium mass balance leading to

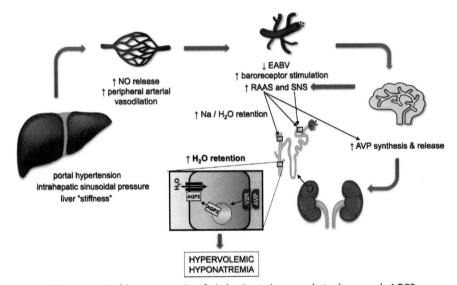

Fig. 2. Pathogenesis of hyponatremia of cirrhosis. ↑, increased; ↓, decreased; AQP2, aquaporin 2; AVP, arginine vasopressin; EABV, effective arterial blood volume; H_2O, water; Na, sodium; NO, nitric oxide; RAAS, renin-angiotensin-aldosterone system; SNS, sympathetic nervous system; V2R, vasopressin 2 receptor.

hyponatremia or its correction.[30] Potassium deficiency could be originated from renal or gastrointestinal losses (see Etiology).

ETIOLOGY
Cirrhosis Itself

Most cases of hyponatremia in cirrhosis encountered in clinical grounds are AVP-dependent (**Fig. 3**). As described earlier, sequential development of cirrhosis, portal hypertension, hyperdynamic circulation, and decrease in EABV lead to adaptive AVP release. Thus, progressive worsening of cirrhosis and portal hypertension is a sufficient factor on its own to cause hyponatremia.

Gastrointestinal Fluid Losses

Another cause of hyponatremia relates to causes of hypovolemic hyponatremia. This category includes scenarios triggered by fluid losses as the primary insult. However, it is the adaptive release of AVP secondary to the decrease in EABV that which ultimately drives the hyponatremia, rather than the sodium depletion itself. Prophylaxis for HE with oral lactulose is commonly used in cirrhosis. Lactulose can cause profuse diarrhea, volume depletion, and lead to clinical presentation with hyponatremia.

Renal Sodium Losses

Diuretic therapy is commonly used to manage ascites in patients with cirrhosis. Loop diuretics are unlikely to cause hyponatremia because blockade of the Na^+-K^+-$2Cl^-$ cotransporter by them leads to the reduction in the renal medullary interstitial tonicity necessary for water reabsorption. However, aldosterone receptor antagonists, such as spironolactone, do not perturb the renal medullary tonicity. Furthermore, they block Na reabsorption in the collecting duct and can potentially lead to significant urinary loss of Na, hypovolemia, and exacerbation in AVP release and water retention.[31]

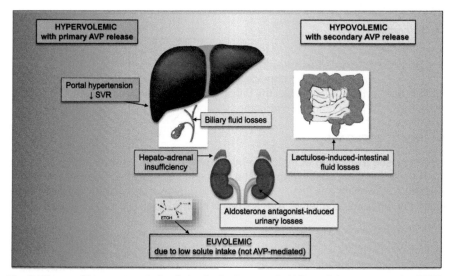

Fig. 3. Cause of hyponatremia in cirrhosis. ↓, decreased; AVP, arginine vasopressin; ETOH, ethanol; SVR, systemic vascular resistance.

Adrenal Insufficiency

The prevalence of adrenal insufficiency in cirrhosis has been reported to be increased, with a prevalence of up to 49%.[32] Thus, the term hepatoadrenal insufficiency has been proposed.[33] Under physiologic conditions, cortisol inhibits AVP release in the hypothalamus. Thus, cortisol deficiency, as seen in adrenal insufficiency, leads to unopposed AVP release. Because AVP release is already augmented in the context of cirrhosis, it might be difficult to ascertain clinically to what extent adrenal insufficiency may contribute to hyponatremia. Supporting a contributing role of adrenal insufficiency, hyponatremia was found to be present in 42% of patients with cirrhosis and adrenal insufficiency compared with only 17% in those without adrenal insufficiency.[32]

Terlipressin

Terlipressin is a vasopressin analogue with greater affinity for the V2 receptor (VR) than that for the V1a receptor. Thus, it can mimic the actions of AVP in the renal collecting duct. Terlipressin is currently used as a vasoconstrictor for the treatment of HRS-1 and acute variceal bleeding in Europe, Asia, and some countries in Latin America, but it is not approved in North America. In a retrospective study of 44 patients treated with terlipressin for acute variceal bleeding, a mean decrease in SNa of 11 mmol/L was observed.[34] In a larger multicenter cohort of patients treated with terlipressin for acute gastrointestinal bleeding, hyponatremia and severe hyponatremia (<125 mmol/L) were present in 26% and 13%, respectively.[35] Notably, in a recent randomized placebo-controlled trial testing the use of terlipressin for HRS-1 in North America (CONFIRM trial), hyponatremia was not reported to be more common in terlipressin-treated subjects.[36]

Low Solute Intake

Individuals with alcoholic cirrhosis may also present with hyponatremia after a period of heavy intake of alcoholic beverages coupled with low solute intake, as seen in beer potomania.[37] In these cases, AVP release is not stimulated. Importantly, complex cases of chronic high AVP state combined with low solute intake may be encountered and may represent a therapeutic challenge.

Pseudohyponatremia

Obstructive cholestasis can be associated with substantial increase in total cholesterol and lipoprotein X. This rare phenomenon has also been described in primary biliary cirrhosis and should be considered in cases of unexplained hyponatremia.[38] The lipid layer artificially increases the denominator in SNa estimate. Sodium determination by direct potentiometry overcomes this problem.

DIAGNOSTIC APPROACH

The diagnostic evaluation of hyponatremia in patients with cirrhosis is similar to the one in the general population (**Fig. 4**). The main goals are to determine whether hyponatremia is hypotonic, and if so, whether hypotonic hyponatremia is mediated by AVP, and in this latter case, whether AVP secretion is physiologically appropriate.[39]

Is the Hyponatremia Hypotonic?

A serum osmolality (SOsm) of less than 275 mOsm/kg confirms hypotonicity. A SOsm of 275 mOsm/kg or greater can represent isotonicity or hypertonicity but in some instances can also represent hypotonicity when ineffective osmoles (eg, urea and ethanol) are present in large concentrations. Therefore, SOsm should be interpreted carefully to

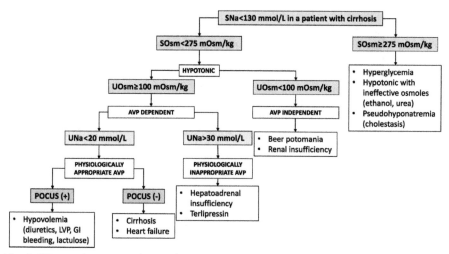

Fig. 4. Diagnostic approach to hyponatremia in cirrhosis. SNa = serum sodium, SOsm = serum osmolality, UOsm = urine osmolality, AVP = arginine vasopressin, UNa = urine sodium, POCUS = point-of-care ultrasound, LVP = large volume paracentesis, and GI = gastrointestinal. POCUS (+): presence of features of intravascular volume depletion. POCUS (−): absence of features of intravascular volume depletion.

prevent misclassification of hyponatremia. Having ruled out the presence of ineffective osmoles, a SOsm concentration of 275 mOsm/kg or greater indicates either hypertonicity usually from hyperglycemia or isotonicity due to pseudohyponatremia.

Is the Hypotonic Hyponatremia Mediated by AVP?

Elevated AVP is the most common mechanism of hypotonic hyponatremia. This is characterized by the presence of urine that is not maximally diluted (UOsm $\geq$ 100 mOsm/kg), whereas a urine that is maximally diluted (UOsm < 100 mOsm/kg) suggests AVP-independent causes such as low-solute intake (eg, beer potomania). Renal insufficiency is also a cause of AVP-independent hyponatremia, and UOsm is typically less than SOsm but not less than 100 mOsm/kg.

Is AVP Secretion in this Hypotonic Hyponatremia Physiologically Appropriate?

The presence of elevated AVP in hyponatremia is physiologically appropriate when the EABV is reduced. States of reduced EABV are characterized by renal sodium avidity manifested by urine sodium (UNa) of less than 20 mmol/L because of RAAS activation.[40] The two main considerations include cirrhosis itself and hypovolemia.[41] Distinguishing between these two possibilities is difficult as the clinical assessment of the volume status in hyponatremia has poor sensitivity and specificity.[42] Point-of-care Ultrasound (POCUS) has emerged as an effective tool to assess the volume status in hyponatremia[43] and may distinguish among patients with cirrhosis who are volume depleted.[44] If the EABV is not reduced, then AVP release is physiologically inappropriate (ie, syndrome of inappropriate antidiuresis [SIAD]). The latter is manifested by UNa greater than 30 mmol/L.

THERAPY
Overview of the Management of Hyponatremia in Cirrhosis

The treatment of hyponatremia in cirrhosis follows the same principles of management in the general population with some caveats. The choice and timing of therapy are guided by the duration of hyponatremia and the severity of symptoms. Hyponatremia can be classified based on its duration as acute (less than 48 hours) or chronic (48 hours or greater) and based on the presence and severity of symptoms as apparently asymptomatic and symptomatic (with mild, moderate, or severe symptoms). The American Expert Panel and European Clinical Practice Guidelines agree that severe symptoms include seizures and coma, whereas there is some disagreement of what constitutes moderate symptoms.[45,46]

The above guidelines recommend that patients with moderately or severely symptomatic hyponatremia, or patients with acute hyponatremia with SNa of less than 130 mmol/L with headache, vomiting, or confusion who are at a risk of brain herniation require emergent therapy with hypertonic saline 3% intravenous (IV) bolus injection 100 or 150 mL, up to three times.[45,46] The goal of correction is to increase SNa by 4 to 6 mmol/L within the first hour. Once symptoms subside, further correction should be postponed for the next day with a limit of no more than 7 mmol/L per day.[47] The American Expert panel alternatively recommends the use of hypertonic saline 3% continuous infusion in patients with moderate symptoms.[46] It is unclear whether bolus injection is superior to continuous infusion. The recent Efficacy and Safety of Rapid Intermittent Correction Compared With Slow Continuous Correction With Hypertonic Saline in Patients With Moderately Severe or Severe Symptomatic Severe Hyponatremia (SALSA) trial, a randomized controlled trial that recruited 178 patients with hyponatremia with moderate or severe symptoms, demonstrated that the rates of overcorrection of hyponatremia with hypertonic saline (3%) were similar among patients treated with bolus injection versus continuous infusion (17.4% vs 24.2%, absolute risk difference, −6.9%, 95% CI: 18.8%–4.9%; $P = .26$).[48]

Hyponatremia in a patient with cirrhosis that is chronic and apparently asymptomatic or mildly symptomatic does not require emergent therapy. In contrast to acute or symptomatic hyponatremia, a SNa correction goal of 4 mmol/L per day should be attained gradually over 24 hours, and similarly, a limit of no more than 7 mmol/L per any 24-h period should be established to prevent the development of complications.[47]

Hypovolemic Hyponatremia

Patients with cirrhosis with hypovolemic hyponatremia need volume expansion with isotonic crystalloids aiming to remove the stimuli for ongoing AVP secretion along with the removal of the precipitating factor (eg, discontinuation of diuretics).

Hyponatremia of Cirrhosis

The treatment of chronic hyponatremia of cirrhosis constitutes a challenge as most treatment modalities have not been extensively studied in this population and/or suffer from limited efficacy or tolerability.

Discontinuation of diuretics
A temporary discontinuation of diuretics is usually recommended in patients with hyponatremia of cirrhosis although this can be challenging as it can lead to worsening ascites requiring repeated paracentesis.

Correction of hypokalemia
As mentioned before, hypokalemia is involved in the pathogenesis of hyponatremia of cirrhosis. In addition, hypokalemia can precipitate HE which underscores the importance of correcting potassium deficits in these patients. Correction of hypokalemia should be done carefully as it can result in (rapid) hyponatremia correction.[30]

Fluid restriction

The goal of fluid restriction (FR) is to create a state of negative free water balance. In several randomized controlled trials comparing vaptans to placebo, the efficacy of FR in the placebo group in improving SNa by greater than 5 mmol/L ranged from 0% to 26%.[49,50] A hyponatremia registry which included 595 patients with cirrhosis showed that only 27% and 36% of patients with moderate (120–125 mmol/L) and severe (less than 120 mmol/L) hyponatremia treated with FR increased their SNa by 5 mmol/L or greater at days 2 and 3, respectively.[51] Nevertheless, FR of 1.0 to 1.5 L/d or less is still recommended although efficacy is limited and patient adherence is difficult.

Albumin

The first clues about the potential effects of albumin on the hyponatremia of cirrhosis came from old studies demonstrating that acute expansion of plasma volume with IV albumin and saline in cirrhosis increases renal free water clearance.[52] Further evidence was provided by a small case series.[53]

In a prospective cohort of 2435 hospitalized patients with cirrhosis, there was significant difference in hyponatremia resolution between those who did and those did not receive albumin (85.41% vs 44.78%, $P = .0057$; OR = 1.50, 95% CI: 1.13–2.00).[54]

Recently, the human albumin for the treatment of ascites in patients with hepatic cirrhosis (ANSWER) trial randomized 431 patients with cirrhosis and uncomplicated ascites to standard medical treatment (SMT) versus SMT and albumin (40 g twice weekly for 2 weeks, and then 40 g weekly for up to 18 months).[55] The incidence of hyponatremia was significantly lower in the SMT and albumin group than SMT alone (incidence rate ratio = 0.51, 95% CI: 0.40–0.67, $P < .001$). Overall, existing evidence suggest a beneficial effect of albumin in the treatment of hyponatremia of cirrhosis, but further evidence from prospective studies is needed.

Urea

Urea is an endogenous product of amino acid metabolism, and it has been used to treat hyponatremia since the early 1980s because of its osmotic diuretic properties causing free water excretion without sodium.[56] Only a few case reports document its efficacy for the hyponatremia of cirrhosis.[57,58] There is a theoretical concern of HE as a small amount of urea may reach the colon where it may be metabolized by urease-producing bacteria, leading to an increased ammonia production.[59] Given the limited evidence, the role of urea in the treatment of hyponatremia of cirrhosis remains unclear.

Vasopressin antagonists

AVP binds to the V2R on the basolateral membrane of principal cells of the collecting duct activating adenylyl cyclase and generating cyclic AMP (cAMP). In turn, cAMP activates protein kinase A, which phosphorylates aquaporin 2 water channels inducing their relocation to the apical membrane, promoting the net free water reabsorption. Vasopressin antagonists (vaptans) work in hyponatremia by penetrating deep into the V2R and altering the affinity of AVP to its receptor. Therefore, water is not reabsorbed, causing the excretion of diluted urine and thereby increasing SNa.[60] There is significant evidence on the efficacy of vaptans in various forms of AVP-dependent hyponatremia; however, the data in cirrhosis is less convincing.[61]

The SALT (Study of Ascending Levels of Tolvaptan in Hyponatremia 1 and 2) trials enrolled 448 adult patients with euvolemic and hypervolemic hyponatremia with the purpose of investigating the efficacy of tolvaptan to increase SNa .[62] The main causes of euvolemic and hypervolemic hyponatremia were SIAD (42.4%), heart failure (30.8%), and cirrhosis (26.7%). Compared with placebo, patients in the tolvaptan group had a significantly higher mean SNa at day 4 (133.9 ± 4.8 vs 128.7 ± 4.1 mmol/L, respectively) and at day 30 (135.7 ± 5 vs 131 ± 6.2 mmol/L, respectively). Adverse events were similar in both groups with dry mouth and thirst being the most common. A subanalysis of the SALT trials that examined only patients with cirrhosis found similar results.[63]

The SALTWATER (The Safety and sodium Assessment of Long-term Tolvaptan With hyponatremia: A year-long, open-label Trial to gain Experience under Real-world conditions) trial was an extension of the SALT trials enrolling 111 patients at least 7 days after the final tolvaptan dose was received and followed for a mean duration of 1.9 years.[64] The main etiologies of hyponatremia were SIAD (52.3%), heart failure (29.7%), and cirrhosis (18%). Normonatremia was achieved and maintained throughout the duration of the study in 57% of patients.

Overall, the above trials enrolled small numbers of patients with cirrhosis. In addition, a less robust response to tolvaptan was observed in these trials and some meta-analyses.[62,64–66] States associated with low GFR and/or enhanced proximal tubular reabsorption of water such as heart failure and cirrhosis display a reduced amount of tubular fluid delivered to distal nephron segments, the site of vaptan action, limiting their efficacy.[67] Additionally, "real-life" experience with tolvaptan in a small case series of patients with cirrhosis suggest limited efficacy.[61]

At present, only tolvaptan and conivaptan have been approved in the United States by the Food and Drug Administration (FDA), whereas only tolvaptan in Europe has been approved for the management of severe hypervolemic hyponatremia. Conivaptan has a significant V1A receptor affinity, and its use in cirrhosis is not recommended because the V1 blockade could exacerbate splanchnic vasodilatation and interfere with platelet aggregation, thus promoting hypotension and variceal bleeding.[68]

A concern with the use of vaptans in cirrhosis is the potential to exacerbate liver injury. In the SALT or SALTWATER trials, no significant elevation of hepatic enzymes was observed.[62,64] However, the use of tolvaptan in the TEMPO (Tolvaptan Efficacy and Safety in Management of Autosomal Dominant Polycystic Kidney Disease and Its Outcomes) 3:4 study,[69] aimed to determine the efficacy and safety of tolvaptan in autosomal dominant polycystic kidney disease, was associated with a significant increase in liver function tests. Based on these concerns, the FDA issued a warning limiting the use of tolvaptan to 30 days and recommending against the use of vaptans in patients with liver disease.[70] Notably, the dose of tolvaptan used in this study was four times the dose commonly used to treat hyponatremia. Thus, it is recommended to limit the use of tolvaptan in cirrhosis when the clinical benefit outweighs the risks, such as in patients who are imminently awaiting liver transplantation (see perioperative management in patients awaiting liver transplant).).

PERIOPERATIVE MANAGEMENT IN PATIENTS AWAITING LIVER TRANSPLANT

Correction of SNa 8 mmol/L or greater in any 24-hour period in patients with chronic hyponatremia can lead to the osmotic demyelination syndrome (ODS),[47] a potentially devastating neurologic complication. In this setting, cirrhosis and other comorbid conditions (SNa 105 mmol/L or lower, alcohol use disorder, hypokalemia, and malnutrition) increase the susceptibility for ODS.[46] Patients undergoing liver transplant are particularly at risk for rapid SNa correction due to fluid shifts that occur during surgery as a consequence of intraoperative administration of IV crystalloids, blood products, and sodium bicarbonate.[22,71,72] The risk of ODS post-LT inversely correlates with the baseline SNa.[73]

The incidence of ODS post-LT ranges from 0.5% to 1.5%.[73–75] Symptom onset usually occur within 1 to 2 weeks after surgery, and it is commonly manifested as encephalopathy (36%–45%), quadriparesis (up to 45%), and seizures (27%–36%).[74,76,77] Diagnosis is clinical although magnetic resonance imaging (MRI) brain demonstrating

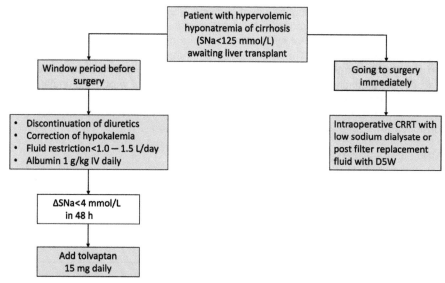

Fig. 5. Perioperative management of hyponatremia in patients awaiting liver transplant. For patients with enough time to correct serum sodium (SNa) slowly (eg, 7-day window before surgery), discontinuation of diuretics, potassium repletion, fluid restriction, and albumin should be attempted for the first 48 hours before moving to tolvaptan. For patients who are immediately going to the operating room where there is no time to correct SNa slowly, intraoperative CRRT with low sodium dialysate or postfilter fluid replacement with dextrose 5% in water could be considered.

the characteristic T2/FLAIR hyperintensity in the central pons ("trident" shaped appearance) supports the diagnosis.[78] MRI changes may not manifest until 4 weeks after symptom onset; hence, serial imaging should be considered.

ODS outcomes post-LT are variable. Although some series showed no difference in mortality,[74,76] two of the largest series demonstrated mortality of 40% at 3 months[77] and 63% at 1 year.[73] In addition, up to 84% of patients that survived remained with permanent sequalae.[76,77]

This heightened risk of ODS in patients with cirrhosis constitutes a real concern for many transplant surgeons who might delay a life-saving surgery until SNa is corrected to an acceptable level, but there is no standardized protocol or SNa threshold across all transplant programs.[22] Some have advocated the short-term use of vaptans to expedite liver transplant surgery. Tolvaptan can be used because the potential for hepatotoxicity is less of a concern in this setting.[79] Intraoperative continuous renal replacement therapy (CRRT) with customized low-sodium dialysate has also been used.[80]

Management of established ODS in liver transplant recipients is mainly supportive with the help of a multidisciplinary team. We suggest correcting SNa to at least 125 mmol/L when the patient can proceed with surgery as the risk of ODS above this SNa becomes negligible. Compulsory frequent SNa checks are recommended. A suggested approach to the perioperative management of hyponatremia in patients awaiting liver transplant is outlined in **Fig. 5**.

SUMMARY

Hyponatremia in cirrhosis is common, and its pathogenesis principally involves non-osmotic AVP release resulting from the circulatory dysfunction associated with later stages of liver disease. Hyponatremia of cirrhosis is associated with poor clinical outcomes including increased mortality and increased risk of cirrhotic complications. The major differential diagnosis for hyponatremia of cirrhosis is hypovolemia and POCUS can help distinguish them. The treatment of hyponatremia of cirrhosis is challenging and involves fluid restriction, discontinuation of diuretics, hypokalemia correction, and possibly albumin. The clinical benefits and risk profile of vaptans is unclear, and its use should be restricted to patients who are imminently awaiting liver transplantation. Patients undergoing liver transplantation are at higher risk for ODS, and slow SNa correction is recommended.

CLINICS CARE POINTS

- POCUS can help distinguish between hyponatremia of cirrhosis and hypovolemia.
- Preoperative management of hyponatremia before liver transplantation surgery should aim to correct SNa by less than 8 mmol/L in any 24-h period to avoid ODS utilizing tools that include tolvaptan and CRRT.

DISCLOSURE

H. Rondon-Berrios is funded by exploratory/developmental research grant R21DK122023 from National Institutes of Diabetes and Digestive and Kidney Diseases of the National Institutes of Health. J.C.Q. Velez has participated in consulting for Mallinckrodt Pharmaceuticals and Bayer, advisory board for Mallinckrodt Pharmaceuticals, Travere, and speaker bureau for Otsuka Pharmaceuticals.

REFERENCES

1. Gines P, Berl T, Bernardi M, et al. Hyponatremia in cirrhosis: from pathogenesis to treatment. Hepatology 1998;28(3):851–64.
2. Angeli P, Wong F, Watson H, et al. Hyponatremia in cirrhosis: results of a patient population survey. Hepatology 2006;44(6):1535–42.
3. Kim JH, Lee JS, Lee SH, et al. The association between the serum sodium level and the severity of complications in liver cirrhosis. Korean J Intern Med 2009; 24(2):106–12.
4. Londono MC, Guevara M, Rimola A, et al. Hyponatremia impairs early posttransplantation outcome in patients with cirrhosis undergoing liver transplantation. Gastroenterology 2006;130(4):1135–43.
5. Ennaifer R, Cheikh M, Romdhane H, et al. Hyponatremia in cirrhosis: risk factors and prognostic value. Tunis Med 2016;94(5):401–5.
6. Velez JCQ, Therapondos G, Juncos LA. Reappraising the spectrum of AKI and hepatorenal syndrome in patients with cirrhosis. Nat Rev Nephrol 2020;16(3): 137–55.
7. Arroyo V, Rodes J, Gutierrez-Lizarraga MA, et al. Prognostic value of spontaneous hyponatremia in cirrhosis with ascites. Am J Dig Dis 1976;21(3): 249–56.
8. Kim WR, Biggins SW, Kremers WK, et al. Hyponatremia and mortality among patients on the liver-transplant waiting list. N Engl J Med 2008;359(10):1018–26.
9. Freeman RB Jr, Wiesner RH, Harper A, et al. The new liver allocation system: moving toward evidence-based transplantation policy. Liver Transpl 2002;8(9): 851–8.

10. Ruf AE, Kremers WK, Chavez LL, et al. Addition of serum sodium into the MELD score predicts waiting list mortality better than MELD alone. Liver Transpl 2005; 11(3):336–43.
11. UNfO Sharing. Changes to OPTN Bylaws and Policies from actions at OPTN/ UNOS Exectuive Committee Meetings. 2015. https://optn.transplant.hrsa.gov/ media/1575/policynotice_20151101.pdf. Accessed May 3, 2021.
12. Guevara M, Baccaro ME, Torre A, et al. Hyponatremia is a risk factor of hepatic encephalopathy in patients with cirrhosis: a prospective study with time-dependent analysis. Am J Gastroenterol 2009;104(6):1382–9.
13. Verbalis JG. Brain volume regulation in response to changes in osmolality. Neuroscience 2010;168(4):862–70.
14. Cordoba J, Alonso J, Rovira A, et al. The development of low-grade cerebral edema in cirrhosis is supported by the evolution of (1)H-magnetic resonance abnormalities after liver transplantation. J Hepatol 2001;35(5):598–604.
15. Haussinger D, Schliess F. Pathogenetic mechanisms of hepatic encephalopathy. Gut 2008;57(8):1156–65.
16. Haussinger D, Laubenberger J, vom Dahl S, et al. Proton magnetic resonance spectroscopy studies on human brain myo-inositol in hypo-osmolarity and hepatic encephalopathy. Gastroenterology 1994;107(5):1475–80.
17. Angeli P, Dalla Pria M, De Bei E, et al. Randomized clinical study of the efficacy of amiloride and potassium canrenoate in nonazotemic cirrhotic patients with ascites. Hepatology 1994;19(1):72–9.
18. Gines A, Escorsell A, Gines P, et al. Incidence, predictive factors, and prognosis of the hepatorenal syndrome in cirrhosis with ascites. *Gastroenterology.* Jul 1993; 105(1):229–36.
19. Deitelzweig S, Amin A, Christian R, et al. Hyponatremia-associated healthcare burden among US patients hospitalized for cirrhosis. Adv Ther 2013;30(1):71–80.
20. Sola E, Watson H, Graupera I, et al. Factors related to quality of life in patients with cirrhosis and ascites: relevance of serum sodium concentration and leg edema. J Hepatol 2012;57(6):1199–206.
21. Dawwas MF, Lewsey JD, Neuberger JM, et al. The impact of serum sodium concentration on mortality after liver transplantation: a cohort multicenter study. Liver Transpl 2007;13(8):1115–24.
22. Leise M, Cardenas A. Hyponatremia in cirrhosis: Implications for liver transplantation. Liver Transpl 2018;24(11):1612–21.
23. Leise MD, Yun BC, Larson JJ, et al. Effect of the pretransplant serum sodium concentration on outcomes following liver transplantation. Liver Transpl 2014;20(6): 687–97.
24. Gines P, Fernandez-Esparrach G, Arroyo V, et al. Pathogenesis of ascites in cirrhosis. Semin Liver Dis 1997;17(3):175–89.
25. Rizvi MR, Tauseef M, Shahid M, et al. Nitric oxide and prostaglandin as mediators in the pathogenesis of hyperkinetic circulatory state in a model of endotoxemia-induced portal hypertension. Hepatol Int 2013;7(2):622–35.
26. Schrier RW, Arroyo V, Bernardi M, et al. Peripheral arterial vasodilation hypothesis: a proposal for the initiation of renal sodium and water retention in cirrhosis. Hepatology 1988;8(5):1151–7.
27. Schrier RW. Water and sodium retention in edematous disorders: role of vasopressin and aldosterone. Am J Med 2006;119(7 Suppl 1):S47–53.
28. Birkenfeld LW, Leibman J, O'Meara MP, et al. Total exchangeable sodium, total exchangeable potassium, and total body water in edematous patients with cirrhosis of the liver and congestive heart failure. J Clin Invest 1958;37(5):687–98.

29. Edelman IS, Leibman J, O'Meara MP, et al. Interrelations between serum sodium concentration, serum osmolarity and total exchangeable sodium, total exchangeable potassium and total body water. J Clin Invest 1958;37(9):1236–56.

30. Berl T, Rastegar A. A patient with severe hyponatremia and hypokalemia: osmotic demyelination following potassium repletion. Am J Kidney Dis 2010;55(4):742–8.

31. Handler J. Well tolerated spironolactone-related hyponatremia. J Clin Hypertens (Greenwich) 2008;10(4):317–21.

32. Singh RR, Walia R, Sachdeva N, et al. Relative adrenal insufficiency in cirrhotic patients with ascites (hepatoadrenal syndrome). Dig Liver Dis 2018;50(11):1232–7.

33. Marik PE, Gayowski T, Starzl TE. Hepatic Cortisol R, Adrenal Pathophysiology Study G. The hepatoadrenal syndrome: a common yet unrecognized clinical condition. Crit Care Med 2005;33(6):1254–9.

34. Han X, Li J, Yang JM, et al. A retrospective analysis of hyponatremia during terlipressin treatment in patients with esophageal or gastric variceal bleeding due to portal hypertension. JGH Open 2020;4(3):368–70.

35. Xu X, Lin S, Yang Y, et al. Development of hyponatremia after terlipressin in cirrhotic patients with acute gastrointestinal bleeding: a retrospective multicenter observational study. Expert Opin Drug Saf 2020;19(5):641–7.

36. Wong F, Pappas SC, Curry MP, et al. Terlipressin plus albumin for the treatment of type 1 hepatorenal syndrome. N Engl J Med 2021;384(9):818–28.

37. Ouellette L, Michel K, Riley B, et al. Beer potomania: Atypical cause of severe hyponatremia in older alcoholics. Am J Emerg Med 2018;36(7):1303.

38. Hickman PE, Dwyer KP, Masarei JR. Pseudohyponatraemia, hypercholesterolaemia, and primary biliary cirrhosis. J Clin Pathol 1989;42(2):167–71.

39. Workeneh BT, Jhaveri KD, Rondon-Berrios H. Hyponatremia in the cancer patient. Kidney Int 2020;98(4):870–82.

40. Schrier RW. Decreased effective blood volume in edematous disorders: what does this mean? J Am Soc Nephrol 2007;18(7):2028–31.

41. Gines P, Guevara M. Hyponatremia in cirrhosis: pathogenesis, clinical significance, and management. Hepatology 2008;48(3):1002–10.

42. Chung HM, Kluge R, Schrier RW, et al. Clinical assessment of extracellular fluid volume in hyponatremia. Am J Med 1987;83(5):905–8.

43. Evins C, Rao A. Point-of-care ultrasound to evaluate volume status in severe hyponatremia. BMJ Case Rep 2020;(6):13.

44. Velez JCQ, Petkovich B, Karakala N, et al. Point-of-Care Echocardiography Unveils misclassification of acute kidney injury as hepatorenal syndrome. Am J Nephrol 2019;50(3):204–11.

45. Spasovski G, Vanholder R, Allolio B, et al. Clinical practice guideline on diagnosis and treatment of hyponatraemia. Nephrol Dial Transpl Apr 2014;29(Suppl 2):i1–39.

46. Verbalis JG, Goldsmith SR, Greenberg A, et al. Diagnosis, evaluation, and treatment of hyponatremia: expert panel recommendations. Am J Med Oct 2013;126(10 Suppl 1):S1–42.

47. Tandukar S, Sterns RH, Rondon-Berrios H. Osmotic demyelination syndrome following correction of hyponatremia by ≤10 mEq/L per day. Kidney360 2021;2(9):1415–23.

48. Baek SH, Jo YH, Ahn S, et al. Risk of overcorrection in rapid Intermittent bolus vs slow continuous infusion therapies of hypertonic saline for patients with symptomatic hyponatremia: the SALSA randomized clinical trial. JAMA Intern Med 1 2021;181(1):81–92.

49. Gerbes AL, Gulberg V, Gines P, et al. Therapy of hyponatremia in cirrhosis with a vasopressin receptor antagonist: a randomized double-blind multicenter trial. Gastroenterology 2003;124(4):933–9.
50. Gines P, Wong F, Watson H, et al. Effects of satavaptan, a selective vasopressin V(2) receptor antagonist, on ascites and serum sodium in cirrhosis with hyponatremia: a randomized trial. Hepatol 2008;48(1):204–13.
51. Sigal SH, Amin A, Chiodo JA 3rd, et al. Management Strategies and outcomes for hyponatremia in cirrhosis in the hyponatremia registry. Can J Gastroenterol Hepatol 2018;2018:1579508.
52. Vlahcevic ZR, Adham NF, Jick H, et al. Renal effects of acute expansion of plasma volume in cirrhosis. N Engl J Med 1965;272:387–90.
53. McCormick PA, Mistry P, Kaye G, et al. Intravenous albumin infusion is an effective therapy for hyponatraemia in cirrhotic patients with ascites. Gut 1990;31(2):204–7.
54. Bajaj JS, Tandon P, O'Leary JG, et al. The impact of albumin Use on resolution of hyponatremia in hospitalized patients with cirrhosis. Am J Gastroenterol 2018;113(9):1339.
55. Caraceni P, Riggio O, Angeli P, et al. Long-term albumin administration in decompensated cirrhosis (ANSWER): an open-label randomised trial. Lancet 2018;391(10138):2417–29.
56. Decaux G, Brimioulle S, Genette F, et al. Treatment of the syndrome of inappropriate secretion of antidiuretic hormone by urea. Am J Med 1980;69(1):99–106.
57. Decaux G, Mols P, Cauchi P, et al. Use of urea for treatment of water retention in hyponatraemic cirrhosis with ascites resistant to diuretics. Br Med J (Clin Res Ed) 1985;290(6484):1782–3.
58. Decaux G, Mols P, Cauchie P, et al. Treatment of hyponatremic cirrhosis with ascites resistant to diuretics by urea. Nephron 1986;44(4):337–43.
59. Rondon-Berrios H. Urea for chronic hyponatremia. Blood Purif 2020;49(1–2):212–8.
60. Berl T. Vasopressin antagonists. N Engl J Med 2015;372(23):2207–16.
61. Pose E, Sola E, Piano S, et al. Limited efficacy of tolvaptan in patients with cirrhosis and severe hyponatremia: real-life experience. Am J Med 2017;130(3):372–5.
62. Schrier RW, Gross P, Gheorghiade M, et al. Tolvaptan, a selective oral vasopressin V2-receptor antagonist, for hyponatremia. N Engl J Med 2006;355(20):2099–112.
63. Cardenas A, Gines P, Marotta P, et al. Tolvaptan, an oral vasopressin antagonist, in the treatment of hyponatremia in cirrhosis. J Hepatol 2012;56(3):571–8.
64. Berl T, Quittnat-Pelletier F, Verbalis JG, et al. Oral tolvaptan is safe and effective in chronic hyponatremia. J Am Soc Nephrol 2010;21(4):705–12.
65. Jaber BL, Almarzouqi L, Borgi L, et al. Short-term efficacy and safety of vasopressin receptor antagonists for treatment of hyponatremia. Am J Med 2011;124(10):977 e1–9.
66. Rozen-Zvi B, Yahav D, Gheorghiade M, et al. Vasopressin receptor antagonists for the treatment of hyponatremia: systematic review and meta-analysis. Am J Kidney Dis 2010;56(2):325–37.
67. Rondon-Berrios H, Berl T. Vasopressin receptor antagonists: Characteristics and clinical role. Best Pract Res Clin Endocrinol Metab 2016;30(2):289–303.
68. Hline SS, Pham PT, Pham PT, et al. Conivaptan: a step forward in the treatment of hyponatremia? Ther Clin Risk Manag 2008;4(2):315–26.

69. Torres VE, Chapman AB, Devuyst O, et al. Tolvaptan in patients with autosomal dominant polycystic kidney disease. N Engl J Med 2012;367(25):2407–18.
70. US Food and Drug Administration. FDA Drug Safety Communication: FDA limits duration and usage of Samsca (tolvaptan) due to possible liver injury leading to organ transplant or death. Available at: https://www.fda.gov/drugs/drug-safety-and-availability/fda-drug-safety-communication-fda-limits-duration-and-usage-samsca-tolvaptan-due-possible-liver. Accessed April 16, 2021.
71. Crismale JF, Meliambro KA, DeMaria S Jr, et al. Prevention of the osmotic demyelination syndrome after liver transplantation: a multidisciplinary Perspective. Am J Transplant 2017;17(10):2537–45.
72. Romanovsky A, Azevedo LC, Meeberg G, et al. Serum sodium shift in hyponatremic patients undergoing liver transplantation: a retrospective cohort study. Ren Fail 2015;37(1):37–44.
73. Yun BC, Kim WR, Benson JT, et al. Impact of pretransplant hyponatremia on outcome following liver transplantation. Hepatology 2009;49(5):1610–5.
74. Crivellin C, Cagnin A, Manara R, et al. Risk factors for central pontine and extrapontine myelinolysis after liver transplantation: a single-center study. Transplant 2015;99(6):1257–64.
75. Singh TD, Fugate JE, Rabinstein AA. Central pontine and extrapontine myelinolysis: a systematic review. Eur J Neurol 2014;21(12):1443–50.
76. Lee EM, Kang JK, Yun SC, et al. Risk factors for central pontine and extrapontine myelinolysis following orthotopic liver transplantation. Eur Neurol 2009;62(6):362–8.
77. Morard I, Gasche Y, Kneteman M, et al. Identifying risk factors for central pontine and extrapontine myelinolysis after liver transplantation: a case-control study. Neurocrit Care 2014;20(2):287–95.
78. Alleman AM. Osmotic demyelination syndrome: central pontine myelinolysis and extrapontine myelinolysis. Semin Ultrasound CT MR 2014;35(2):153–9.
79. Lenci I, Milana M, Angelico M, et al. Short-term, low-dose Use of tolvaptan as a Bridge therapy to expedite liver transplant for severe hyponatremic, cirrhotic patients with high model for end-stage liver disease scores. Exp Clin Transpl 2017;15(6):689–92.
80. Nagai S, Moonka D, Patel A. Novel intraoperative management in the model for end-stage liver disease-sodium era: continuous venovenous hemofiltration for severe hyponatremia in liver transplantation. Liver Transpl 2018;24(2):304–7.

Hepatorenal Syndrome
Pathophysiology

Timea Csak, MD, PhD[a],*,
David Bernstein, MD, FAASLD, MACG, FACP, AGAF[b]

KEYWORDS

- Hepatorenal syndrome • Pathophysiology • Kidneys • Mortality
- Systemic inflammation

KEY POINTS

- Renal hypoperfusion due to intense vasoconstriction as a compensatory mechanism secondary to peripheral arterial vasodilation and effective hypovolemia remains the cornerstone of HRS.
- Cirrhotic cardiomyopathy, defined as systolic and/or diastolic dysfunction, with or without electrophysiological abnormalities in cirrhotic patients in absence of other cardiac disease, contributes to the circulatory dysfunction.
- Cirrhosis is a pro-inflammatory state and a distinct inflammatory profile has been reported depending on the severity and the associated organ failures, including renal failure.
- PAMPs and DAMPs activate immune responses and the extensive production of inflammatory cytokines, chemokines, upregulation of their receptors either directly contribute to tissue damage or effect vascular reactivity.
- Relative adrenal insufficiency, cholemic or bile cast nephropathy and increased intra-abdominal pressure are some of the additional mechanisms in the development of hepatorenal syndrome.

INTRODUCTION

Hepatorenal syndrome (HRS), defined as "functional" renal failure in patients with severe liver disease, is one of the major complications of cirrhosis and portal hypertension, but can also occur in severe alcoholic hepatitis, acute fulminant liver failure and rare reports exist in metastatic liver disease[1]. Initial reports date back to the late 19th

a Sandra Atlas Bass Center for Liver Diseases, Northwell Health, 400 Community Drive, Manhasset, NY 11030, USA; b Division of Hepatology and Sandra Atlas Bass Center for Liver Diseases, Northwell Health, Zucker School of Medicine at Hofstra/Northwell, 400 Community Drive, Manhasset, NY 11030, USA
* Corresponding author.
E-mail address: tcsak@northwell.edu

Clin Liver Dis 26 (2022) 165–179
https://doi.org/10.1016/j.cld.2022.01.013
1089-3261/22/© 2022 Elsevier Inc. All rights reserved.

liver.theclinics.com

century and its functional nature was demonstrated by the lack of major histologic changes in the kidneys[2]. Recovery of renal function in patients with end-stage liver disease after liver transplant supports its functional nature[3]. Renal hypoperfusion due to intense vasoconstriction as a result of complex circulatory dysfunction has been suggested to be the cornerstone of HRS [1]. Selective renal angiography shows beading and tortuosity of the intrarenal arteries, along with marked impairment of vascular filling in the cortical vessels. Reversal of all the vascular abnormalities has been observed during postmortem angiography [1]. Renal vasoconstriction along with near-normal kidney histology differentiates HRS from other types of renal injuries in patients with cirrhosis, such as intrinsic kidney disease and acute tubular necrosis (ATN) often related to shock or nephrotoxic agents. The diagnosis, however, remains challenging, as no specific diagnostic markers exist[4]. Furthermore, renal recovery and the response rate to the current therapeutic strategies with vasoconstrictors plus albumin, based on correcting the circulatory dysfunction, is limited[5,6]. HRS remains a major cause of death in patients with cirrhosis[4]. Thus, a better understanding of the pathogenesis is crucial. Increasing evidence suggests that HRS is more than just the consequence of circulatory dysfunction and a substantial role systemic inflammation has been implicated.

Here we aim to summarize the current understanding of the pathophysiology of HRS.

CIRCULATORY DYSFUNCTION: "PERIPHERAL ARTERIAL VASODILATION HYPOTHESIS"

Peripheral arterial vasodilation hypothesis (PAVH) was proposed in the 1980s to be the initiating and cardinal step of renal dysfunction in cirrhosis[7]. The concept is based on that arterial vasodilation in the splanchnic circulation results in increased splanchnic blood flow and contributes to portal hypertension, while arterial vasodilation in the systemic circulation decreases the arterial pressure leading to effective arterial hypovolemia and hypotension. The latter one triggers the activation of the vasoconstrictor mechanisms, such as renin–angiotensin–aldosterone system (RAAS), sympathetic nervous system (SNS), and arginine–vasopressin (AVP) system [4]. As a result of this, the marked renal vasoconstriction leads to decreased glomerular filtration rate (GFR) and HRS.

An abnormal distribution of total blood volume with an increase in the splanchnic circulation has been observed even in compensated cirrhosis in the absence of ascites, but in a posture dependent manner[8]. Bernardi and colleagues[9] found splanchnic arterial vasodilation in the supine, but not in the upright position in patients with compensated cirrhosis. These patients usually do not have overt renal dysfunction, but they can have abnormalities in sodium excretion[10]. Sodium retention, however, occurred only in the upright position. The authors suggested that in preascitic sodium retention in the upright posture the main mechanism is splanchnic venous pooling due to portal hypertension[11]. Notably, vasoconstrictor mechanisms were not activated in the early compensated state, measured by normal plasma renin activity, aldosterone and norepinephrine levels [8].

In contrary, patients with decompensated cirrhosis with ascites have significant splanchnic arterial vasodilation, significant effective hypovolemia and persistent activation of the vasoconstrictor mechanisms, irrespective of posture [11]. The presence of functional renal abnormalities in decompensated cirrhosis is well established.

Paracentesis-induced circulatory dysfunction (PCID), a unique entity characterized by increased venous return immediately after large-volume paracentesis (LVP), followed by prolonged arterial vasodilation and compensatory activation of vasocon-strictor mechanisms, further increases the risk of AKI and HRS development[12].

The vasodilatory state is a result of increased levels of circulating vasodilators and reduced vascular responsiveness to vasoconstrictors. These changes can be observed in the systemic and splanchnic circulation, but not in the hepatic microcir-culation.[13] On the other hand, the dominance of vasoconstriction forces over vasodi-lation is reported in the renal vasculature[14] but the mechanisms leading to it is not fully characterized yet.

Increased Level of Circulating Vasodilators

Numerous vasodilators have been implicated in the pathogenesis of cirrhotic circula-tory dysfunction[15], including nitric oxide (NO)[16], carbon monoxide (CO)[17], endocanna-binoids[18], prostacyclin[19], endothelin[20], calcitonin gene-related peptide[21] and many others. NO is the most extensively studied vasodilator in both animal models and in human cirrhosis.

Patients with cirrhosis and ascites have higher plasma NO concentration compared with control subjects, and it is higher in the portal venous plasma than in peripheral venous blood[22]. The activity of nitric oxide synthetase (NOS) in polymorphonuclear cells and monocytes was increased in patients with cirrhosis with ascites[23], suggest-ing a potential role of the inducible NOS (iNOS). Other studies rather suggested a path-ogenic role of the endothelial NOS (eNOS)[24]. Genetic studies using NOS2 or NOS3 knock out mice also provided contradictory data[11]. However, further pharmacologic studies showed that eNOS hyperactivity and not iNOS overproduction is responsible for the increased NO production in the splanchnic vasculature [24]. Increased eNOS expression, increased phosphorylation, increased availability of its cofactor tetrahy-drobiopterin and enhanced interaction with heat shock protein 90 (HSP 90) were all reported[25]. The initiating step was thought to be the mechanical shear force, but now substantial evidence supports the role of systemic inflammation in NO production as discussed later . Notably, increased NO production was reported in portal hyper-tensive rats preceding hyperdynamic circulation[26].

Reduced Vascular Responsiveness to Vasoconstrictors

The marked decrease of vascular resistance due to vasodilation leads to the activation of various vasoconstrictor mechanisms, including the activation of the SNS, RAAS, and AVP [4]. However, despite the activation of vasoconstrictors, arterial hypotension still occurs because of reduced vascular responsiveness to vasoconstrictors [11]. The reduced response to vasoconstrictors can be restored by the inhibition of NOS and is endothelial dependent [11].

Renal Vasoconstriction

The response to vasoconstrictors might differ in renal and systemic vasculature. Renal hemodynamic changes were elegantly demonstrated by *Kew and colleagues*[27]. Using Xenon-133 washout technique, the authors found reduced mean renal blood flow, particularly affecting the outer cortex and the poor cortical perfusion was associated with lower GFR [27]. Prominent renal vasoconstriction has also been demonstrated by selective renal arteriogram and resolution of the vascular changes has been observed in postmortem studies, confirming reversibility [1]. The studies of *Maroto A* and col-leagues[28] using Doppler ultrasound to estimate intrarenal arteriolar vascular resis-tance suggested significantly increased resistive index in cirrhotic patients with ascites and a correlation was found with renal function (GFR, free water clearance), arterial pressure and plasma renin activity. The mechanism of renal vasoconstriction in cirrhosis is yet to be fully characterized. Increased renal vascular reactivity has been related to the presence of endothelin-1 (ET-1), contributing to the dominance of renal vasoconstriction over vasodilation [14].

In summary, the PAVH identifies splanchnic arterial vasodilation and effective hypovolemia as central mechanisms leading to renal dysfunction in cirrhosis. The efficacy of vasoconstrictors, especially terlipressin, in combination with albumin, does support the PAVH. On other hand, effective hypovolemia leads to an increase in cardiac output which compensates for the hemodynamic changes, but with disease progression, this compensatory mechanism fails. Thus, impaired cardiac function is also a key player in cirrhotic circulatory dysfunction, eventually predisposing for the development of HRS.

CIRCULATORY DYSFUNCTION: CIRRHOTIC CARDIOMYOPATHY

In patients with cirrhosis, hyperdynamic circulation was described in the 1950s[29], and cases of sudden cardiac death due to heart failure after TIPS or liver transplantation have been reported in the 1980s[30], but the definition of cirrhotic cardiomyopathy (CCM) was first proposed in 2005 during the World Congress of Gastroenterology[13]. CCM is defined as systolic and/or diastolic dysfunction, with or without electrophysiological abnormalities in cirrhotic patients with no other known cardiac disease. Impaired β-adrenergic pathway, altered membrane fluidity, enhanced endocannabinoid pathway, negative inotropic factors including NO, CO, and certain cytokines (TNFα, IL-1β) and the activation RAAS, all contribute to its development[31].

CCM manifests in early cirrhosis, but it becomes more evident at the time of stress, including during bacterial infections, such as spontaneous bacterial peritonitis (SBP). An insufficient chronotropic and inotropic response to stress situations leading to submaximal cardiac output contributes to the development of the HRS as the cirrhotic heart is unable to compensate for the arterial vasodilation [13]. Patients who develop HRS have been shown to have lower cardiac output even before the onset of HRS[32], suggesting that CCM increases the risk of HRS.

While the role of circulatory dysfunction is well established (**Fig. 1**), the limitations of current treatment options that are based on improving renal perfusion, the observation that renal dysfunction can progress even without progression of the circulatory dysfunction, lead to tremendous research to explore other mechanisms.

SYSTEMIC INFLAMMATION

The role of innate immunity in acute kidney injury (AKI) in sepsis has been established[33]. Increasing evidence suggests that the persistent inflammatory state in cirrhosis contributes to the development of AKI-HRS.

The CANONIC study revealed that ACLF (acute on chronic liver failure) which is defined by the presence of 2 or more extrahepatic organ failures, including renal failure, is associated with increased nonspecific inflammatory markers, such as WBC count and C-reactive protein[34]. Systemic inflammation is now thought to be the primary driver of ACLF in cirrhosis[35,36].

Higher pro-inflammatory cytokine levels were found in ACLF compared with chronic liver disease (CLD) without ACLF[37]. Increased inflammatory biomarkers have been already observed in compensated cirrhosis, but acute decompensation with or without ACLF results in further enhancement of systemic inflammation. In a multicenter European study, the inflammatory profile of 3 distinct phenotypes of acutely decompensated (AD) cirrhosis was studied by measuring 15 cytokines and chemokines such as TNFα, IL-6, IL-8, MCP-1, IP-10, MIP-1β, G-CSF, GM-CSF, IL-10, IL-1ra, IFNγ, IL-17A, IL-7, and eotaxin. The study showed progression of systemic

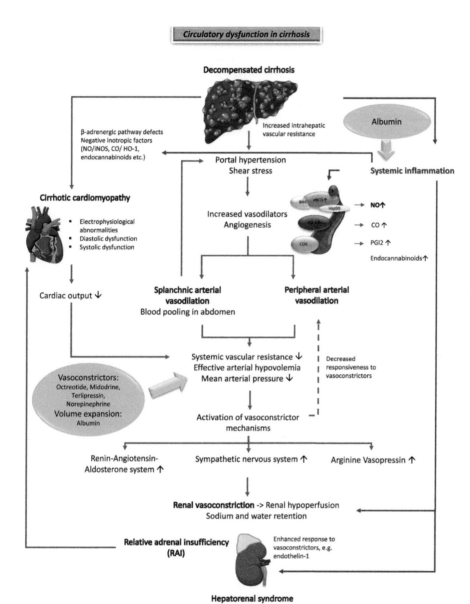

Fig. 1. Increased intrahepatic vascular resistance and portal hypertension lead to splanchnic and peripheral arterial vasodilation via the increased production of vasodilator molecules. The effective arterial hypovolemia results in the activation of vasoconstrictor mechanisms, including the renin–angiotensin–aldosterone system (RAAS), sympathetic nervous system (SNS) and arginine–vasopressin (AVP) system. Renal vasoconstriction leads to decreased glomerular filtration rate and hepatorenal syndrome. Cirrhotic cardiomyopathy with insufficient chronotropic and inotropic response and decreased cardiac output contributes to the circulatory dysfunction. Relative adrenal insufficiency plays role affecting beta-adrenergic response. Systemic inflammation affects most of the steps involved in the development of hepatorenal syndrome. Current therapeutic strategies target the circulatory dysfunction, but albumin also has an immunmodulatory effect.

inflammation, suggesting a continuum, from compensated cirrhosis through AD without renal, cerebral or any other organ dysfunction (AD-1 phenotype) to patients with AD with isolated renal and/or cerebral dysfunction (AD-2 phenotype) or with isolated nonrenal organ failure (AD-3 phenotype) and finally to ACLF[38].

The pattern of elevated inflammatory markers was different in AD-2 and AD-3. Some of the markers, including TNFα, HNA1, IP-10, were elevated in AD-2 but not in states of acute decompensation without renal dysfunction (AD-3 or AD-1). Thus, systemic inflammation is strongly associated with the severity of cirrhosis and organ dysfunction, including renal impairment. Similarly, Sole and colleagues[39] showed different cytokine profiles in patients with AKI-HRS compared with patients with prerenal AKI and compared with patients with acute decompensation but without AKI. Patients with AKI-HRS had higher levels of MCP-1 in the urine and IL-6, TNFα, IL-8, VCAM-1 in the plasma, but lower MIP-1α and fractalkine levels [39]. There was no difference in the above cytokine levels in patients with AKI-HRS with or without infection, except in IL-6 levels. The authors also suggested that the cytokine levels are related to AKI-HRS rather than ACLF, as they found no significant differences between patients with ACLF with and without AKI-HRS, although the small sample size limits the interpretation. The cytokine profile in HRS-AKI was comparable to other nonhepatic conditions, such as rheumatoid arthritis, systemic lupus erythematosus, inflammatory bowel disease, cystic fibrosis [39].

Interestingly, HRS treatment led to the reduction of TNFα and RANTES levels but has not affected the other cytokines. On other hand, patients who have not responded to terlipressin plus albumin, which counts about 50% of the cases, had higher levels of Interferon gamma-induced protein 10 (IP-10) and Vascular cell adhesion molecule −1 (VCAM-1) [40]. IP-10 is a chemokine playing role in chemoattraction for various immune cells, while VCAM-1 mediates the adhesion of those immune cells to the vascular endothelium.

In summary, there is robust evidence that cirrhosis is a proinflammatory state and a distinct inflammatory profile has been reported depending on its severity and associated organ failures, including renal failure.

Factors Leading to the Systemic Inflammatory State

It is well known that acute decompensation and HRS development are often triggered by bacterial infections, such as SBP or urinary tract infection (UTI), but renal failure can persist or progress even after the resolution of the infection and it can also occur without active infection. Precipitating factors were identified in 38% of patients with acute decompensation without ACLF, and 71% of patients with ACLF in the PREDICT study[40].

Inflammation can be driven by pathogen-associated molecular patterns (PAMPs), including bacterial products in the presence or absence of active infection, or by damage-associated molecular patterns (DAMPs) released during tissue damage (**Fig. 2**). In cirrhosis, bacterial overgrowth, impaired intestinal peristalsis, dysbiosis and enhanced gut permeability, all contribute to the bacterial translocation and increased serum endotoxin levels[41]. Both PAMPs and DAMPs are recognized by pattern recognition receptors (PRRs), such as the membrane-bound Toll-like receptors (TLRs) and C-type lectin receptors (CLRs) or the cytoplasmic nucleotide-binding oligomerization domain-like receptors (NLRs) and retinoic acid inducible gene (RIG)-I-like receptors (RLRs). Activation of these PRRs leads to the production of various inflammatory molecules, including several cytokines and chemokines[42].

How Does Systemic Inflammation Affect the Kidneys in Cirrhosis?

Extensive production of inflammatory cytokines, chemokines, upregulation of their receptors and release of reactive oxygen species (ROS) from the activated immune cells

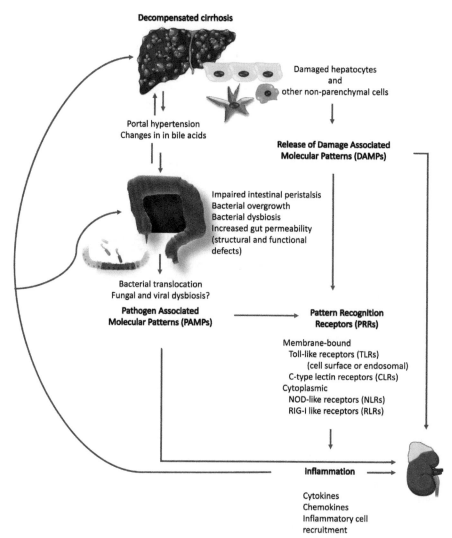

Fig. 2. Systemic inflammation triggered by pathogen-associated molecular patterns (PAMPs) or damage-associated molecular patterns (DAMPs) can affect the kidneys directly or via contribution to the circulatory dysfunction.

all contribute to tissue damage[43]. Beyond tissue damage, cytokines affect vascular reactivity[44].

Direct renal effects
TLRs are expressed both in immune and nonimmune cells of the kidneys. Cirrhosis is linked to increased TLR4 expression in renal tubules, especially in case of acute decompensation[45]. Peng and colleagues[46] recently summarized the role of endotoxemia in cirrhosis related renal dysfunction. Endotoxemia results in increased TLR4 expression in proximal renal tubules, leading to proinflammatory cytokine production and thus renal tubular damage, which is further enhanced by the impaired peritubular

capillary flow[47]. TLR4 and its coreceptor CD14 are also present on podocytes, thus LPS can lead to podocyte damage via TNFα and oxidative stress[48]. The reduced GFR in LPS injected mice can be partially prevented by pretreatment with TNF-soluble receptor p55[49]. TLR4 knock out mice are protected against renal ischemia-reperfusion injury (IRI)[50].

In a bile duct ligated (BDL) model of cirrhosis norfloxacin used for selective gut decontamination prevented renal tubular injury and development of AKI[51]. This was associated with reduced plasma and renal TNFα levels, and attenuation of the increased renal TLR4, NFκB and caspase-3 expression [51]. The role of TLRs in CKD-HRS is uncertain.

These observations are further supported by human studies. SBP primary prophylaxis with norfloxacin in case of low protein ascites and advanced cirrhosis not only reduced the risk of SBP and improved survival but also reduced the 1-year probability of developing HRS, irrespective of its effect on SBP prevention[52]. Rifaximin, another antibiotic, was suggested to play role in gut barrier repair, ameliorating bacterial translocation and thus systemic inflammation[53]. Rifaximin suppressed the growth of orally originating bacteria in the feces in patients with cirrhosis, preventing gut mucin barrier degradation [53]. Rifaximin did ameliorate endotoxemia and systemic inflammation shown by the reduced plasma TNFα levels and neutrophil TLR-4 expression [53]. Rifaximin has been shown to decrease the incidence and severity of AKI and AKI-HRS in patients with cirrhosis[54].

Further supporting the role of intestinal homeostasis and the role of the gut–kidney axis, *Park and colleagues*[55] showed that the depletion of intestinal Paneth cells attenuates renal dysfunction in hepatic IRI model, possibly via decreased IL-17A production.

Similarly, a direct bidirectional relationship exists between the gut and liver. PAMPs directly reach the liver via the portal circulation and can exert an overwhelming proinflammatory response augmenting liver damage. The role of various DAMPs released from dying liver cells has been implicated in the development of hepatorenal injury. Dying cells release DNA, called cell-free or extracellular DNA that contains both nuclear and mitochondrial DNA (mtDNA), latter one recognized by TLR9. Increased cell-free DNA level was reported in thioacetamide (TAA)-induced liver injury, and the authors speculated that this extracellular DNA is involved in the pathogenesis of associated renal dysfunction, as treatment with deoxyribonuclease improved serum creatinine[56].

Schulz and colleagues suggested that biglycan, an extracellular matrix (ECM) component, released from the cirrhotic liver promotes hepatorenal cross-talk, and can elicit both pro- and anti-inflammatory responses. Biglycan triggers proinflammatory responses via the TLR2/TLR4 and CD14 receptor complex and by promoting NLRP3 inflammasome activation, the latter leading to IL-1β production[57]. Biglycan also leads to immune cell recruitment to the kidneys, especially proinflammatory type, including M1 macrophages and neutrophils[58]. In return, the proinflammatory cytokines, for example, TNFα have been shown to induce apoptosis of renal tubular cells[59]. Biglycan can also trigger autophagy, via the TLR4/CD44 receptor complex, and promote anti-inflammatory M2 macrophage polarization. *Poluzzi and colleagues*[60] showed that during renal IRI, the biglycan/TLR4/CD44-induced autophagy ameliorates renal tubular injury.

Mitochondrial dysfunction is the hallmark of AKI in cirrhosis in animal experiments and metabolomic profile in ACLF also suggests decreased mitochondrial ATP production[61]. Mitophagy, which is the selective degradation of mitochondria by autophagy, prevents apoptosis of renal tubular cells by removal of the damaged mitochondria[62].

Inflammation and circulatory dysfunction

Inflammatory pathways might contribute to HRS development not only by directly affecting the renal tubular cells but also via circulatory dysfunction, both renal and systemic.

It has been suggested that bacterial translocation, particularly endotoxemia does affect vascular endothelium and decreases peritubular capillary flow [46]. Rats injected with LPS had impaired cortical and medullary renal perfusion[63]. LPS enhanced renal vascular reactivity to endothelin-1 (ET-1), contributing to the dominance of renal vaso-constriction over vasodilation [14]. Pretreatment with an endothelin receptor type A (ET_A) antagonist, but not with a type B (ET_B) antagonist, ameliorated the LPS-induced enhanced renal vascular response in cirrhotic rats using CBDL model [14].

Furthermore, selective decontamination with norfloxacin decreased vascular NO production, and partially reversed the hyperdynamic circulatory state with increased SVR, increased MAP, decreased cardiac output, but without the alteration of GFR.[64]

RELATIVE ADRENAL INSUFFICIENCY

Relative adrenal insufficiency (RAI), reported overall in 25% to 30% of patients with decompensated cirrhosis, is more common in patients with severe sepsis, but also observed in the noncritically ill patient[65]. The mechanisms leading to RAI are not fully characterized, but adrenal hypoperfusion, systemic inflammation leading to decreased hormone synthesis and decreased cholesterol availability as a precursor due to liver failure, have been implicated[66]. Interestingly, the prevalence of RAI does not necessarily correlate with the severity of liver disease[67].

Patients with RAI have a higher probability to develop HRS and an increased 3-month mortality [67]. RAI affects β-adrenergic receptors and thus contributes to cardio-myopathy via their downregulation [65]. RAI was shown to be associated with lower mean arterial pressure (MAP), and activation of the vasoconstrictor mechanisms, supported by higher baseline plasma renin activity and noradrenaline concentration compared with patients with intact adrenal function. Beyond the characteristic circulatory changes leading to HRS, RAI also increased the risk of infections [67], possibly via the intestinal effects of the overactive SNS.

OTHER MECHANISMS OF RENAL DYSFUNCTION IN CIRRHOSIS
Cholemic or Bile Cast Nephropathy

Jaundice in advanced liver disease contributes to AKI via renal tubular damage due to the toxic effect of bile constituents and via intratubular bile cast formation[68]. It is supported by the observation that HRS treatment is less effective in patients with high serum bilirubin levels[69]. Kidney biopsies of patients with liver disease suggested that cholemic nephropathy occurs only in AKI, and not in CKD[70]. Its mechanism is yet to be fully clarified. Intratubular bile cast formation is associated with irreversible kidney injury, while the bile acid-induced tubulopathy without cast formation is less severe and potentially reversible[71]. Bile acids are thought to cause renal tubular damage via oxidative stress, with distal and proximal tubule vacuolization and necrosis as seen in autopsies, along with interstitial edema, inflammatory cell infiltration and glomerular congestion. Basement membrane damage leads to leaky tubules[72]. Oxidative stress and production of ROS influence vascular function via release of vasoactive molecules, and thus indirectly affect renal function[73]. More recently, cholemic nephropathy was found to be associated with loss of Aquaporin-2 in renal collecting ducts[74]. In contrast to bile acids, the role of bilirubin in kidney injury is less clear [72].

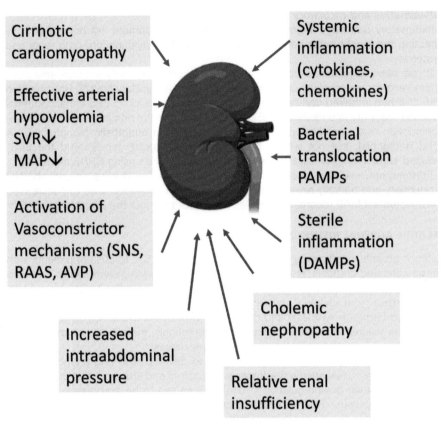

Fig. 3. Summarizing the mechanisms contributing to the development of hepatorenal syndrome.

Nonetheless, jaundice and bile acids are important players in the development of AKI in advanced liver disease, and are potentially reversible depending on the severity, by treating the underlying cause and limiting the bile cast promoting factors. Bile cast formation has been observed in severe prolonged jaundice. Nor-ursodeoxycholic acid has been shown to inhibit renal tubular injury in BDL mice[75]. Cholemic nephropathy is still often underdiagnosed.

Cholemic nephropathy when associated with bile cast formation needs to be distinguished from HRS. However, bile acids can directly affect crucial steps in the development of HRS, thus contributing to kidney injury even in the absence of bile cast formation. A direct vasodilatory effect of bile acids leading to hypotension has been also speculated[76] which along with suspected negative inotropic and chronotropic effects on the heart[77] can lead to reduced renal perfusion.

Patients with advanced cirrhosis have lower total fecal bile acids and reduced ratio of secondary to primary bile acids. This change in bile acid composition contributes to the enhanced bacterial translocation and endotoxemia in cirrhosis [77], enhancing systemic inflammation, a major pillar of HRS development.

Abdominal Compartment Syndrome

The normal intraabdominal pressure (IAP) is 0 to 5 mm Hg. Accumulation of a large amount of ascites increases IAP, leading to intraabdominal hypertension, defined as persistently or repeatedly elevated IAPs greater than 12 mm Hg. This predisposes to renal dysfunction, particularly when IAP is higher than 20 mm Hg, leading to the development of the abdominal compartment syndrome. Structural changes in the kidneys have been reported in a mouse model of cirrhosis with IAP greater than 10 mm Hg, including interstitial inflammatory infiltrates, constrictive renal tubular lumen, and hyperemia with cast formation once IAP was higher than 20 mm Hg[78]. Reduction of IAP is associated with the improvement of renal function[79]. A sudden drop of IAP, such as that seen after LVP, may precipitate AKI.

Biomarkers

A better understanding of the pathogenesis of AKI-HRS can lead to the advancement of therapeutic options and for the development of biomarkers to detect subclinical AKI and differentiate other causes of non-HRS AKIs. The research on these biomarkers is beyond the focus of this review, but multiple potential candidates have been investigated, such as urinary NGAL, IL-18, KIM-1, L-FABP and are summarized in recent reviews[80]. Urinary NGAL has been suggested to differentiate between ATN and AKI-HRS or prerenal AKI. Interestingly, urinary NGAL levels in patients with HRS associated with infection were comparable to those seen in ATN, suggesting some degree of tubular injury in those selected patients with HRS[81].

SUMMARY

Hepatorenal syndrome remains a major cause of mortality in patients with cirrhosis. Our understanding of the underlying mechanism (**Fig. 3**) has changed in the recent decade, suggesting a substantial role of systemic inflammation beyond the well-established circulatory dysfunction. Large number of patients fails to respond to current treatments with vasoactive agents plus albumin, despite that the albumin's theraputic effect extends beyond volume expansion, as it modulates the immune system [82]. Thus a better understanding of pathomechanism can help to develop new or additional therapeutic strategies.

REFERENCES

1. Epstein M. Hepatorenal syndrome: emerging perspectives of pathophysiology and therapy. J Am Soc Nephrol 1994;4:1735–53.
2. Wadei HM, Mai ML, Ahsan N, et al. Hepatorenal syndrome: pathophysiology and management. Clin J Am Soc Nephrol 2006;1(5):1066–79.
3. Wong F, Leung W, Al Beshir M, et al. Outcomes of patients with cirrhosis and hepatorenal syndrome type 1 treated with liver transplantation. Liver Transplantation 2014;21(3):300–7.
4. Gines P, Sola E, Angeli P, et al. Hepatorenal syndrome. Nat Rev 2018;4:23.
5. Cavallin M, Kamath PS, Merli M, et al. Terlipressin plus albumin versus midodrine and octreotide plus albumin in the treatment of hepatorenal syndrome: a randomized trial. Hepatology 2015;62:567–74.
6. Sanyal AJ, Boyer T, Garcia-Tsao G, et al. A randomized, prospective, double-blind, placebo-controlled trial of terlipressin for type 1 hepatorenal syndrome. Gastroenterology 2008;134:1360–8.
7. Schrier RW, Arroyo V, Bernardi M, et al. Peripheral arterial vasodilation hypothesis: a proposal for the initiation of renal sodium and water retention in cirrhosis. Hepatology 1988;8:1151–7.

8. Iwao T, Toyonaga A, Sato M, et al. Effect of posture-induced blood volume expansion on systemic and regional hemodynamics in patients with cirrhosis. J Hepatol 1997;27:484–91.

9. Bernardi M, Di Marco C, Trevisani F, et al. The hemodynamic status of preascitic cirrhosis: an evaluation under steady-state conditions and after postural change. Hepatology 1992;16(2):341–6.

10. Martin PY, Gines P, Schrier RW. Nitric oxide as a mediator of hemodynamic abnormalities and sodium and water retention in cirrhosis. Mechanism Dis 1998;339(8): 533–41.

11. Bernardi M, Moreau R, Angeli P, et al. Mechanisms of decompensation and organ failure in cirrhosis: from peripheral arterial vasodilation to systemic inflammation hypothesis. J Hepatol 2015;63:1272–84.

12. Adebayo D, Neong SF, Wong F. Ascites and hepatorenal syndrome. Clin Liver Dis 2019;23:659–82.

13. Moller S, Henriksen JH. Cardiovascular complications of cirrhosis. Gut 2008; 57(2):268–78.

14. Chuang CL, Chang CC, Hsu SJ, et al. Endotoxinemia-enhanced renal vascular reactivity to endothelin-1 in cirrhotic rats. Am J Physiol Gastrointest Liver Physiol 2018;315:G752–61.

15. Iwakiri Y, Groszmann RJ. The hyperdynamic circulation of chronic liver disease: from the patient to the molecule. Hepatology 2006;43:S121–31.

16. Wiest R, Groszmann RJ. The paradox of nitric oxide in cirrhosis and portal hypertension: too much, not enough. Hepatology 2002;35:478–91.

17. Bolognesi M, Sacerdoti D, Piva A, et al. Carbon monoxide-mediated activation of large conductance calcium-activated potassium channels contributes to mesenteric vasodilation in cirrhotic rats. J Pharmacol Exp Ther 2007;321:187–94.

18. Mallat A, Lotersztajn S. Endocannabinoids and their receptors in the liver. Am J Physiol Gastrointest Liver Physiol 2008;294(1):G9–12.

19. Oberti F, Sogni P, Cailmail S, et al. Role of prostacyclin in hemodynamic alterations in conscious rats with extrahepatic or intrahepatic portal hypertension. Hepatology 1993;18(3):621–7.

20. Moore K. Endothelin and vascular function in liver disease. Gut 2004;53(2): 159–61.

21. Gupta S, Morgan TR, Gordan GS. Calcitonin gene-related peptide in hepatorenal syndrome. A possible mediator of peripheral vasodilation? J Clin Gastroenterol 1992;14(2):122–6.

22. Battista S, Bar F, Mengozzi G, et al. Hyperdynamic circulation in patients with cirrhosis: direct measurement of nitric oxide levels in hepatic and portal veins. J Hepatol 1997;26:75–80.

23. Laffy G, Foschi M, Masini E, et al. Increased production of nitric oxide by neutrophils and monocytes from cirrhotic patients with ascites and hyperdynamic circulation. Hepatology 1995;22(6):1666–73.

24. Wiest R, Das S, Cadelina G, et al. Bacterial translocation in cirrhotic rats stimulates eNOS-derived NO production and impairs mesenteric vascular contractility. J Clin Invest 1999;104:1223–33.

25. Martell A, Coll M, Ezkurdia N, et al. Pathophysiology of splanchnic vasodilation in portal hypertension. World J Hepatol 2010;2(6):208–20.

26. Wiest R, Shah V, Sessa WC, et al. NO overproduction by eNOS precedes hyperdynamic splanchnic circulation in portal hypertensive rats. Am J Physiol 1999; 276:G1043–51.

27. Kew MC, Varma RR, Williams HS, et al. Renal and intrarenal blood flow in the cirrhosis of the liver. Lancet 1971;2:504–10.
28. Maroto A, Gines A, Salo J, et al. Diagnosis of functional kidney failure of cirrhosis with Doppler sonography: prognostic value of resistive index. Hepatology 1994; 20:839–44.
29. Kowalski HJ, Abelmann WH. The cardiac output at rest in Laennec cirrhosis. J Clin Invest 1953;32:1025–33.
30. Wong F. Cirrhotic cardiomyopathy. Hepatol Int 2009;3:294–304.
31. Chayanupatkul M, Liangpunsakul S. Cirrhotic cardiomyopathy: review of pathophysiology and treatment. Hepatol Int 2014;8(3):308–15.
32. Ruiz-del-Arbol L, Monescillo A, Arocena C, et al. Circulatory function and hepatorenal syndrome in cirrhosis. Hepatology 2005;42(2):439–47.
33. Chousterman BG, Boissonnas A, Poupel L. Ly6C high monocytes protects against kidney damage during sepsis via a CX3CR-1-dependent adhesion mechanism. J Am Soc Nephrol 2016;27(3):792–803.
34. Moreau R, Jalan R, Gines P, et al. Acute-on chronic liver failure is a distinct syndrome that develops in patients with acute decompensation of cirrhosis. Gastroenterology 2013;144:1426–37.
35. Engelmann C, Claria J, Szabo G, et al. Pathophysiology of decompensated cirrhosis: portal hypertension, circulatory dysfunction, inflammation, metabolism and mitochondrial dysfunction. J Hepatol 2021;75(S1):S49–66.
36. Arroyo V, Angeli P, Moreau R, et al. The systemic inflammation hypothesis: towards a new paradigm of acute decompensation and multiorgan failure in cirrhosis. J Hepatol 2021;74(3):670–85.
37. Claria J, Stauber RE, Coenradd MJ, et al. Systemic inflammation in decompensated cirrhosis: characterization and role in acute-on-chronic liver failure. Hepatology 2016;64(4):1249–64.
38. Trebicka J, Amoros A, Pitarch C, et al. Addressing profiles of systemic inflammation across the different clinical phenotypes of acutely decompensated cirrhosis. Front Immunol 2019;1:476.
39. Sole C, Sola E, Huelin P, et al. Characterization of inflammatory response in hepatorenal syndrome, relationship with kidney outcome and survival. Liver Int 2019; 39:1246–55.
40. Trebicka J, Fernandez J, Papp M, et al. PREDICT identifies precipitating events associated with the clinical course of acutely decompensated cirrhosis. J Hepatol 2021;74(5):1097–108.
41. West R, Garcia-Tsao G. Bacterial translocation (BT) in cirrhosis. Hepatology 2005; 41:422–33.
42. Li D, Wu M. Pattern recognition receptors in health and disease. Signal Transduct Target Ther 2021;6(1):291.
43. Khanam A, Kottilil S. Acute-on-Chronic liver failure pathophysiological mechanisms and management. Front Med 2021;8:752875.
44. Vila E, Salaices M. Cytokines and vascular reactivity in resistance arteries. Am J Physiol Heart Circ Physiol 2005;288(3):H1016–21.
45. Shah N, Mohamed FE, Jover-Cobos M, et al. Increased renal expression and urinary excretion of TLR4 in acute kidney injury associated with cirrhosis. Liver Int 2013;33:398–409.
46. Peng J, Techasatian W, Hato T, et al. The role of endotoxemia in causing renal dysfunction in cirrhosis. J Investig Med 2020;68(1):26–9.

47. Cunningham PN, Dyanov HM, Park P, et al. Acute renal failure in endotoxemia is caused by TNF acting directly on TNF receptor-1 in kidney. J Immunol 2002;168: 5817–23.
48. Banas MC, Banas B, Hudkins KL, et al. TLR4 links podocytes with the innate immune system to mediate glomerular injury. J Am Soc Nephrol 2008;19:704–13.
49. Knotek M, Rogachev B, Wang W, et al. Endotoxemic renal failure in mice: role of tumor necrosis factor independent of inducible nitric oxide synthase. Kidney Int 2001;59:2243–9.
50. Wu H, Chen G, Wyburn KR, et al. TLR4 activation mediates kidney ischemia/reperfusion injury. J Clin Invest 2007;117:2847–59.
51. Shah N, Dhar D, El Zahraa Mohammed F, et al. Prevention of acute kidney injury in a rodent model of cirrhosis following selective gut decontamination is associated with reduced renal TLR4 expression. J Hepatol 2012;56:1047–53.
52. Fernandez J, Navasa M, Planas R, et al. Primary prophylaxis of spontaneous bacterial peritonitis delays hepatorenal syndrome and improves survival in cirrhosis. Gastroenterology 2007;133:818–24.
53. Patel VC, Lee S, McPhail MJW, et al. Rifaximin-α reduces gut-derived inflammation and mucin degradation in cirrhosis and encephalopathy: RIFSYS randomized controlled trial. J Hepatol 2021;76(2):332–42.
54. Dong T, Aronsohn A, Reddy KG, Te HS. Rifaximin Decreases the Incidence and Severity of Acute Kidney Injury and Hepatorenal Syndrome in Cirrhosis.
55. Park SW, Kim M, Brown KM, et al. Paneth cell-derived interleukin-17A causes multiorgan dysfunction after hepatic ischemia nd reperfusion injury. Hepatology 2011;53:162–1675.
56. Vokalova L, Laukova L, Conka J, et al. Deoxyribonuclease partially ameliorates thioacetamide-induced hepatorenal injury. Am J Physiol Gastrointest Liver Physiol 2017;312:G457–63.
57. Schulz M, Diehl V, Trebicka J, et al. Biglycan: a regulator of hepatorenal inflammation and autophagy. Matrix Biol 2021;100-101:150–61.
58. Nastase MV, Janicova A, Roedig H, et al. Small leucine-rich proteoglycans in renal inflammation: two sides of the coin. J Histochem Cytochem 2018;66: 261–72.
59. Jo SK, Cha DR, Cho WJ, et al. Inflammatory cytokines and lipopolysaccharide induce fas-mediated apoptosis in renal tubular cells. Nephron 2002;91:406–15.
60. Poluzzi C, Nastase MV, Zeng-Brouwers JZ, et al. Biglycan evokes autophagy in macrophages via novel CD44/Toll-lie receptor 4 signaling axis in ischemia-reperfusion injury. Kidney Int 2019;95:540–62.
61. Moreau R, Claria J, Aguilar F, et al. Blood metabolomics uncovers inflammation-associated mitochondrial dysfunction as a potential mechanism underlying ACLF. J Hepatol 2020;72(4):688–701.
62. Fu ZJ, Wang ZY, Xu L, et al. HIF-1α-BNIP3-mediated mitophagy in tubular cells protects against renal ischemia/reperfusion injury. Redox Biol 2020;36:1–16.
63. Millar CG, Thimermann C. Intrarenal haemodynamic and renal dysfunction in endotoxemia: effects of nitric oxide synthase inhibition. Br J Pharmacol 1997;121: 1824–30.
64. Rasaratnam B, Kaye D, Jennings D, et al. The effect of selective intestinal decontamination on the hyperdynamic circulatory state in cirrhosis. A randomized trial. Ann Intern Med 2003;139:186–93.
65. Chancharoenthana W, Leelahavanichkul A. Acute kidney injury spectrum in patients with chronic liver disease: where do we stand? World J Gastroenterol 2019;25(28):3684–703.

66. Fede G, Spadaro L, Tomaselli T, et al. Adrenocortical dysfunction in liver disease: as systematic review. Hepatology 2012;55:1282–91.
67. Acevedo J, Fernandez J, Prado V, et al. Relative adrenal insufficiency in decompensated cirrhosis: relationship to short-term risk of severe sepsis, hepatorenal syndrome, and death. Hepatology 2013;58:1757–65.
68. Fickert P, Rosenkranz AR. Cholemic nephropathy reloaded. Semin Liver Dis 2020;40(1):91–100.
69. Nazar A, Pereira GH, Guevara M, et al. Predictors of response to therapy with terlipressin and albumin in patients with cirrhosis and type 1 hepatorenal syndrome. Hepatology 2010;51:219–26.
70. Maiwall R, Pasupuleti SSR, Bihari C, et al. Incidence, risk factors, and outcomes of transition of acute kidney injury to chronic kidney disease in cirrhosis: a prospective cohort study. Hepatology 2020;71:1009–22.
71. vanSlambrouck CM, Salem F, Meehan SM, et al. Bile cast nephropathy is a common pathologic finding for kidney injury associated with severe liver dysfunction. Kidney Int 2013;84(1):192–7.
72. Tinti F, Umbro I, D'Allessandro M, et al. Cholemic nephropathy as cause of acute and chronic kidney disease. update on an under-diagnosed disease. Life (Basel) 2021;11(11):1200.
73. Li J, Qu J, Chen H, et al. The pathogenesis of renal injury in obstructive jaundice: a review of underlying mechanisms, inducible agents and therapeutic strategies. Pharmacol Res 2021;163:105311.
74. Brasen JH, Mederacke YS, Schmitz J, et al. Cholemic nephropathy causes acute kidney injury and is accompanied by loss of aquaporin 2 in collecting ducts. Hepatology 2019;69(5):2107–19.
75. Eckert P, Krones E, Pollheimer MJ, et al. Bile acids trigger cholemic nephropathy in common bile duct ligated mice. Hepatology 2013;58(6):2056–69.
76. Sauerbuch T, Hennenberg M, Trebicka J, et al. Bile acids, liver cirrhosis, and extrahepatic vascular dysfucntion. Front Physiol 2021;12:718783.
77. El Chediak A, Janom K, Koubar SH. Bile cast nephropathy: when the kidneys turn yellow. Ren Replace Ther 2020;6:15.
78. Chang Y, Qi X, Li Z, et al. Hepatorenal syndrome: insights into the mechanisms of intra-abdominal hypertension. Int J Clin Exp Pathol 2013;6(11):2523–8.
79. Umgelter A, Reindl W, Wagner KS, et al. Effects of plasma expansion with albumin and paracentesis on haemodynamics and kidney function in critically ill cirrhotic patients with tense ascites and hepatorenal syndrome: a prospective uncontrolled trial. Crit Care 2008;12:R4.
80. Menez S, Parikh CR. Assessing the health of the nephron in AKI: biomarkers of kidney function and injury. Curr Opin Nephrol Hypertens 2019;28(6):560–6.
81. Angeli P, Tonon M, Pilutti C, et al. Sepsis-induced acute kidney injury in patients with cirrhosis. Hepatol Int 2016;10:115–23.
82.. Jagdish RK, Maras JS, Sarin SK. Albumin in Advanced Liver Diseases: The Good and the Bad of a Drug. Hepatology 2021;74(5):2848–62.

Hepatorenal Syndrome
Definitions, Diagnosis, and Management

Sebastiano Buccheri, MD[a], Ben L. Da, MD[b],*

KEYWORDS

- Hepatorenal syndrome • Terlipressin • Liver transplantation • Norepinephrine
- Octreotide

INTRODUCTION

Hepatorenal syndrome (HRS) is a hemodynamically mediated, rapidly progressive decline in renal function without clear parenchymal injury.[1] Our understanding of HRS has evolved from simply a diagnosis of exclusion driven by the vasodilatory theory to a spectrum disease encompassing HRS-AKI to HRS-AKI on chronic kidney disease (CKD).[2,3] Conventional management involves volume expansion with albumin and vasoconstriction. There are no Food and Drug Administration (FDA)-approved treatments for HRS currently, although major liver societies are coming to consensus about what should be first-line therapy.[4] Renal replacement therapy (RRT) is a bridge to definitive therapy with orthotopic liver transplantation (OLT) or simultaneous liver kidney transplant (SLK). However, HRS remains a complex condition that is in need for further innovations in management.

DEFINITIONS AND DIAGNOSIS

Our understanding of HRS derives from the criteria set by the International Club of Ascites and various liver societies (**Tables 1–3**). Traditional definitions of HRS include such definitions as greater than 100% increase in serum creatinine (sCr) to a value greater than 2.5 mg/dL within less than 2 weeks for HRS-1 or a gradually progressive renal impairment to greater than 1.5 mg/dL, which is usually accompanied by refractory ascites for HRS-2.[2,5,6] Strictly creatinine-based definitions have yielded to newer definitions that delineate multiple subtypes of HRS disease ranging from HRS-AKI to HRS-AKI on CKD as shown on **Table 2**.[3,6–8] Because much of the

[a] Department of Internal Medicine, Donald and Barbara Zucker School of Medicine at Hofstra/Northwell Health, 400 Community Drive, Manhasset, NY 11030, USA; [b] Department of Internal Medicine, Division of Hepatology, Sandra Atlas Bass Center for Liver Diseases & Transplantation, Donald and Barbara Zucker School of Medicine at Hofstra/Northwell Health, 400 Community Drive, Manhasset, NY 11030, USA
* Corresponding author. Donald and Barbara Zucker School of Medicine/Northwell Health, 400 Community Drive, Manhasset, NY 11030.
E-mail address: bda@northwell.edu

Clin Liver Dis 26 (2022) 181–201
https://doi.org/10.1016/j.cld.2022.01.002
1089-3261/22/© 2022 Elsevier Inc. All rights reserved.

liver.theclinics.com

Table 1
Selected criteria for hepatorenal syndrome diagnosis

Classification Criteria	Sassari[92]	ICA 1996[92]	ICA 2007[5]	ICA 2015[5]
Extent of liver disease	Severe liver disease	Chronic or acute liver disease with hepatic failure and portal hypertension	Cirrhosis with ascites, acute liver failure, or alcoholic hepatitis	Cirrhosis with ascites
Renal function	sCr >1.5 mg/dL progressing over days to weeks	sCr >1.5 mg/dL or 24 hour CrCl <40 mL/min	sCr >1.5 mg/dL CrCl excluded	Diagnosis of AKI per ICA-AKI criteria
Fluid responsiveness	No sustained improvement with fluids to CVP >10 cm H_2O	No sustained renal function improvement with diuretic withdrawal and fluids	No improvement after two days of diuretic withdrawal and albumin volume expansion	Lack of response after two consecutive days of: (1) Diuretic withdrawal (2) Volume expansion with albumin 1 g/kg body weight
Presence of other intrarenal pathology	Trace amounts of protein may be present	(1) Proteinuria <0.5 g/day (2) No obstructive uropathy or renal parenchymal disease on US	(1) Proteinuria >500 mg/day (2) Abnormal renal US	(1) No macroscopic structural injury (2) Normal findings on US
Presence of systemic illness	Renal failure may occur spontaneously in liver disease or associated with infection, paracentesis, diuresis, and volume loss generally	Absence of shock or ongoing bacterial infection. Absence of excessive fluid losses (gastrointestinal losses, renal losses)	Absence of shock	Absence of shock
Treatment with nephrotoxic drugs	Absence of nephrotoxic agents	No recent treatment	No current or recent treatment	No current or recent treatment
Urine volume	<800 mL/day, with some variation	<500 mL/day	Removed	Removed
Urine sodium	<10 mEq/L and often <5 mEq/L	<10 mEq/L	Removed	Removed

		Absence of microhematuria (<50 RBC per HPF)	Absence of microhematuria (<50 RBC per HPF)	Absence of microhematuria (<50 RBC per HPF)
Urine RBC	Not discussed			
Casts	May or may not contain hyaline or granular casts	Not discussed	Not discussed	Not explicitly discussed
Histology	Variable, nonspecific, and may be normal	Not discussed	Not discussed	Structural damage possible

Abbreviations: CrCl, creatinine clearance; CVP, central venous pressure; HPF, high-power field; ICA-AKI, International Club of Ascites-Acute Kidney Injury; RBC, red blood cells; sCr, serum creatinine; US, ultrasound.

Table 2
Spectrum of hepatorenal syndrome pathophysiology

Old Classification	HRS-1		HRS-NAKI/HRS-2	
New classification	HRS-AKI	HRS-AKD	HRS-CKD	HRS-AKI on CKD
Serum creatinine	Absolute sCr increase: 1 >0.3 mg/dL within 48 hours or 2 ≥50% from 3-month baseline	sCr increase <50% from 3-month baseline	Not defined	Not defined
Other measures of renal function	UOP <.5 mL/kg in ≥6 hours	eGFR <60 mL/min/ 1.73 m² for <3 months	eGFR <60 mL/min/ 1.73 m² for ≥3 months	Not defined
Evidence of structural damage	No	No	No	Yes/No[a]

Abbreviations: eGFR, estimated glomerular filtration rate; HRS-1, hepatorenal syndrome type I; HRS-2, hepatorenal syndrome type II; HRS-AKD, hepatorenal syndrome-acute kidney disease; HRS-AKI on CKD, hepatorenal syndrome-acute kidney injury on chronic kidney disease; HRS-AKI, hepatorenal syndrome-acute kidney injury; HRS-CKD, hepatorenal syndrome-chronic kidney disease; HRS-NAKI, hepatorenal syndrome-nonacute kidney injury; sCr, serum creatinine; UOP, urine output.
[a] There may be evidence of chronic structural damage with high suspicion for HRS-AKI.

Table 3
Hepatorenal syndrome definitions across organizations

Society	EASL[6]	AASLD[49]	APASL[50,51]
Functional renal failure?	Partially. Definition will likely need revision	Yes	Yes, primarily. Urinary biomarkers to differentiate from structural disease
Pathogenesis	Hemodynamic/ inflammatory	Hemodynamic/ inflammatory	Hemodynamic/ Inflammatory
Histology	Absence of renal parenchymal damage not biopsy proven	HRS-AKI: no significant abnormalities Structural damage with repeated episodes of HRS	Not discussed
Serum creatinine	Revised classification	ICA-AKI criteria	Not discussed
HRS subtypes	HRS-AKI, HRS-NAKI, and HRS-CKD	HRS-AKI HRS-NAKI (HRS-AKD and HRS-CKD) not explicitly discussed	Spectrum of AKI in ACLF
Diagnosis of exclusion	Yes, although renal parenchymal damage may be present thus superimposed disease	Yes, although may change with urinary biomarkers	Not discussed

Abbreviations: AASLD, American Association for the Study of Liver Diseases; ACLF, acute on chronic liver failure; APASL, Asian Pacific Association for the Study of the Liver; EASL, European Association for the Study of the Liver; HRS, hepatorenal syndrome; HRS-AKD, hepatorenal syndrome-acute kidney disease; HRS-AKI, hepatorenal syndrome-acute kidney injury; HRS-CKD, hepatorenal syndrome-chronic kidney disease; HRS-NAKI, hepatorenal syndrome-nonacute kidney injury; ICA-AKI, International Club of Ascites-Acute Kidney Injury.

literature involves using the older classification of HRS-1 and HRS-2, the authors still use that nomenclature in this review knowing, for example, that HRS-1 and HRS-AKI are synonymous.

HEPATORENAL SYNDROME PREVENTION
Albumin

Albumin infusion increases oncotic pressure, which serves to preserve effective circulating volume, sodium retention, and renal perfusion. Another proposed mechanism for albumin in HRS prevention involves antiinflammatory properties with reversible inhibition of cytokines such as tumor necrosis factor alpha and complement factors.[9] Short-term albumin use has resulted in positive renal-related outcomes and decreased mortality in spontaneous bacterial peritonitis (SBP), which is highlighted in **Table 4**.[8,10–14] Limited evidence exists for albumin administration for HRS prevention with non-SBP infections.[15] Furthermore, albumin may mitigate the effects of post-paracentesis circulatory dysfunction, which results in decreased peripheral vascular resistance, effective circulating volume, and arterial pressure, thereby increasing HRS risk.[9,16] Long-term albumin administration may reduce rates of HRS, SBP,

Table 4
Studies on the prevention of hepatorenal syndrome

Therapy	Study	Design	Results
Long term albumin	Caraceni et al,[13] 2018 (ANSWER study)	Randomized, open-label, multicenter, parallel trial	18-month survival higher in albumin group (77% vs 66%, $P = .028$)
			Reduced incidence of HRS-1: RR 0.39 (95% CI 0.19–0.76, $P = .004$)
			Reduced episodes of renal dysfunction: RR 0.50 (95% CI 0.39–0.64, $P < .001$)
	China et al,[19] 2021 (ATTIRE study)	Randomized, multicenter, open-label, parallel-group trial	No difference in kidney dysfunction, new infection, or death
			Composite HR 1.04 (95% CI: 0.81–1.35) for infection, kidney dysfunction, or death
	Di Pascoli et al,[18] 2019	Nonrandomized, prospective study	Reduction in mortality at 24 months (41.6% vs 65.5%, $P = .032$)
			Nonsignificant trend toward decrease in HRS (57.7% vs 22.5%, $p = NS$)

(continued on next page)

Table 4
(continued)

Therapy	Study	Design	Results
Short term albumin	Sort et al,[10] 1999	Double-blinded, randomized controlled trial	Decreased incidence of renal impairment (10% vs 33%, $P = .002$) Reduction in mortality (10% vs 29%, $P = .01$)
	Fernandez et al,[22] 2020	Open-label, multicenter randomized controlled trial	No between group improvement in: sCr ($P = .18$) MAP ($P = .18$) No difference in mortality between groups (13.1% vs 10.5%, $P = .66$)
NSBB and HRS prevention	Bhutta et al,[29] 2018	Subanalysis of NACSELD database	No change in MAP between groups Not difference in mortality
	Mandorfer et al,[30] 2014	Retrospective analysis	Higher proportion on NSBB developed HRS (24% vs 11%, $P = .027$) and grade C acute kidney injury (20% vs 8%, $P = .021$)
	Scheiner et al,[33] 2017	Retrospective analysis	Over a 3-year follow-up: No association with an increased incidence of AKI (p = NS, 0.323)
	Serste et al,[32] 2010	Single-center, observational, case-only, prospective	Decreased survival at 1year (19% vs 64%, $P < .0001$)
Antibiotics use in SBP and non-SBP infections	Kamal et al,[23] 2017	Meta-analysis	Protective against HRS (pooled OR 0.25, 95% CI: 0.13–0.50, I = 0%)
	Menshawy et al,[24] 2019	Meta-analysis	Rifaximin plus norfloxacin prevented SBP (RR 0.58, 95% CI 0.37–0.92, $P = .02$)
	Fernandez et al,[14] 2007	Randomized controlled trial	Reduced the probability of HRS at 1 year (28% vs 41%, $P = .02$)

Abbreviations: AKI, acute kidney injury; HR, hazard ratio; HRS, hepatorenal syndrome; HRS-1, hepatorenal syndrome type I; MAP, mean arterial pressure; NACSELD, North American consortium for the study of end-stage liver disease; NSBB, nonselective β-blocker; RR, risk ratio; SBP, spontaneous bacterial peritonitis; sCr, serum creatinine readmissions/hospital length of stay, and improve survival, although studies have been conflicted.[8,13,17,18] However, recent evidence have suggested that tailoring therapy to serum albumin goals do not reduce infection, kidney dysfunction, or death.[19]

Antibiotics

Bacterial infection is an identifiable trigger for HRS in decompensated and compensated cirrhosis whereby acute on chronic liver failure (ACLF) can develop, mediated by a systemic inflammatory state.[20,21] Bacterial translocation is one of the main mechanisms by which bacterial infection, systemic inflammation, and decompensation can occur in cirrhosis. Selective intestinal decontamination with fluoroquinolones and other antibiotics may prevent bacterial translocation and sequelae such as HRS.[21] Antibiotic prophylaxis with antibiotics such as rifaximin and norfloxacin in certain high-risk populations with low total protein concentrations in the ascites seems to be effective in the prevention of SBP and HRS[14,22–24] (see **Table 4**). However, patients with SBP receiving antibiotics may still develop HRS with resultant morbidity and mortality.[10,25,26] The use of preventative antibiotics needs to be balanced against an increased risk of multidrug resistant organisms (MDRO) with prophylactic antibiotics, which could theoretically place patients at higher risk of infection and by corollary HRS.[21] Probiotics, bile acids, statins, and hematopoietic growth factors have been proposed as potential alternatives to antibiotics for prophylaxis in cirrhosis to mitigate deleterious effects such as MDRO but further investigation is needed.[27]

β-Blocker Therapy

There is no consensus regarding whether β-blocker (BB) therapy is beneficial or potentially harmful in HRS prevention. BB therapy must be selectively chosen and tailored to particular populations. BB therapy may precipitate HRS by causing cardiac index (CI) reduction.[28–30] In addition, BB therapy remains disputed in ACLF and contraindicated in SBP due to a risk of hemodynamic compromise.[30–32] However, there has also been studies that have reported that BB use is not associated with an increased incidence of AKI or mortality.[33,34] Certain select patients with decompensated liver cirrhosis are likely to benefit from BB therapy, wherein BB therapy can reduce portal pressures and the chances of variceal bleed and bacterial translocation, whereas the CI remains relatively intact. Nonetheless, careful monitoring for the development of HRS is required.[35]

HEPATORENAL SYNDROME MANAGEMENT: EFFICACY AND ADVERSE EFFECTS

The initial step in the management of HRS involves treating the cause of hepatic decompensation, which may include management of the primary disease process (ie, alcohol cessation in severe alcoholic hepatitis or antiviral therapy in hepatitis B infection), judicious use of antibiotics, and holding diuretic therapy if present. Pharmacologic treatment of HRS can vary depending on local practices. There are currently no FDA-approved treatments for HRS.[4] The combination of midodrine, octreotide, and albumin is perhaps the most commonly used regimen in the United States for the treatment of HRS, despite norepinephrine and terlipressin being often seen as superior.[7,36–39] Although there have been new advances, there is still much room for improvement, as clinical outcomes have not improved for HRS in clinical trials since 2002. A recent meta-analysis of 14 randomized controlled trials involving 778 participants from 2002 to 2018 reported that there has been no improvement in survival (odds ratio [OR] 1.02 95% confidence interval [CI] 0.94–1.11, $P = .66$) or HRS reversal rates (OR 1.03, 95% CI 0.96–1.11, $P = .41$) with more recent clinical trials.[1] **Table 5**

Table 5
Medical therapy for hepatorenal syndrome

Pharmacologic Agent	Mechanism of Action	Dose	Adverse Effects
Terlipressin	V1/V2 agonism	Start: 2 mg/d continuous infusion Titrate: every 24–48 h to a maximum of 12 mg/d until creatinine decreases	Abdominal pain, digit ischemia, nausea, and respiratory failure
Midodrine	α agonism	7.5–15.0 PO 3 times a day	Hypertension when supine and sitting, paresthesia, chills, bradycardia, and urinary frequency and urgency
Octreotide	Somatostatin analogue	100 μg SC 3 times a day to a maximum of 200 μg SC 3 times a day	Nausea, diarrhea, headache, arthralgia, peripheral edema, and tachyphylaxis
Norepinephrine	α and β agonism	Start: 0.5 mg/h infusion Titrate: 0.5 mg/h every 4 h to maximum 3 mg/h Titrated to a goal MAP increase of 10 mm Hg or UOP increase >200 mL/4h	Anxiety, atypical angina, and tissue hypoxia
Albumin	Volume expansion	1 g/kg (up to 100 g) initially followed by 40–50 g/d Can be administered to maintain CVP between 4–10 mm Hg	Urticaria, flushing, hypotension, volume overload, and respiratory failure

Abbreviations: CVP, central venous pressure; PO, orally; SC, subcutaneously; UOP, urine output.

outlines the most used therapies in current HRS management with mechanism of action, dosage, and potential adverse effects.

Midodrine and Octreotide

Therapies that are currently available in the United States for HRS are often thought to be ineffective or inferior by many experts. The primary example of this is midodrine/octreotide, which has traditionally been first-line therapy in the United States for the management of HRS. This combination has limited efficacy with trials reporting conflicting results. Data supporting the use of midodrine/octreotide for HRS is also limited compared with that of norepinephrine and terlipressin. Positive studies have been predominantly retrospective and small in nature (**Table 6**).

Despite limited data, this combination is still the most administered HRS therapy, as it can be easily administered outside the intensive care unit (ICU). Common side effects of midodrine include supine and sitting hypertension, bradycardia, paresthesia, chills, and urinary urgency/frequency. Common side effects for octreotide include nausea, diarrhea, headache, arthralgia, hyperhidrosis, and peripheral swelling. In addition, octreotide therapy is hampered by tachyphylaxis with repeated boluses.

In a nonrandomized, comparison trial of 13 patients with HRS type 1, midodrine/octreotide with albumin was found to improve renal plasma flow, glomerular filtration rate, and urinary sodium compared with dopamine drip with albumin.[2,36] A retrospective

Table 6
Studies on the medical treatment of hepatorenal syndrome

	Study	Design	Results
Midodrine, octreotide, and albumin	Pomier-Layrargues et al.,[42] 2003	Double-blinded, randomized, cross-over trial	Octreotide with albumin was not effective for HRS treatment in cirrhotic patients
	Esrailian et al,[40] 2007	Retrospective analysis	Sustained reduction in sCr (40% vs 10%, $P < .05$)
	Skagen et al,[41] 2009	Nonrandomized, controlled trial	Improved survival in HRS-I and HRS-2 ($P = .0003$ and $P = .009$) Improved renal function at 1 mo ($P = .03$)
Norepinephrine	Nassar et al,[93] 2014	Meta-analysis	No difference in HRS reversal with norepinephrine vs terlipressin (RR = 0.97, 95% CI 0.76–1.23) No difference in HRS recurrence with norepinephrine vs terlipressin (RR = 0.72, 95% CI 0.36–1.45)
	Singh et al,[43] 2012	Randomized controlled trial	No difference in HRS reversal with terlipressin vs norepinephrine (39.1% vs 43.4%, p = NS, 0.764)
	Saif et al,[44] 2018	Randomized controlled trial	No difference in HRS reversal with norepinephrine vs terlipressin (53% vs 57%, p = NS)
	El-Desoki Mahmoud et al,[45] 2021	Randomized controlled trial	Higher rate of full response with norepinephrine vs midodrine/octreotide (57.6% vs 20.0%, $P = .006$)
Terlipressin	Gluud et al,[94] 2010	Meta-analysis	Terlipressin plus albumin reduced mortality compared with albumin (RR 0.81, 95% CI 0.68–0.97) in type I but not type II HRS
	Gifford et al,[57] 2017	Meta-analysis	Terlipressin and albumin had more frequent reversal of HRS compared with albumin alone or placebo (RR 2.54 95% CI: 1.51–4.26)
	Facciorusso et al,[38] 2017	Meta-analysis	Terlipressin improved HRS reversal compared with midodrine/octreotide (OR 26.25, 95% CI: 3.07–224.21)
	Nanda et al,[39] 2018	Meta-analysis	Terlipressin and albumin had improved HRS reversal compared with 1 .Placebo plus albumin (OR 4.72, 95% CI: 1.72–12.93, $P = .003$) or

(*continued on next page*)

Table 6 (continued)		
		2 .Midodrine/octreotide plus albumin (OR 5.94, 95% CI: 1.69–20.85, P = .005)
Solanki et al,[52] 2003	Randomized, controlled, single-blind trial	Terlipressin improved systemic hemodynamics and renal function compared with placebo
Martin-Llahi et al,[53] 2008	Randomized, controlled	Terlipressin improved renal function compared with albumin alone (43.5% vs 8.7%, P = .017)
Sanyal et al,[54] 2008	Prospective, double-blind, placebo controlled trial	Terlipressin improved sCr from baseline to day 14 compared with placebo (−0.7 mg/dL vs 0 mg/dL, P < .009) Terlipressin was superior to placebo for HRS reversal (34% vs 13%, P = .008)
Boyer et al,[55] 2016 (REVERSE trial)	Randomized controlled trial	Terlipressin plus albumin was superior to placebo and albumin in reducing sCr (−1.1 mg/dL vs −0.6 mg/dL, P < .001) There was no difference in HRS reversal with terlipressin plus albumin compared with placebo and albumin (23.7% vs 15.2%, P = .13)
Wong et al,[56] 2021 (CONFIRM study)	Randomized controlled trial	Terlipressin plus albumin improved HRS reversal compared with placebo and albumin (32% vs 17%, P = .006) No mortality benefit was seen with terlipressin (51% vs 45%, p = NS)

Abbreviations: HRS, hepatorenal syndrome; HRS-1, hepatorenal syndrome type I; HRS-2, hepatorenal syndrome type II; sCr, serum creatinine.

study examining survival of patients with HRS-1 found that midodrine and octreotide therapy significantly lowered 30-day mortality in the treatment group compared with placebo (43% vs 71%, P < .05) with sustained improvement in sCr.[40] In another retrospective study including 75 patients with HRS-1 and HRS-2, midodrine/octreotide and albumin therapy improved short-term overall and transplant-free survival compared with a group of 87 historical controls.[41] Octreotide therapy without midodrine seems to have no effect as shown in a randomized, double-blind, cross-over study from 2003, which found no improvement in renal function compared with albumin alone.[42]

Norepinephrine

Norepinephrine may be comparable to terlipressin and superior to midodrine/octreotide in the management of HRS-AKI.[43–45] Adverse effects such as arrhythmia and ischemia often necessitate ICU level monitoring, limiting widespread utilization. Although available literature is limited, norepinephrine and terlipressin were comparable in the management of HRS.[46,47] Advantages of norepinephrine over terlipressin include reduced drug cost and wide availability; however, this must be weighed against costs incurred with ICU monitoring.[48] In addition, norepinephrine seems to be superior to midodrine/octreotide in HRS. In a randomized trial of 60 ICU patients with HRS, norepinephrine with albumin was found to be more effective than midodrine and octreotide in improving renal function.[45]

Terlipressin

Terlipressin is a vasopressin analogue selective for V1/V2 receptors, which, administered with albumin, has long been considered first-line therapy for HRS in Europe and Asia and most recently in the United States[6,49-51] (**Table 7**). The mechanism of action is thought to be via V1 receptor agonism resulting in splanchnic and extrarenal vasoconstriction, leading to improved effective circulating volume and renal perfusion pressures.[37]

Initial studies include a prospective, randomized, placebo-controlled clinical trial of 24 patients with HRS comparing terlipressin, administered 1 mg intravenous (IV) every 12 hours versus placebo.[52] Terlipressin resulted in significant improvement in urine output, creatinine clearance, sCr, and mean arterial pressure (MAP). Five of the twelve patients in the treatment group survived with reversal of HRS at day 15 compared with no patients in the placebo group with HRS reversal in all survivors ($P < .05$).[52] A follow-up study of 46 patients with HRS compared terlipressin (1-2 mg IV every 4 hours) and albumin (1 g/kg) followed by albumin (20-40 g/d) versus albumin alone (1 g/kg followed by 20-40 g/d) for 15 days.[53] The combination of terlipressin/albumin resulted in improved renal function recovery compared with albumin alone (43.5% and 8.7%, $P = .017$). However, there was no difference in survival between the 2 groups at 3 months (27% terlipressin/albumin vs 19% albumin, $P = .7$).[53]

In 2008, Sanyal and colleagues conducted a randomized, prospective, double-blind, placebo-controlled trial in 112 patients with HRS-1 comparing terlipressin versus placebo.[54] Terlipressin was associated with a significant decrease in sCr; however, a benefit in overall and transplant-free survival extending to 180 days of follow-up was not seen.[54] More recently, multiple phase 3 studies have shown efficacy with terlipressin compared with placebo with both primary and secondary endpoints.[54-56] The CONFIRM trial enrolled 300 patients randomized 2:1 to terlipressin versus placebo for up to 14 days. Terlipressin was shown to be more effective than placebo for reversal of HRS (32% vs 17%, $P = .006$) and reducing the need for RRT compared with placebo (19.6% vs 44.8%, $P = .03$). However, this did not translate into an improvement in mortality between the 2 groups with a higher number of patients in the terlipressin group dying from respiratory failure. The lack of difference in mortality is possibly partially attributed to a higher rate of liver transplantation in the placebo group.[56]

Terlipressin is associated with several adverse effects, including abdominal pain, nausea, diarrhea, and respiratory failure, which is mediated by cardiac overload (increased afterload due to terlipressin and preload due to albumin). A meta-analysis demonstrated about a 4-fold increased risk of adverse events with terlipressin therapy but did show about a 3-fold improvement in HRS reversal.[57] Factors that are predictive of terlipressin response include lower baseline sCr (<3.0 mg/dL) and total bilirubin (<10 mg/dL), model for end-stage liver disease (MELD) score, and improvement in MAP by greater than 5 mm Hg at day 3 of therapy.[58,59] Continuous monitoring, careful selection of candidates for therapy, and dosing titration are ways that the adverse side effects of terlipressin can be mitigated.

Terlipressin remains unavailable in the United States and Canada outside of clinical trials, but approval was considered in the treatment of HRS-1 (HRS-AKI) based on

Table 7
Management of hepatorenal syndrome by International Society

Organization	AASLD Guidance[49]	EASL Guidelines[6]	APASL[50,51]
Pharmacologic management	1st line: terlipressin 2nd line: norepinephrine 3rd line: midodrine/octreotide	1st line: terlipressin 2nd line: norepinephrine 3rd line: midodrine/octreotide All in association with albumin	Terlipressin superior to norepinephrine in HRS-AKI
Response	sCr decreases to <1.5 mg/dL or returns to within 0.3 mg/dL of baseline over a maximum of 14 d	Complete response: return to within 0.3 mg/dL from baseline Partial response: final Scr $\geq$0.3 mg/dL of baseline	Not discussed
Transplant	Urgent OLT evaluation SLK if renal recovery not expected with OLT	OLT is best therapeutic option for HRS SLK for treatment refractory AKI including HRS-AKI	OLT may be required
RRT	Consider RRT in: (1) Nonresponders with worsening laboratory abnormalities	Consider RRT in: (1) HRS-AKI nonresponders to vasoconstrictors (2) ESRD and ATN	Initiate RRT those with volume overload or worsening metabolic abnormalities with a lower threshold in multiorgan failure RRT modality based on hemodynamic status and equipment availability
TIPS	Insufficient data	May improve renal function in HRS-1, shown to improve in HRS-2	Not discussed
Liver support systems	No recommendation	Requires further investigation	Improves HRS but not transplant-free survival in ACLF

Abbreviations: ACLF, acute chronic liver failure; ATN, acute tubular necrosis; ESRD, end-stage renal disease; HRS-1, hepatorenal syndrome type 1; HRS-2, hepatorenal syndrome type 2; HRS-AKI, hepatorenal syndrome-acute kidney injury; OLT, orthotopic liver transplant; RRT, renal replacement therapy; sCr, serum creatinine; SLK, simultaneous liver kidney transplant; TIPS, transjugular portosystemic shunt.

data from the CONFIRM trial among others. However, in September of 2020, a complete response letter was issued by the FDA rejecting approval.[4]

Dopamine

The premise for dopamine treatment in HRS centers on theory that HRS is mediated by decreased cardiac output and therefore inotropic medications can be used for HRS treatment.[26,60] One of the first studies from 1975 found that patients with HRS who were treated with low doses of dopamine had improved cortical blood flow rates;

however, urine flow rate and glomerular filtration rate (GFR) did not consistently improve.[61] In a subsequent study of 7 patients with HRS type 1 refractory to albumin treated with low-dose dopamine, promising results were seen with ornipressin and dopamine. HRS reversed in 4 of 7 patients within 1 month, supporting the use of dopamine in combination therapy.[62] The first randomized controlled study with dopamine was done in 40 patients with HRS-1 and HRS-2 comparing the combination of dopamine, albumin, and low-dose furosemide to terlipressin and albumin by assessing markers of renal response such as urine output and urinary excretion of sodium. Study findings suggested that dopamine-containing regimen was noninferior to terlipressin; however, this study was limited by a lack of meaningful long-term outcomes and low terlipressin dosing (compared with prior terlipressin trials).[63]

Pentoxifylline

There has also been interest in the use of pentoxifylline in HRS due to its protective effect against oxidative renal cell injury and clinical efficacy in preventing HRS as shown in several alcoholic hepatitis trials.[64,65] Tyagi and colleagues conducted a randomized trial in 70 patients with sCr less than 1.5 mg/dL without renal disease comparing pentoxifylline versus placebo in preventing HRS. Improvements in renal function, serum sodium, and MAP were seen in the pentoxifylline group extending to 6 months of follow-up, whereas the placebo group demonstrated worsening of those parameters. Only 2 patients developed HRS in the pentoxifylline group compared with 10 patients in the placebo group.[65] However, a recent small randomized controlled trial comparing pentoxifylline versus placebo in addition to the combination regimen of albumin with midodrine/octreotide in HRS-1 showed no clinical significance in HRS resolution or survival.[66] Based on limited evidence, pentoxifylline may be an effective prophylaxis but this needs to be investigated further.

ASSESSING RESPONSE TO THERAPY

Studies across therapeutic modalities in HRS prevention and management have commonly used HRS reversal as a primary endpoint. Reversal and incomplete response are typically measured as change in sCr. Translatability across studies may be limited, as HRS definitions have evolved and previous researchers had applied criteria contemporary to the study period (see **Tables 1–3**). For example, use of a prior criterion for HRS in the CONFIRM trial may have led to a "sicker" population with more advanced disease.[67] The use of a sCr cut-off has significant limitations because sCr is often low at baseline in patients with cirrhosis due to decreased muscle mass and hepatic creatinine production. Thus, a sCr less than 1.5 mg/dL may still represent clinically significant renal dysfunction in these patients.[68–70] In addition, severely elevated serum bilirubin, which is often found in decompensated liver disease, can also affect creatinine assays.[37]

Other potential solutions include using GFR calculations such as the Cockcroft-Gault and Modification of Diet in Renal Disease equations although they may overestimate the true GFR in patients with cirrhosis.[69] For this purpose, cystatin C–based equations are promising in estimating the true GFR and may be used to assess reversal or incomplete response.[8,68,69] Outside of laboratory markers, urine output, central venous pressure (CVP) monitoring, and MAP measurement can be used as a measure for fluid or vasoconstrictor response and likelihood of HRS reversal.[58] The main limitation of surrogate markers is that although they are expected to correlate with RRT-free survival, posttransplant outcomes, and length of ICU stay, this may not always be the case.

Secondary endpoints that have been used in assessing response to therapies in HRS trials have included all-cause mortality, RRT-free survival, transplant-free survival, post-OLT survival, and requirement for post-OLT dialysis. Mortality may have limited application as a primary endpoint due to the large sample sizes needed to ensure that there is adequate power to detect statistical significance between populations. RRT-free survival may no longer be as valuable a metric, as HRS is no longer a contraindication to RRT and patients who receive pre-OLT RRT can have similar outcomes to patients who do not require RRT.[71–73] However, post-OLT dialysis is associated with worse outcomes and therefore pharmacotherapies or interventions that can modulate dialysis requirements in the post-LT setting are worth evaluating.[3,74,75]

MANAGEMENT OF PATIENTS WITHOUT RESPONSE TO MEDICAL THERAPY
Use of Renal Replacement Therapy in Hepatorenal Syndrome

The utilization of RRT in HRS needs to be made on a case-by-case basis, especially in patients who are not considered OLT candidates.[72] There remains limited data surrounding RRT in cirrhotic patients with comorbid kidney injury.[72,73,76,77] A trial of RRT can be indicated in pharmacologically refractive HRS where the subtype of renal injury is unclear (on the spectrum of acute tubular necrosis to HRS).[73] RRT can be used as a bridge to OLT or SLK; however, patients need to be carefully selected, and those who are the most critically ill, such as mechanically ventilated patients, can be poor candidates.[78] A recent meta-analysis demonstrated that patients with HRS receiving pre-LT continuous renal replacement therapy can have similar outcomes to LT recipients without renal failure.[71]

Liver Transplant and Simultaneous Liver-Kidney Transplant

Definitive HRS treatment remains OLT.[3,79–81] Because organ allocation is based on the MELD score, patients who develop HRS receive a MELD score boost that enables them to move up the transplant list. Meanwhile, reversal of HRS via pharmacotherapy lowers the MELD score and waitlist position. Fair allocation with prepharmacotherapy baseline MELD and consideration for pharmacologic failure would be ideal in HRS but implementation of such a concept is difficult.[82] Pretransplant and posttransplant sCr levels are associated with successful post-OLT outcomes.[79] Current SLK criteria focuses on allowing for the opportunity for those patients heading into OLT on RRT to undergo combined liver and kidney transplant and potentially have better posttransplant outcomes; however, future optimization of this criteria should focus on identification of patients that will require long-term HD after OLT.[3,74,75] Persistent kidney dysfunction after OLT and the presence of structural disease on autopsy may guide future strategies for prevention, pharmacotherapy, and definitive therapy with transplant.[75,83]

Alternative and Emerging Therapies

Transjugular intrahepatic portosystemic shunt
Transjugular intrahepatic portosystemic shunt (TIPS) is a procedure that creates a low-resistance shunt between the portal vein and hepatic vein, thereby reducing portal hypertension and improving renal function via decreased renal autoregulation and improved central venous system filling.[84,85] TIPS may have a role as a salvage therapy in HRS in patients who fail to respond to medical therapy and can serve as a bridge to LT in those with acceptable liver function.[85,86] The role for TIPS in HRS is controversial, especially considering the severity of liver failure that is often copresent, as TIPS can lead to hepatic decompensation. Evidence of TIPS efficacy for HRS is conflicted and limited to small, primarily retrospective studies. For example, a study of 7 patients who

underwent TIPS for HRS-1 found that there was a significant improvement in renal function and renal perfusion, as well as a reduction in plasma renin activity, aldosterone, and norepinephrine. However, the mean survival in this study was only about 2 months following TIPS.[87]

Molecular Adsorbent Recirculating System

Liver support systems such as molecular adsorbent recirculating system (MARS) have been used as a bridge to OLT.[88–90] MARS uses charcoal and anion-exchanger columns to selectively remove albumin bound substances and is used in series with RRT.[89,90] Toxin and cytokine production mediating inflammatory response may be mitigated with MARS.[88] Plasma nitric oxide is removed with MARS, a compound that is thought to contribute to splanchnic and systemic vasodilation in liver failure. However, results for MARS in HRS thus far have been mixed.[91]

SUMMARY

Despite the relative stagnation of treatment advancement in previous years, there has recently been a revival of HRS interest culminating in the recent FDA consideration of terlipressin approval; this has triggered spirited discussion among hepatologists, nephrologists, and intensivists, as terlipressin is considered first-line therapy among all liver societies and its rejection by the FDA represents a setback in HRS management within the United States. Regardless, further advances need to be made with this crippling complication of decompensated liver disease, as the treatment options remain very limited. RRT and even TIPS have a role in bridging a patient with HRS to definite therapy with LT. With renewed interest in HRS, we must ensure that these patients undergo fair organ allocation. A diagnosis of exclusion cannot mean less attention for this still misunderstood and lethal condition.

CLINICS CARE POINTS

- HRS is defined by hemodynamic and inflammatory changes causing potentially reversible renal dysregulation that is associated with high morbidity and mortality.
- HRS can be further subtyped into HRS-AKI (hepatorenal syndrome-acute kidney injury), HRS-AKD (hepatorenal syndrome-acute kidney disease), HRS-CKD (hepatorenal syndrome-chronic kidney disease), and HRS-AKI on CKD.
- Prevention of HRS involves short-term albumin use in SBP and large-volume paracentesis, antibiotics use in SBP-related indications, and NSBB therapy within a therapeutic window that is based on cirrhosis severity.
- Terlipressin is validated as first-line pharmacotherapy for HRS in the United States, although it lacks FDA approval.
- RRT, liver dialysis, and TIPS are potential bridging strategies to definitive therapy with OLT or SLK.

CONFLICT OF INTEREST STATEMENT

The authors declare that there is no conflict of interest.

AUTHOR INVOLVEMENT

The authors were involved equally in drafting this article.

REFERENCES

1. Thomson MJ, Taylor A, Sharma P, et al. Limited progress in hepatorenal syndrome (HRS) reversal and survival 2002-2018: a systematic review and meta-analysis. Dig Dis Sci 2020;65:1539–48.
2. Angeli P, Volpin R, Piovan D, et al. Acute effects of the oral administration of midodrine, an alpha-adrenergic agonist, on renal hemodynamics and renal function in cirrhotic patients with ascites. Hepatology 1998;28:937–43.
3. Angeli P, Garcia-Tsao G, Nadim MK, et al. News in pathophysiology, definition and classification of hepatorenal syndrome: a step beyond the International Club of Ascites (ICA) consensus document. J Hepatol 2019;71:811–22.
4. Association FaD. FDA briefing document cardiovascular and renal drugs Advisory Committee Meeting july 15,2020 NDA 22231 terlipressin. 2020. Available at: https://www.fda.gov/media/139963/download. Accessed September 10, 2021.
5. Angeli P, Gines P, Wong F, et al. Diagnosis and management of acute kidney injury in patients with cirrhosis: revised consensus recommendations of the International Club of Ascites. Gut 2015;64:531–7.
6. easloffice@easloffice.eu EAftSotLEa, Liver EAftSot. EASL Clinical Practice Guidelines for the management of patients with decompensated cirrhosis. J Hepatol 2018;69:406–60.
7. Cavallin M, Kamath PS, Merli M, et al. Terlipressin plus albumin versus midodrine and octreotide plus albumin in the treatment of hepatorenal syndrome: a randomized trial. Hepatology 2015;62:567–74.
8. Francoz C, Durand F, Kahn JA, et al. Hepatorenal syndrome. Clin J Am Soc Nephrol 2019;14:774–81.
9. Bernardi M, Caraceni P, Navickis RJ, et al. Albumin infusion in patients undergoing large-volume paracentesis: a meta-analysis of randomized trials. Hepatology 2012;55:1172–81.
10. Sort P, Navasa M, Arroyo V, et al. Effect of intravenous albumin on renal impairment and mortality in patients with cirrhosis and spontaneous bacterial peritonitis. N Engl J Med 1999;341:403–9.
11. Narula N, Tsoi K, Marshall JK. Should albumin be used in all patients with spontaneous bacterial peritonitis? Can J Gastroenterol 2011;25:373–6.
12. Caraceni P, Domenicali M, Tovoli A, et al. Clinical indications for the albumin use: still a controversial issue. Eur J Intern Med 2013;24:721–8.
13. Caraceni P, Riggio O, Angeli P, et al. Long-term albumin administration in decompensated cirrhosis (ANSWER): an open-label randomised trial. Lancet 2018;391:2417–29.
14. Fernández J, Navasa M, Planas R, et al. Primary prophylaxis of spontaneous bacterial peritonitis delays hepatorenal syndrome and improves survival in cirrhosis. Gastroenterology 2007;133:818–24.
15. Zaccherini G, Tufoni M, Bernardi M. Albumin administration is efficacious in the management of patients with cirrhosis: a systematic review of the literature. Hepat Med 2020;12:153–72.
16. Salerno F, Guevara M, Bernardi M, et al. Refractory ascites: pathogenesis, definition and therapy of a severe complication in patients with cirrhosis. Liver Int 2010;30:937–47.
17. Romanelli RG, La Villa G, Barletta G, et al. Long-term albumin infusion improves survival in patients with cirrhosis and ascites: an unblinded randomized trial. World J Gastroenterol 2006;12:1403–7.

18. Di Pascoli M, Fasolato S, Piano S, et al. Long-term administration of human albumin improves survival in patients with cirrhosis and refractory ascites. Liver Int 2019;39:98–105.

19. China L, Freemantle N, Forrest E, et al. A randomized trial of albumin infusions in hospitalized patients with cirrhosis. N Engl J Med 2021;384:808–17.

20. Salerno F, Monti V. Hepatorenal syndrome type 1 and bacterial infection: a catastrophic association in patients with cirrhosis. Hepatology 2014;59:1239–41.

21. Garcia-Tsao G. Prophylactic antibiotics in cirrhosis: are they promoting or preventing infections? Clin Liver Dis (Hoboken) 2019;14:98–102.

22. Fernández J, Angeli P, Trebicka J, Merli M, Gustot T, Alessandria C, Aagaard NK, et al. Efficacy of albumin treatment for patients with cirrhosis and infections unrelated to spontaneous bacterial peritonitis. Clin Gastroenterol Hepatol 2020;18: 963–73.e4.

23. Kamal F, Khan MA, Khan Z, et al. Rifaximin for the prevention of spontaneous bacterial peritonitis and hepatorenal syndrome in cirrhosis: a systematic review and meta-analysis. Eur J Gastroenterol Hepatol 2017;29:1109–17.

24. Menshawy A, Mattar O, Barssoum K, et al. Safety and efficacy of rifaximin in prophylaxis of spontaneous bacterial peritonitis: a systematic review and meta-analysis. Curr Drug Targets 2019;20:380–7.

25. Follo A, Llovet JM, Navasa M, et al. Renal impairment after spontaneous bacterial peritonitis in cirrhosis: incidence, clinical course, predictive factors and prognosis. Hepatology 1994;20:1495–501.

26. Ruiz-del-Arbol L, Urman J, Fernández J, et al. Systemic, renal, and hepatic hemodynamic derangement in cirrhotic patients with spontaneous bacterial peritonitis. Hepatology 2003;38:1210–8.

27. Fernández J, Tandon P, Mensa J, et al. Antibiotic prophylaxis in cirrhosis: good and bad. Hepatology 2016;63:2019–31.

28. Krag A, Bendtsen F, Henriksen JH, et al. Low cardiac output predicts development of hepatorenal syndrome and survival in patients with cirrhosis and ascites. Gut 2010;59:105–10.

29. Bhutta AQ, Garcia-Tsao G, Reddy KR, et al. Beta-blockers in hospitalised patients with cirrhosis and ascites: mortality and factors determining discontinuation and reinitiation. Aliment Pharmacol Ther 2018;47:78–85.

30. Mandorfer M, Bota S, Schwabl P, et al. Nonselective β blockers increase risk for hepatorenal syndrome and death in patients with cirrhosis and spontaneous bacterial peritonitis. Gastroenterology 2014;146:1680–90.e1.

31. Runyon BA, AASLD. Introduction to the revised American Association for the Study of Liver Diseases Practice Guideline management of adult patients with ascites due to cirrhosis 2012. Hepatology 2013;57:1651–3.

32. Sersté T, Melot C, Francoz C, et al. Deleterious effects of beta-blockers on survival in patients with cirrhosis and refractory ascites. Hepatology 2010;52: 1017–22.

33. Scheiner B, Parada-Rodriguez D, Bucsics T, et al. Non-selective beta-blocker treatment does not impact on kidney function in cirrhotic patients with varices. Scand J Gastroenterol 2017;52:1008–15.

34. Mookerjee RP, Pavesi M, Thomsen KL, et al. Treatment with non-selective beta blockers is associated with reduced severity of systemic inflammation and improved survival of patients with acute-on-chronic liver failure. J Hepatol 2016;64:574–82.

35. Krag A, Wiest R, Albillos A, et al. The window hypothesis: haemodynamic and non-haemodynamic effects of β-blockers improve survival of patients with cirrhosis during a window in the disease. Gut 2012;61:967–9.

36. Angeli P, Volpin R, Gerunda G, et al. Reversal of type 1 hepatorenal syndrome with the administration of midodrine and octreotide. Hepatology 1999;29:1690–7.

37. Flamm SL, Brown K, Wadei HM, et al. The current management of hepatorenal syndrome-acute kidney injury in the United States and the potential of terlipressin. Liver Transpl 2021;27:1191–202.

38. Facciorusso A, Chandar AK, Murad MH, et al. Comparative efficacy of pharmacological strategies for management of type 1 hepatorenal syndrome: a systematic review and network meta-analysis. Lancet Gastroenterol Hepatol 2017;2:94–102.

39. Nanda A, Reddy R, Safraz H, et al. Pharmacological therapies for hepatorenal syndrome: a systematic review and meta-analysis. J Clin Gastroenterol 2018;52:360–7.

40. Esrailian E, Pantangco ER, Kyulo NL, et al. Octreotide/Midodrine therapy significantly improves renal function and 30-day survival in patients with type 1 hepatorenal syndrome. Dig Dis Sci 2007;52:742–8.

41. Skagen C, Einstein M, Lucey MR, et al. Combination treatment with octreotide, midodrine, and albumin improves survival in patients with type 1 and type 2 hepatorenal syndrome. J Clin Gastroenterol 2009;43:680–5.

42. Pomier-Layrargues G, Paquin SC, Hassoun Z, et al. Octreotide in hepatorenal syndrome: a randomized, double-blind, placebo-controlled, crossover study. Hepatology 2003;38:238–43.

43. Singh V, Ghosh S, Singh B, et al. Noradrenaline vs. terlipressin in the treatment of hepatorenal syndrome: a randomized study. J Hepatol 2012;56:1293–8.

44. Saif RU, Dar HA, Sofi SM, et al. Noradrenaline versus terlipressin in the management of type 1 hepatorenal syndrome: a randomized controlled study. Indian J Gastroenterol 2018;37:424–9.

45. El-Desoki Mahmoud EI, Abdelaziz DH, Abd-Elsalam S, et al. Norepinephrine is more effective than midodrine/octreotide in patients with hepatorenal syndrome-acute kidney injury: a randomized controlled trial. Front Pharmacol 2021;12:675948.

46. Alessandria C, Ottobrelli A, Debernardi-Venon W, et al. Noradrenalin vs terlipressin in patients with hepatorenal syndrome: a prospective, randomized, unblinded, pilot study. J Hepatol 2007;47:499–505.

47. Sharma P, Kumar A, Shrama BC, et al. An open label, pilot, randomized controlled trial of noradrenaline versus terlipressin in the treatment of type 1 hepatorenal syndrome and predictors of response. Am J Gastroenterol 2008;103:1689–97.

48. Ghosh S, Choudhary NS, Sharma AK, et al. Noradrenaline vs terlipressin in the treatment of type 2 hepatorenal syndrome: a randomized pilot study. Liver Int 2013;33:1187–93.

49. Biggins SW, Angeli P, Garcia-Tsao G, et al. Diagnosis, evaluation, and management of ascites, spontaneous bacterial peritonitis and hepatorenal syndrome: 2021 Practice Guidance by the American Association for the Study of Liver Diseases. Hepatology 2021;74:1014–48.

50. Sarin SK, Kedarisetty CK, Abbas Z, et al. Acute-on-chronic liver failure: consensus recommendations of the Asian Pacific Association for the study of the liver (APASL) 2014. Hepatol Int 2014;8:453–71.

51. Sarin SK, Choudhury A, Sharma MK, et al. Correction to: acute-on-chronic liver failure: consensus recommendations of the Asian Pacific association for the study of the liver (APASL): an update. Hepatol Int 2019;13:826–8.

52. Solanki P, Chawla A, Garg R, et al. Beneficial effects of terlipressin in hepatorenal syndrome: a prospective, randomized placebo-controlled clinical trial. J Gastroenterol Hepatol 2003;18:152–6.

53. Martín-Llahí M, Pépin MN, Guevara M, et al. Terlipressin and albumin vs albumin in patients with cirrhosis and hepatorenal syndrome: a randomized study. Gastroenterology 2008;134:1352–9.

54. Sanyal AJ, Boyer T, Garcia-Tsao G, et al. A randomized, prospective, double-blind, placebo-controlled trial of terlipressin for type 1 hepatorenal syndrome. Gastroenterology 2008;134:1360–8.

55. Boyer TD, Sanyal AJ, Wong F, et al. Terlipressin plus albumin is more effective than albumin alone in improving renal function in patients with cirrhosis and hepatorenal syndrome type 1. Gastroenterology 2016;150:1579–89.e2.

56. Wong F, Pappas SC, Curry MP, et al. Terlipressin plus albumin for the treatment of type 1 hepatorenal syndrome. N Engl J Med 2021;384:818–28.

57. Gifford FJ, Morling JR, Fallowfield JA. Systematic review with meta-analysis: vasoactive drugs for the treatment of hepatorenal syndrome type 1. Aliment Pharmacol Ther 2017;45:593–603.

58. Boyer TD, Sanyal AJ, Garcia-Tsao G, et al. Predictors of response to terlipressin plus albumin in hepatorenal syndrome (HRS) type 1: relationship of serum creatinine to hemodynamics. J Hepatol 2011;55:315–21.

59. Nazar A, Pereira GH, Guevara M, et al. Predictors of response to therapy with terlipressin and albumin in patients with cirrhosis and type 1 hepatorenal syndrome. Hepatology 2010;51:219–26.

60. Piano S, Angeli P. Dopamine and furosemide for the treatment of hepatorenal syndrome: a reappraisal or just smoke and mirrors? J Clin Exp Hepatol 2015;5: 273–5.

61. Bennett WM, Keeffe E, Melnyk C, et al. Response to dopamine hydrochloride in the hepatorenal syndrome. Arch Intern Med 1975;135:964–71.

62. Gülberg V, Bilzer M, Gerbes AL. Long-term therapy and retreatment of hepatorenal syndrome type 1 with ornipressin and dopamine. Hepatology 1999;30:870–5.

63. Srivastava S, Shalimar VS, Prakash S, et al. Randomized controlled trial comparing the efficacy of terlipressin and albumin with a combination of concurrent dopamine, furosemide, and albumin in hepatorenal syndrome. J Clin Exp Hepatol 2015;5:276–85.

64. Ozturk H, Cetinkaya A, Firat TS, et al. Protective effect of pentoxifylline on oxidative renal cell injury associated with renal crystal formation in a hyperoxaluric rat model. Urolithiasis 2019;47:415–24.

65. Tyagi P, Sharma P, Sharma BC, et al. Prevention of hepatorenal syndrome in patients with cirrhosis and ascites: a pilot randomized control trial between pentoxifylline and placebo. Eur J Gastroenterol Hepatol 2011;23:210–7.

66. Stine JG, Wang J, Cornella SL, et al. Treatment of Type-1 hepatorenal syndrome with pentoxifylline: a randomized placebo controlled clinical trial. Ann Hepatol 2018;17:300–6.

67. Jamie W, Alicja R-R, Joel T, et al. CONFIRMing hepatorenal syndrome management: #NephJC Editorial. 2021. Available at: https://www.kidneymedicinejournal. org/article/S2590-0595(21)00175-8/fulltext. Accessed August 28, 2021.

68. De Souza V, Hadj-Aissa A, Dolomanova O, et al. Creatinine- versus cystatine C-based equations in assessing the renal function of candidates for liver transplantation with cirrhosis. Hepatology 2014;59:1522–31.

69. Francoz C, Prié D, Abdelrazek W, et al. Inaccuracies of creatinine and creatinine-based equations in candidates for liver transplantation with low creatinine: impact on the model for end-stage liver disease score. Liver Transpl 2010;16:1169–77.

70. Schrier RW, Shchekochikhin D, Ginès P. Renal failure in cirrhosis: prerenal azotemia, hepatorenal syndrome and acute tubular necrosis. Nephrol Dial Transplant 2012;27:2625–8.

71. Thorat A, Jeng LB. Management of renal dysfunction in patients with liver cirrhosis: role of pretransplantation hemodialysis and outcomes after liver transplantation. Semin Vasc Surg 2016;29:227–35.

72. Keller F, Heinze H, Jochimsen F, et al. Risk factors and outcome of 107 patients with decompensated liver disease and acute renal failure (including 26 patients with hepatorenal syndrome): the role of hemodialysis. Ren Fail 1995;17:135–46.

73. Belcher JM. Is there a role for dialysis in patients with hepatorenal syndrome who are not liver transplant candidates? Semin Dial 2014;27:288–91.

74. Marik PE, Wood K, Starzl TE. The course of type 1 hepato-renal syndrome post liver transplantation. Nephrol Dial Transpl 2006;21:478–82.

75. van Slambrouck CM, Salem F, Meehan SM, et al. Bile cast nephropathy is a common pathologic finding for kidney injury associated with severe liver dysfunction. Kidney Int 2013;84:192–7.

76. Capling RK, Bastani B. The clinical course of patients with type 1 hepatorenal syndrome maintained on hemodialysis. Ren Fail 2004;26:563–8.

77. Allegretti AS, Parada XV, Eneanya ND, et al. Prognosis of patients with cirrhosis and AKI who initiate RRT. Clin J Am Soc Nephrol 2018;13:16–25.

78. Witzke O, Baumann M, Patschan D, et al. Which patients benefit from hemodialysis therapy in hepatorenal syndrome? J Gastroenterol Hepatol 2004;19:1369–73.

79. Eason JD, Gonwa TA, Davis CL, et al. Proceedings of consensus Conference on simultaneous liver kidney transplantation (SLK). Am J Transplant 2008;8:2243–51.

80. Davis CL, Feng S, Sung R, et al. Simultaneous liver-kidney transplantation: evaluation to decision making. Am J Transpl 2007;7:1702–9.

81. Nadim MK, Sung RS, Davis CL, et al. Simultaneous liver-kidney transplantation summit: current state and future directions. Am J Transpl 2012;12:2901–8.

82. Angeli P, Gines P. Hepatorenal syndrome, MELD score and liver transplantation: an evolving issue with relevant implications for clinical practice. J Hepatol 2012;57:1135–40.

83. Velez JC, Nietert PJ. Therapeutic response to vasoconstrictors in hepatorenal syndrome parallels increase in mean arterial pressure: a pooled analysis of clinical trials. Am J Kidney Dis 2011;58:928–38.

84. Acevedo JG, Cramp ME. Hepatorenal syndrome: update on diagnosis and therapy. World J Hepatol 2017;9:293–9.

85. Allaire M, Walter A, Sutter O, et al. TIPS for management of portal-hypertension-related complications in patients with cirrhosis. Clin Res Hepatol Gastroenterol 2020;44:249–63.

86. Testino G, Ferro C, Sumberaz A, et al. Type-2 hepatorenal syndrome and refractory ascites: role of transjugular intrahepatic portosystemic stent-shunt in eighteen patients with advanced cirrhosis awaiting orthotopic liver transplantation. Hepatogastroenterology 2003;50:1753–5.

87. Guevara M, Ginès P, Bandi JC, et al. Transjugular intrahepatic portosystemic shunt in hepatorenal syndrome: effects on renal function and vasoactive systems. Hepatology 1998;28:416–22.
88. García Martínez JJ, Bendjelid K. Artificial liver support systems: what is new over the last decade? Ann Intensive Care 2018;8:109.
89. Mitzner SR. Extracorporeal liver support-albumin dialysis with the molecular adsorbent recirculating system (MARS). Ann Hepatol 2011;10(Suppl 1):S21–8.
90. Mitzner SR, Stange J, Klammt S, et al. Improvement of hepatorenal syndrome with extracorporeal albumin dialysis MARS: results of a prospective, randomized, controlled clinical trial. Liver Transpl 2000;6:277–86.
91. Bañares R, Nevens F, Larsen FS, et al. Extracorporeal albumin dialysis with the molecular adsorbent recirculating system in acute-on-chronic liver failure: the RELIEF trial. Hepatology 2013;57:1153–62.
92. Arroyo V, Ginès P, Gerbes AL, et al. Definition and diagnostic criteria of refractory ascites and hepatorenal syndrome in cirrhosis. International Ascites Club. Hepatology 1996;23:164–76.
93. Nassar Junior AP, Farias AQ, D'Albuquerque LA, et al. Terlipressin versus norepinephrine in the treatment of hepatorenal syndrome: a systematic review and meta-analysis. PLoS One 2014;9:e107466.
94. Gluud LL, Christensen K, Christensen E, et al. Systematic review of randomized trials on vasoconstrictor drugs for hepatorenal syndrome. Hepatology 2010;51:576–84.

Glomerular Disease in Liver Disease

Purva Sharma, MD[a],*, Medha Airy, MD, MPH[b]

KEYWORDS

• Hepatitis • Liver disease • Kidney • Nephropathy

KEY POINTS

- Glomerular Diseases are an important cause of kidney disease in patients with liver disease.
- IgA nephropathy is the most common glomerulonephritis noted in patients with liver disease. Membranoproliferative glomerulonephritis, membranous nephropathy and polyarteritis nodosa are also common.
- Treatment of glomerular diseases associated with liver disease typically entails treatment of the underlying disorder but glomerulonephritis targeted immunosuppression may be needed in some cases.

GLOMERULAR DISEASE IN LIVER DISEASE

Glomerular diseases are an important cause of kidney disease in patients with liver disease. **Fig. 1** Although kidney involvement due to tubular or vascular disease is more common, glomerular diseases became more prevalent as hepatitis infections increased and then subsequently decreased with the widespread availability of hepatitis A and B vaccines and the development of effective antiviral treatments for hepatitis B and C. Ideally, a kidney biopsy is needed to make the diagnosis of these glomerulopathies; however, practically this is not possible owing to the coagulopathy and thrombocytopenia that is associated with advanced liver disease. In this review, we discuss the common glomerular pathologies that are seen in patients with liver disease and the current treatment options available to them.

IgA Nephropathy

IgA nephropathy is the most common glomerulonephritis seen in patients with liver disease. Chronic liver disease, in particular alcoholic cirrhosis, is commonly

[a] Division of Kidney Disease and Hypertension, The Glomerular Disease Center at Northwell Health Donald and Barbara Zucker School of Medicine at Hofstra/Northwell, 100 Community Drive, 2nd floor, Great Neck, NY 11021, USA; [b] Selzman Kidney Institute, Baylor College of Medicine, 7200 Cambridge Street, 8th Floor Suite 8B, Houston, TX 77030, USA
* Corresponding author.
E-mail address: Psharma7@northwell.edu
Twitter: @purvasharma821 (P.S.); @NephDr (M.A.)

Clin Liver Dis 26 (2022) 203–212
https://doi.org/10.1016/j.cld.2022.01.007
1089-3261/22/© 2022 Elsevier Inc. All rights reserved.

liver.theclinics.com

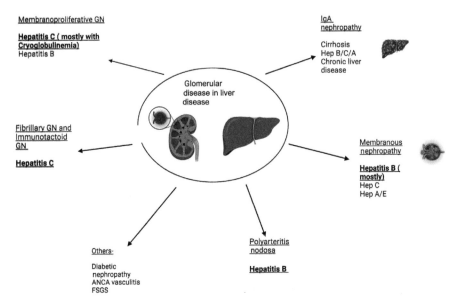

Fig. 1. Glomerular Disease Eiologies in Liver Diseases.

associated with benign mesangial IgA deposition.[1,2] However, it can also present as acute glomerulonephritis in patients with chronic hepatitis B and C[3,4] as well as acute hepatitis A infection.[5,6]

The pathophysiology involves impaired removal of IgA complexes by Kupffer cells in the liver leading to IgA deposition in the kidney.[7] The predominant isoform of IgA deposited is IgA1, although IgA2 can also be found.

A typical kidney biopsy shows the classic finding on immunofluorescence of dominant or codominant deposits of IgA with IgG, IgM, or both. As in primary IgA nephropathy, the primary IgA deposited is IgA1, with a predominance for lambda light chains. Acute glomerulonephritis is associated with subendothelial capillary wall IgA deposits and higher histologic activity (mesangial and endocapillary hypercellularity) with poorer renal outcome.[8] Other histologic findings may include glomerular deposition of C3, absence of C1q, mesangial expansion, and hypercellularity.

Despite the presence of glomerular IgA deposits in patients with liver disease, oftentimes these patients do not have any overt manifestations of glomerular disease.[1,2,4] In a biopsy series of 18 children in whom kidney biopsy was performed at the time of liver transplantation, there was hematuria and proteinuria in one-third of these patients and evidence of glomerulonephritis in all, with most patients having IgA nephropathy.[9]

Immunosuppressive therapy is not indicated in patients with secondary IgA nephropathy due to liver disease.

Membranous Nephropathy

Membranous nephropathy most commonly occurs in association with hepatitis B infection, although it has been reported with hepatitis C and less commonly with hepatitis A and E infections. Hepatitis infections occur mostly in children in endemic areas who are Hep B carriers,[10–13] but it may occur at any age. Hepatitis B-associated membranous nephropathy occurs mostly in males.[14] Serology is positive for the hepatitis B e antigen (HBeAg), surface antigen, and anti-hepatitis B core antibody. Spontaneous resolution of disease can happen in children as they seroconvert from HBeAg to HBeAb.[15] However, spontaneous resolution rarely occurs in adults, with some patients having progressively worse kidney disease.[12,16,17] There was persistent proteinuria in 60% of patients at 1 year in a randomized study in the absence of treatments other than corticosteroids.[17]

The pathogenetic mechanisms of hepatitis B virus (HBV)-associated membranous nephropathy remain controversial. The two postulated mechanisms are direct cytopathic effects of the virus and immune complex deposition.[18] The hepatitis B e antigen and the anti-Hep B e antibody are primarily deposited in the glomeruli.[10,12,19] Hepatitis B DNA has been reported in glomerular and tubular cells suggesting a cytopathogenic effect of the virus. HBeAg has a very low molecular weight and may pass through the glomerular basement membrane inciting an immune response.[18] Some HLA associations have also been found with membranous nephropathy and HBV. HLA-DR or a related genetic factor was associated with disease susceptibility to HBV-associated glomerulonephritis in Korean patients.[20] HLA DQB1 has been associated with membranous nephropathy and HBV.[21]

HBV-associated secondary membranous nephropathy commonly presents with nephrotic range proteinuria and frequently hematuria and hypocomplementemia.[14] Most specific for this lesion in a kidney biopsy is the typical "spike formation" by projection of the glomerular basement membrane material in between the immune complexes, which causes formation of the signature "sawtooth" appearance.

Immunofluorescent staining of biopsy is often positive for granular IgG, C3, and some IgM as well in the subepithelial region of glomerular basement membrane.[22] Subendothelial and mesangial immune deposits in addition to the typical subepithelial location are clues to a secondary form of membranous nephropathy. Additional changes include effacement of podocyte foot processes and occasionally presence of viral particles.[23]

phospholipase A2 receptor (PLA2R) antibody in serum or anti-phospholipase A2 receptor staining on kidney biopsy is typically not found in hepatitis B-associated membranous nephropathy. However, there was one retrospective study of 39 Chinese patients with hepatitis B associated with membranous nephropathy that found 64% cases showing PLA2R staining of immune deposits with colocalization with hepatitis B surface antigen (HBsAg). Serum titers were positive in only 6 patients.[24]

Treatment of chronic hepatitis B in children includes the use of either pegylated interferon alpha or nucleoside/nucleotide analogues. A recent meta-analysis by Yang and colleagues[25] showed that interferon and nucleoside analogues are both effective in HBV clearance and reducing proteinuria. Complete remission (odds ratio [OR] = 26.87, 95% confidence interval [CI]: 8.06–89.52) and total remission (OR = 10.31, 95% CI: 3.59–29.63) of proteinuria and HBeAg clearance (OR = 20.91, 95% CI: 6.90–63.39) increased significantly after antiviral therapy.[25] Entecavir and tenofovir alafenamide seem to be promising medications for HBV-related glomerulopathy, especially in interferon-resistant cases.[26] Other agents, such as tenofovir disoproxil fumarate and adefovir, are not preferred due to nephrotoxic adverse effects.

Cases of membranous nephropathy with hepatitis C have been reported, although this is a less common association and conflicting data exist. One of the earlier studies done by Yamabe and colleagues[27] had showed that 8.3% of patients with membranous nephropathy had anti-hepatitis C virus (HCV) antibodies or detectable HCV RNA. Several small studies additionally have suggested a correlation, although the data are conflicting.[28–32] A Spanish study reported a higher prevalence of membranous nephropathy in hepatitis C-positive kidney transplant recipients compared with those who were negative.[33] However, in another study, only 5% of the 19 patients with membranous nephropathy had anti-HCV antibodies, which was not different than that observed in control patients with diabetic nephropathy.[30]

Pathologic changes in cases of membranous nephropathy associated with hepatitis C are often similar to the primary forms; however, immunofluorescence staining often has IgM, IgG, and IgA as well as complement distribution similar to HCV particles noted on electron microscopy.[34]

Antiviral treatment remains the mainstay of therapy. This is particularly true among children with membranous nephropathy in whom spontaneous recovery over 6 months to 2 years is common.[10,16,35] There may be a role for immunosuppressive therapy for patients with refractory membranous nephropathy. Rituximab may be used in association with antiviral therapy in cases with PLA2R autoimmunization induced by HBV and under the cover of antiviral therapy. There has been description in the literature of patients who remained persistently nephrotic despite effective treatment with antivirals and needed immunosuppression.[36,37] However, the generalizability of this approach remains to be established.[38]

Aside from infection, there are few reports of membranous nephropathy with autoimmune hepatitis and primary biliary cholangitis. These cases also demonstrated electron-dense immune deposits that stained positive for IgG and C3 on immunofluorescence. These cases were treated with immunosuppression and reported resolution of proteinuria.

Membranoproliferative Glomerulonephritis

Membranoproliferative glomerulonephritis (MPGN) is most commonly associated with hepatitis C infection, although it has been reported with hepatitis B infection as well.

The most common cause of HCV-related kidney damage is mixed cryoglobulinemia, which is a systemic vasculitis involving small vessels and presents with fever, nonspecific systemic symptoms such as arthralgias, palpable purpura, neuropathy, and kidney involvement with hematuria, proteinuria, and worsening kidney function. In a review of 146 patients with HCV-related mixed essential cryoglobulinemia, 41% patients had microscopic hematuria and subnephrotic proteinuria with or without chronic kidney disease, 14% had acute glomerulonephritis, 65% had hypertension, and 13% had chronic kidney disease without significant urinalysis abnormalities.[39]

Cryoglobulins are defined as polyclonal immunoglobulin G (IgG) bound to another immunoglobulin that acts as anti-IgG rheumatoid factor (RF), which together precipitate in serum cooled to 4 °C. Mixed essential cryoglobulinemia is classified as type II and comprises polyclonal IgG and IgM RF of monoclonal origin.

Laboratory tests indicate low complement levels with reduction in C4 that is greater than the reduction of C3. Kidney biopsy shows mesangial proliferation and diffuse and global endocapillary hypercellularity. Cryoglobulin deposits can also lead to vasculitis and fibrinoid necrosis of glomeruli, with acute phase showing neutrophilic infiltration and crescent formation in severe cases.[40] Classic double contours of glomerular basement membrane along with subendothelial deposits of IgM, IgG, and complement components are typically seen on electron microscopy and immunofluorescence, respectively. Type II cryoglobulins are most common, but type III mixed cryoglobulinemia has been described.

Compared with hepatitis C, hepatitis B is a rare cause of mixed cryoglobulinemia that may be associated with MPGN.[41–43] In an observational study of 12 patients with HBV-associated cryoglobulinemia, all patients had nephrotic-range proteinuria and microscopic hematuria and 9 (75%) had impaired kidney function. All patients had low complements and histologic features of MPGN on kidney biopsies. Almost

50% of these patients died or developed end-stage kidney disease during follow-up despite immunosuppressive and antiviral treatments.

Both HBsAg and HBeAg deposition have been implicated in this disorder, although the relationship needs to be further studied.[15]

HCV-related MPGN that is not associated with cryoglobulinemia is also described and is related to deposition of HCV-IgG immune complexes, and viral nonstructural protein-3 (NS3) has been detected in the glomeruli as well as the capillary wall and mesangial deposits.[44] These patients subsequently develop measurable cryoglobulins and may be underrecognized.

Similar to the treatment mentioned in earlier sections, the underlying treatment strategy for HCV-related MPGN involves direct-acting antiviral (DAA) treatment with sofosbuvir/ledipasvir, sofosbuvir/velpatasvir, or glecaprevir/pibrentasvir with the goal of achieving sustained virologic response, defined as no viremia for 24 weeks after ending the antiviral therapy. Several small-scale studies indicate that response to DAA in cryoglobulin-associated MPGN is associated with complete resolution of glomerulonephritis and improvement in laboratory test results. In addition, B-cell-depleting therapies, specifically, rituximab, have been shown to play an important role in cryoglobulinemic disease, especially in cases in which DAA therapy did not achieve remission. These therapies have also been used as add-on therapy to DAA treatment with positive results. Last, plasma exchange (for cryoglobulinemic vasculitis with or without renal involvement), which aims at removing circulating cryoglobulins, has been widely used due to lack of definitive therapy.

Immunosuppressive agents such as cyclophosphamide, mycophenolate mofetil, and steroids need to be used with caution because they may increase HCV RNA levels in infection.[40] Treatment of HBV-related MPGN disease is similar to that described in the Membranous Nephropathy section and involves pegylated interferon in children and nucleoside/nucleotide analogue as antiviral therapy in adults.

Polyarteritis Nodosa

Polyarteritis nodosa (PAN) is a necrotizing vasculitis affecting the small- and medium-sized blood vessels. HBV-associated PAN occurs typically within a few months after the initial presentation of hepatitis B[45] and is estimated to account for less than 8% of PAN cases, which is a significant decline after widespread use of hepatitis B vaccines. Antigen-antibody immune complexes are thought to play a role.[10,16] Inflammation and thickening of the vessel wall causes reduced blood flow, thrombosis, and ischemia or infarction of the affected organ.

The clinical features of PAN include systemic manifestations such as fever, weight loss, fatigue, and arthralgias. Kidney involvement is seen with a variable degree of reduced kidney function and hypertension. Narrowing of the inflamed arteries leads to ischemia, but not inflammation or necrosis. A urinalysis can show subnephrotic proteinuria and hematuria, but the presence of red blood cell casts should prompt the search for an alternative diagnosis. Hypertension is a common finding and occurs due to kidney infarction leading to renin-angiotensin system activation.[46] Last, rupture of renal arterial aneurysms can lead to perirenal hematomas.

PAN can be suspected from clinical and radiological features but should ideally be confirmed by biopsy of the affected organ. A kidney biopsy when performed can reveal inflammation of the medium-sized arteries; however, it is prone to sampling error. Besides, the presence of microaneurysms in the kidney increases the chances of bleeding from a kidney biopsy, and hence it is reserved for patients in whom the diagnosis cannot be confirmed on arteriography. Renal arteriography demonstrates multiple aneurysms and irregular constrictions in the larger vessels with occlusion of smaller penetrating arteries. Computed tomography and magnetic resonance angiography can also be used. Wedge-shaped infarcts of the kidney can also be found; however, they are less specific for PAN than the microaneurysms detected by conventional arteriography. A search for concomitant hepatitis C infection should always be performed.

Treatment of hepatitis B- or C-associated PAN consists initially of treating the underlying liver disease with antivirals. Patients with severe manifestations of hepatitis B-associated PAN may benefit from short-term treatment with glucocorticoids and plasma exchange. No randomized control trials exist in this particular subset of patients to guide treatment.[47] A very limited literature exists on the use of mycophenolate mofetil in refractory cases.[48]

Fibrillary Glomerulonephritis and Immunotactoid Glomerulopathy

Fibrillary glomerulonephritis and immunotactoid glomerulopathy have been described with hepatitis C.[49,50] In one case series,[50] findings at presentation included proteinuria, renal insufficiency, and hematuria. Renal biopsy revealed a membranoproliferative pattern of glomerular disease in 5 cases, and a membranous glomerulopathy with mesangial proliferative features in 1. On immunofluorescence, all cases stained with IgG4 and C3. Electron microscopy revealed fibrils of the expected diameter, 16 to 28 nm in fibrillary glomerulonephritis and 33 to 45 nm in immunotactoid glomerulopathy. In only 1 case were cryoglobulins detected (at low titer and on only 1 of 3 assays). Antiviral therapy was not given in any of the 6 cases. Outcomes were mixed, with progression to renal failure occurring in 2 patients and persistent proteinuria with stable or improved renal function in 3.

Diabetic Nephropathy

Diabetes is commonly found in association with HCV.[51,52] In patients with type 2 diabetes, more rapid renal function loss is seen in HCV-infected compared with uninfected patients.[53] However, the impact of diabetes on kidney function in HCV-infected individuals remains to be established.

ANCA Vasculitis

Anti neutrophil Cytoplasmic Antibiodies (ANCA) vasculitis has been described in association with alpha-1 antitrypsin (AAT) deficiency and primary sclerosing cholangitis. AAT variants, homozygous ZZ and SS, heterozygous Z, and SZ, occur in higher-than-expected frequency among individuals with multisystem vasculitides.[54–57] AAT plays an important role as an inhibitor of proteinase-3, a neutrophil elastaselike serine protease located in the primary granules of the neutrophil. If unchecked, proteinase-3 can destroy tissues, so a deficiency of AAT could conceivably trigger an autoimmune response by allowing increased extracellular exposure to proteinase-3.[58] Systemic vasculitis with perinuclear ANCA and specificity for myeloperoxidase has been described in patients with AAT deficiency.[57,59]

Focal Segmental Glomerulosclerosis

Hepatic failure, independent of cause, also has been associated with renal histologic changes. These changes have been called hepatic glomerulosclerosis.[60–62] Hepatic glomerulosclerosis is characterized by variable degrees of mesangial expansion, thickening of capillary walls, a modest increase in endothelial and epithelial cell size and number, and deposits of immunoglobulins and electron-dense material in the mesangium and capillary walls. There is nonspecific mesangial deposition of macromolecules, such as abnormal IgA aggregates, that are normally cleared by interaction with hepatic and white blood cell receptors in the presence of good hepatic function. Furthermore, HCV can directly injure podocytes and lead to glomerulosclerosis as well.

SUMMARY

There is a strong causal relationship between glomerular diseases and certain types of liver diseases especially hepatitis B and C infections and cirrhosis. It is important to understand this association and the progression of disease in these patients. The main treatment is disease-specific therapy, but immunosuppression is used in specific clinical situations with severe or progressive disease.

CLINICS CARE POINTS

- A variety of glomerular diseases are associated with cirrhosis, hepatitis B and C infections, and it is important to keep a low threshold for a kidney biopsy for diagnosis of these conditions.

- The primary treatment involves treating the underlying disease but immunosuppression is used in specific clinical situations with severe or progressive disease.

REFERENCES

1. Newell GC. Cirrhotic glomerulonephritis: incidence, morphology, clinical features, and pathogenesis. Am J Kidney Dis 1987;9(3):183–90.
2. Pouria S, Feehally J. Glomerular IgA deposition in liver disease. Nephrol Dial Transplant 1999;14(10):2279–82.
3. Wang N-S, Wu Z-L, Zhang Y-E, et al. Role of hepatitis B virus infection in pathogenesis of IgA nephropathy. World J Gastroenterol 2003;9(9):2004–8.
4. McGuire BM, Julian BA, Bynon JS Jr, et al. Brief communication: glomerulonephritis in patients with hepatitis C cirrhosis undergoing liver transplantation. Ann Intern Med 2006;144(10):735–41.
5. Cheema SR, Arif F, Charney D, et al. IgA-dominant glomerulonephritis associated with hepatitis A. Clin Nephrol 2004;62(2):138–43.
6. Han SH, Kang EW, Kie JH, et al. Spontaneous remission of IgA nephropathy associated with resolution of hepatitis A. Am J Kidney Dis 2010;56(6):1163–7.
7. Amore A, Coppo R, Roccatello D, et al. Experimental IgA nephropathy secondary to hepatocellular injury induced by dietary deficiencies and heavy alcohol intake. Lab Invest 1994;70(1):68–77.
8. Bellur SS, Troyanov S, Cook HT, et al, Working Group of International IgA Nephropathy Network and Renal Pathology Society.. Immunostaining findings in IgA nephropathy: correlation with histology and clinical outcome in the Oxford classification patient cohort. Nephrol Dial Transplant 2011;26(8):2533–6.
9. Noble-Jamieson G, Thiru S, Johnston P, et al. Glomerulonephritis with end-stage liver disease in childhood. Lancet 1992;339(8795):706–7.
10. Johnson RJ, Couser WG. Hepatitis B infection and renal disease: clinical, immune pathogenetic and therapeutic considerations. Kidney Int 1990;37(2):663–76.
11. Yoshikawa N, Ito H, Yamada Y, et al. Membranous glomerulonephritis associated with hepatitis B antigen in children: a comparison with idiopathic membranous glomerulonephritis. Clin Nephrol 1985;23(1):28–34.

12. Lai KN, Li PK, Lui SF, et al. Membranous nephropathy related to hepatitis B virus in adults. N Engl J Med 1991;324(21):1457–63.

13. Seggie J, Davies PG, Ninin D, et al. Patterns of glomerulonephritis in Zimbabwe: survey of disease characterised by nephrotic proteinuria. Q J Med 1984;53(209): 109–18.

14. Li P, Wei R-B, Tang L, et al. Clinical and pathological analysis of hepatitis B virus-related membranous nephropathy and idiopathic membranous nephropathy. Clin Nephrol 2012;78(6):456–64.

15. Takekoshi Y, Tochimaru H, Nagata Y, et al. Immunopathogenetic mechanisms of hepatitis B virus-related glomerulopathy. Kidney Int Suppl 1991;35:S34–9.

16. Lai KN, Lai FM. Clinical features and the natural course of hepatitis B virus-related glomerulopathy in adults. Kidney Int Suppl 1991;35:S40–5.

17. Lin CY. Treatment of hepatitis B virus-associated membranous nephropathy with recombinant alpha-interferon. Kidney Int 1995;47(1):225–30.

18. He XY, Fang LJ, Zhang YE, et al. In situ hybridization of hepatitis B DNA in hepatitis B-associated glomerulonephritis. Pediatr Nephrol 1998;12(2):117–20.

19. Jennette JC, Iskandar SS, Dalldorf FG. Pathologic differentiation between lupus and non lupus membranous glomerulopathy. Kidney Int 1983;24(3):377–85.

20. Park MH, Song EY, Ahn C, et al. Two subtypes of hepatitis B virus-associated glomerulonephritis are associated with different HLA-DR2 alleles in Koreans. Tissue Antigens 2003;62(6):505–11.

21. Bhimma R, Coovadia M, Hammond MG, et al. HLA associations with HBV carriage and proteinuria. Pediatr Nephrol 2002;17(9):724–9.

22. Shah AS, Amarapurkar DN. Spectrum of hepatitis B and renal involvement. Liver Int 2018;38(1):23–32.

23. Chan TM, Hepatitis B, Disease Renal. Curr Hepat Rep 2010;9(2):99–105.

24. Xie Q, Li Y, Xue J, et al. Renal phospholipase A2 receptor in hepatitis B virus-associated membranous nephropathy. Am J Nephrol 2015;41(4–5):345–53.

25. Yang Y, Ma Y-P, Chen D-P, et al. A meta-analysis of antiviral therapy for hepatitis B virus-associated membranous nephropathy. PLoS One 2016;11(9):e0160437.

26. Mahajan V, D'Cruz S, Nada R, et al. Successful use of entecavir in hepatitis B-associated membranous nephropathy. J Trop Pediatr 2018;64(3):249–52.

27. Yamabe H, Johnson RJ, Gretch DR, et al. Hepatitis C virus infection and membranoproliferative glomerulonephritis in Japan. J Am Soc Nephrol 1995;6(2):220–3.

28. Uchiyama-Tanaka Y, Mori Y, Kishimoto N, et al. Membranous glomerulonephritis associated with hepatitis C virus infection: case report and literature review. Clin Nephrol 2004;61(2):144–50.

29. Stehman-Breen C, Alpers CE, Couser WG, et al. Hepatitis C virus associated membranous glomerulonephritis. Clin Nephrol 1995;44(3):141–7.

30. Cosio FG, Roche Z, Agarwal A, et al. Prevalence of hepatitis C in patients with idiopathic glomerulopathies in native and transplant kidneys. Am J Kidney Dis 1996;28(5):752–8.

31. Johnson RJ, Willson R, Yamabe H, et al. Renal manifestations of hepatitis C virus infection. Kidney Int 1994;46(5):1255–63.

32. Johnson RJ, Gretsch DR, Yamabe H, et al. Membranoproliferative glomerulonephritis associated with hepatitis C virus infection. N Engl J Med 1993;328(7): 465–70.

33. Morales JM, Pascual-Capdevila J, Campistol JM, et al. Membranous glomerulonephritis associated with hepatitis C virus infection in renal transplant patients. Transplantation 1997;63(11):1634–9.

34. Appel GB. Immune-complex glomerulonephritis–deposits plus interest. N Engl J Med 1993;328(7):505–6.

35. Guillevin L, Lhote F. Treatment of polyarteritis nodosa and microscopic polyangiitis. Arthritis Rheum 1998;41(12):2100–5.

36. Berchtold L, Zanetta G, Dahan K, et al. Efficacy and safety of rituximab in hepatitis B virus-associated PLA2R-positive membranous nephropathy. Kidney Int Rep 2018;3(2):486–91.

37. Kataoka H, Mochizuki T, Akihisa T, et al. Successful entecavir plus prednisolone treatment for hepatitis B virus-associated membranoproliferative glomerulonephritis: a case report. Medicine 2019;98(2):e14014.

38. Mazzaro C, Maso LD, Gragnani L, et al. Hepatitis B virus-related cryoglobulinemic vasculitis: review of the literature and long-term follow-up analysis of 18 patients treated with nucleos(t)ide analogues from the Italian study group of cryoglobulinemia (GISC). Viruses 2021;13(6):1032.

39. Roccatello D, Fornasieri A, Giachino O, et al. Multicenter study on hepatitis C virus-related cryoglobulinemic glomerulonephritis. Am J Kidney Dis 2007;49(1): 69–82.

40. Angeletti A, Cantarelli C, Cravedi P. HCV-associated nephropathies in the Era of direct acting antiviral agents. Front Med 2019;6:20.

41. Enríquez R, Sirvent AE, Andrada E, et al. Cryoglobulinemic glomerulonephritis in chronic hepatitis B infection. Ren Fail 2010;32(4):518–22.

42. Perez GO, Pardo V, Fletcher M. Renal involvement in essential mixed cryoglobulinemia. Am J Kidney Dis 1987;10(4):276–80.

43. Li S-J, Xu S-T, Chen H-P, et al. Clinical and morphologic spectrum of renal involvement in patients with HBV-associated cryoglobulinemia. Nephrology 2017;22(6):449–55.

44. Barsoum RS, William EA, Khalil SS. Hepatitis C and kidney disease: a narrative review. J Advert Res 2017;8(2):113–30.

45. Guillevin L, Lhote F, Cohen P, et al. Polyarteritis nodosa related to hepatitis B virus. A prospective study with long-term observation of 41 patients. Medicine 1995;74(5):238–53.

46. Stockigt JR, Topliss DJ, Hewett MJ. High-renin hypertension in necrotizing vasculitis. N Engl J Med 1979;300(21):1218.

47. Guillevin L, Mahr A, Cohen P, et al. Short-term corticosteroids then lamivudine and plasma exchanges to treat hepatitis B virus-related polyarteritis nodosa. Arthritis Rheum 2004;51(3):482–7.

48. Fernanda F, Serena C, Giustina R, et al. Mycophenolate mofetil treatment in two children with severe polyarteritis nodosa refractory to immunosuppressant drugs. Rheumatol Int 2012;32(7):2215–9.

49. Nasr SH, Valeri AM, Cornell LD, et al. Fibrillary glomerulonephritis: a report of 66 cases from a single institution. Clin J Am Soc Nephrol 2011;6(4):775–84.

50. Markowitz GS, Cheng JT, Colvin RB, et al. Hepatitis C viral infection is associated with fibrillary glomerulonephritis and immunotactoid glomerulopathy. J Am Soc Nephrol 1998;9(12):2244–52.

51. Kendrick EA, McVicar JP, Kowdley KV, et al. Renal disease in hepatitis C-positive liver transplant recipients. Transplantation 1997;63(9):1287–93.

52. Zein NN, Abdulkarim AS, Wiesner RH, et al. Prevalence of diabetes mellitus in patients with end-stage liver cirrhosis due to hepatitis C, alcohol, or cholestatic disease. J Hepatol 2000;32(2):209–17.

53. Soma J, Saito T, Taguma Y, et al. High prevalence and adverse effect of hepatitis C virus infection in type II diabetic-related nephropathy. J Am Soc Nephrol 2000; 11(4):690–9.
54. Esnault VL, Testa A, Audrain M, et al. Alpha 1-antitrypsin genetic polymorphism in ANCA-positive systemic vasculitis. Kidney Int 1993;43(6):1329–32.
55. Mahr AD, Edberg JC, Stone JH, et al. Alpha₁-antitrypsin deficiency-related alleles Z and S and the risk of Wegener's granulomatosis. Arthritis Rheum 2010;62(12): 3760–7.
56. O'Donoghue DJ, Guckian M, Blundell G, et al. Alpha-1-proteinase inhibitor and pulmonary haemorrhage in systemic vasculitis. Adv Exp Med Biol 1993;336: 331–5.
57. Rahmattulla C, Mooyaart AL, van Hooven D, et al. Genetic variants in ANCA-associated vasculitis: a meta-analysis. Ann Rheum Dis 2016;75(9):1687–92.
58. Esnault VL, Audrain MA, Sesboüé R. Alpha-1-antitrypsin phenotyping in ANCA-associated diseases: one of several arguments for protease/antiprotease imbalance in systemic vasculitis. Exp Clin Immunogenet 1997;14(3):206–13.
59. Voorzaat BM, van Schaik J, Crobach SLP, et al. Alpha-1 antitrypsin deficiency presenting with MPO-ANCA associated vasculitis and aortic dissection. Case Rep Med 2017;2017:8140641.
60. Lis R. Pathology: state of the art reviews. In: Ferrell LD, editor. Diagnostic problems in liver pathology. Philadelphia: Hanley & Belfus; 1994. p. 258 $42. Hepatology. 1995;22(6):1892. doi, 1016/0270 doi:10.1016/0270-9139(95)90223–90226.
61. Axelsen RA, Crawford DH, Endre ZH, et al. Renal glomerular lesions in unselected patients with cirrhosis undergoing orthotopic liver transplantation. Pathology 1995;27(3):237–46.
62. Sakaguchi H. Hepatic glomerulosclerosis : an electron microscopic study of renal biopsies of liver disease. Lab Invest 1965;14:533–45.

The Interplay Between Nonalcoholic Fatty Liver Disease and Kidney Disease

Emily Truong, MD[a,b], Mazen Noureddin, MD, MHSc[c,d],*

KEYWORDS

- Chronic kidney disease • Hepatocellular carcinoma • Nonalcoholic fatty liver disease
- Type 2 diabetes mellitus

KEY POINTS

- Recent studies support strong connections between increased prevalence and incidence of chronic kidney disease (CKD) and increased prevalence and severity of nonalcoholic fatty liver disease (NAFLD).
- Proposed mechanisms linking CKD and NAFLD include metabolic syndrome, fructose and uric acid accumulation, oxidative stress, intestinal dysbiosis, platelet activation, and genetic predispositions.
- Certain pharmacological treatment choices such as glucagon-like peptide-1 receptor agonists or sodium-glucose cotransporter-2 inhibitors are first-line therapies in coexisting CKD and NAFLD.

INTRODUCTION

Nonalcoholic fatty liver disease (NAFLD) is the most common cause of chronic liver disease worldwide, involving approximately 25% of the general population and increasing in prevalence in patient populations afflicted with metabolic syndrome and type 2 diabetes (T2DM).[1] The spectrum of histologic changes in NAFLD ranges from steatosis to nonalcoholic steatohepatitis (NASH), fibrosis, and even cirrhosis. Not only does NAFLD remain one of the leading causes for liver transplantation but

Grant support: None.
[a] Department of Medicine, 8700 Beverly Boulevard, #5512, Los Angeles, CA 90048, USA;
[b] Cedars-Sinai Medical Center, 8900 Beverly Boulevard, Los Angeles, CA 90048, USA;
[c] Department of Medicine, Karsh Division of Gastroenterology and Hepatology, Comprehensive Transplant Center, Cedars-Sinai Medical Center, Los Angeles, CA, USA; [d] Cedars-Sinai Fatty Liver Program, Division of Digestive and Liver Diseases, Department of Medicine, Comprehensive Transplant Center, Cedars-Sinai Medical Center, 8900 Beverly Boulevard, Los Angeles, CA 90048, USA
* Corresponding author. Cedars-Sinai Fatty Liver Program, Division of Digestive and Liver Diseases, Department of Medicine, Comprehensive Transplant Center, Cedars-Sinai Medical Center, 8900 Beverly Boulevard, Los Angeles, CA 90048.
E-mail address: Mazen.Noureddin@cshs.org

Clin Liver Dis 26 (2022) 213–227
https://doi.org/10.1016/j.cld.2022.01.008
1089-3261/22/© 2022 Elsevier Inc. All rights reserved.

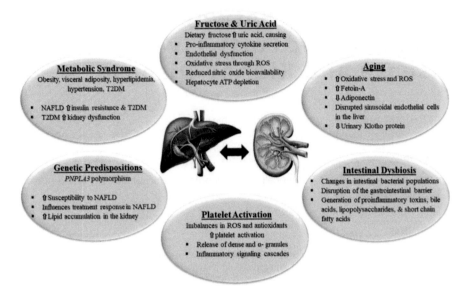

Fig. 1. Potential mechanisms connecting nonalcoholic fatty liver disease (NAFLD) and kidney disease. NAFLD shares numerous cardiometabolic risk factors that may promote CKD. However, NAFLD is an independent risk factor for CKD even after adjusting for traditional cardiometabolic risk factors. Other mechanisms linking NAFLD and kidney disease include fructose and uric acid accumulation, oxidative stress inherent in the aging process, intestinal dysbiosis, platelet activation, and genetic predispositions. Fructose-induced hepatic disease and uric acid-induced renal disease, respectively, contribute to the burden of NAFLD and CKD. Aging-related changes and oxidative stress stimulate inflammatory cascades that significantly contribute to end-organ damage. Imbalances in antioxidants and oxidative stress may also activate platelets to release proinflammatory mediators that further contribute to the vicious cycle of inflammation and tissue damage. Intestinal dysbiosis alters bacterial populations in the gastrointestinal tract, disrupts the gastrointestinal barrier, and generates molecules harmful to the liver and kidneys. An independent risk factor for NAFLD and a modulator of NAFLD treatment response, the PNPLA3 polymorphism has been implicated in the development of both hepatic and renal damage through lipid accumulation. ATP, adenosine triphosphate; NAFLD, nonalcoholic fatty liver disease; PNPLA3, patatinlike phospholipase domain containing 3 gene; ROS, reactive oxygen species; T2DM, type 2 diabetes.

also there is growing evidence that NAFLD is a driver for the development of chronic kidney disease (CKD).[2,3]

Defined as decreased estimated glomerular filtration (eGFR) and/or the presence of significant proteinuria (>500 mg), CKD was the tenth leading cause of death in the Western adult population in 2019.[4,5] T2DM, hypertension, and obesity are the most common risk factors for CKD.[6] Although NAFLD and CKD share similar risk factors, there is a strong association between CKD and NAFLD regardless of the presence of potential confounding diseases such as T2DM, obesity, or hypertension.

This article discusses the complex interplay between NAFLD and CKD, as well as the underlying pathogenesis and mechanisms through which NAFLD and CKD are linked. Exploration of these sophisticated relationships and causative factors is essential to accurately assessing kidney function in patients with NAFLD, recommending pharmacologic treatment of disease, and identifying favorable avenues for future investigation.

Nonalcoholic Fatty Liver Disease: Definition and Staging

NAFLD is defined as the presence of hepatic steatosis in the absence of competing causes for hepatic fat accumulation, including but not limited to alcohol use disorder, viral hepatitis, or long-term use of steatogenic medications.[7] NAFLD is histologically categorized into nonalcoholic fatty liver, defined as greater than or equal to 5% liver steatosis without hepatocellular injury in the form of hepatocyte ballooning or fibrosis, and nonalcoholic steatohepatitis (NASH), defined as greater than or equal to 5% liver steatosis with evidence of hepatocyte injury with or without fibrosis.[7] The presence of NASH is associated with higher risk of cirrhosis, hepatocellular carcinoma (HCC), and liver-related mortality.[7] The most important histologic factor associated with long-term mortality in patients with NAFLD is fibrosis (F2 or stage 2: zone 3 sinusoidal fibrosis plus periportal fibrosis, F3 or stage 3: bridging fibrosis, F4 or stage 4: cirrhosis).[7]

Diagnosis of NAFLD requires evidence of hepatic steatosis by imaging or histology and exclusion of significant alcohol consumption, secondary causes of hepatic steatosis, and coexisting causes for chronic liver diseases.[7] Although NAFLD is frequently detected via abdominal ultrasonography, liver biopsy remains the most definitive approach for identifying NASH and fibrosis. However, liver biopsy is an invasive procedure often limited by associated complications, cost, and sampling error. Noninvasive imaging techniques to identify advanced fibrosis in patients with NAFLD include vibration-controlled transient elastography ([VCTE], Fibroscan), which determines controlled attenuation parameter and liver stiffness to, respectively, assess liver steatosis and fibrosis, and MRI-based assessment, which uses MRI-derived proton density fat fraction and magnetic resonance elastography (MRE) to, respectively, detect liver steatosis and fibrosis.[8,9] Although MRE exhibits superior performance than VCTE in identifying fibrosis stage 2 or greater, both MRE and VCTE perform equally well in identifying fibrosis stage 3 or greater.[10] Apart from imaging, other novel methods for identifying patients with NAFLD at higher risk of progressive NASH (steatohepatitis with NAFLD Activity Score $\geq$4 and fibrosis stage $\geq$2) include biomarkers and composite clinical decision aids, such as the NAFLD fibrosis score (NFS), fibrosis-4 (FIB-4) index, and FibroScan-AST (FAST) score.[11] Both NFS and FIB-4 are blood-based multivariate indices, but NFS uses age, body mass index (BMI), presence or absence of hyperglycemia, platelet count, albumin, aspartate aminotransferase (AST), and alanine aminotransferase (ALT), whereas FIB-4 is based on age, platelet count, AST, and ALT and encompasses dual cutoff values.[12,13] The FAST score identifies patients with NAFLD at higher risk of progressive NASH through a combination of Fibro-Scan and AST.[11]

Interconnections Between Nonalcoholic Fatty Liver Disease and Chronic Kidney Disease

The prevalence and incidence of CKD is higher in patients with NAFLD (assessed via liver biopsy, abdominal ultrasonography, or Fibroscan) independently of demographic characteristics such as gender, age, BMI, or comorbid diseases including obesity, hypertension, or diabetes.[14–16] CKD prevalence in patients with NAFLD ranged from 20% to 55%, whereas patients without NAFLD had 5% to 35% prevalence of CKD.[14] A meta-analysis by Mantovani and colleagues[17] found that NAFLD was associated with a 2-fold increased risk of prevalent CKD and an approximate 40% increase in the long-term risk of incident CKD.

In addition, increased CKD prevalence and severity (based on albuminuria and eGFR) positively correlated with increased severity of NAFLD disease, even after adjusting for features related to metabolic syndrome including BMI, waist circumference, hemoglobin A_{1c} (HgA$_{1c}$), insulin resistance, systolic blood pressure, cholesterol levels, alcohol/tobacco use, and medications used to treat diabetes, hypertension, or hyperlipidemia.[18–21] A retrospective cohort study of 41,430 adults without CKD at baseline demonstrated that, compared with those without NAFLD, the fully adjusted hazard ratios (HRs) for CKD in those with less severe NAFLD (NAFLD fibrosis score <−1.455) and more severe NAFLD (NAFLD fibrosis score ≥−1.455) were 1.09 (95% confidence interval [CI], 0.91–1.32) and 1.58 (95% CI, 1.30–1.92), respectively.[18]

Progressively higher prevalence of CKD correlating with NAFLD disease severity becomes an especial burden in those with cirrhosis, for whom liver transplants are often lifesaving. However, pre–liver transplant CKD has been shown to be significantly associated with post–liver transplant mortality (HR 1.16, $P < .001$) even after adjusting for confounding factors (age, donor risk index, model for end-stage liver disease score (MELD), cause, hepatic encephalopathy, simultaneous liver-kidney transplantation, and diabetes) in 39,719 transplant recipients who were listed for liver transplant in the United States from January 2002 to December 2017.[22] These sobering findings illustrate the growing importance of understanding and appropriately managing the burden of CKD in those with NAFLD.

On the other hand, studies investigating the impact of NAFLD on prognosis and significant adverse clinical outcomes in those with CKD are conflicting.[23] A study involving the Third National Health and Nutrition Examination Survey demonstrated a significant association between NAFLD and all-cause (NAFLD 54.7% vs no NAFLD 46.5%, $P < .05$), but not cardiovascular, mortality in those with CKD, yet this association vanished with adjustments for metabolic features. Another study of 1148 patients with CKD who had undergone liver ultrasound imaging over a 15-year period found that NAFLD did not have a significant effect on all-cause (NAFLD 27.3% vs no NAFLD 33.0%, $P = .14$; unadjusted HR = 0.79; 95% CI, 0.58–1.08) or cardiovascular mortality (NAFLD 31.3% vs no NAFLD 40.5%, $P = .36$) in patients with CKD.[23] Possible mechanisms connecting NAFLD and CKD are shown in **Fig. 1**.

Potential Mechanisms Linking Nonalcoholic Fatty Liver Disease and Chronic Kidney Disease

Metabolic syndrome and type 2 diabetes

Based on current epidemiologic evidence, NAFLD is an independent risk factor for CKD, whose prevalence, incidence, and degree of severity are associated with the histologic severity of NAFLD. Teasing apart causal factors and accounting for potential confounders, such as metabolic syndrome and T2DM, that are interbedded into these closely linked diseases sharing common risk factors is difficult.

Numerous cardiometabolic risk factors are shared among NAFLD, CKD, T2DM, and metabolic syndrome. Metabolic syndrome encompasses a cluster of cardiometabolic features including obesity, visceral adiposity, insulin resistance, high blood pressure, and dyslipidemia that frequently coexist together and heighten the risk of NAFLD, cardiovascular disease, stroke, and T2DM. The risk of T2DM is increased by the presence of metabolic syndrome, and fatty liver also exacerbates insulin resistance and is significantly associated with a 2-fold increased risk of incident diabetes.[16] As assessed in 4 observational studies using either ultrasonographic steatosis scores (n = 3) or NAFLD fibrosis score (n = 1), the risk of incident diabetes in NAFLD progressively increases with higher NAFLD severity.[16] In turn, those with T2DM may develop renal dysfunction due to microvascular and macrovascular damage dealt to the renal glomeruli, respectively, causing abnormal albuminuria and decreased eGFR.

In addition to T2DM, obesity is an independent risk factor for CKD even in the absence of hypertension and diabetes, driving liver and kidney injury through oxidative stress, lipotoxicity, proinflammatory cytokines, and activation of the renin-angiotensin-aldosterone system.[15] Furthermore, NAFLD promotes atherogenic dyslipidemia and oversecretion of very-low-density lipoprotein, both of which may stimulate mesangial cell proliferation and renal glomerular injury.[15] NAFLD thus shares numerous cardiometabolic risk factors that may promote CKD.

However, as previously discussed, NAFLD is an independent risk factor for CKD even after adjusting for traditional cardiometabolic risk factors and the presence or absence of diabetes.[15] Apart from these traditional risk factors, recent evidence suggests that unhealthy diets, the aging process, dysbiosis, platelet activation, and genetic polymorphisms may be contributing mechanisms linking NAFLD and CKD.[4,24]

Dietary Choices: Fructose and Uric Acid Accumulation

Higher dietary intake of fructose, the main constituent of sugar sweeteners, is linked with an increased risk of NAFLD, NASH, and progressive CKD.[4] Fructose fails to promote satiety and decreases resting metabolic rates, thereby provoking unnecessary feeding, excessive caloric intake, and fat accumulation.[25] In addition, fructose is phosphorylated via liver fructokinase to fructose-1-phosphate, which results in buildup of uric acid. Uric acid accumulation may then contribute to the development and progression of insulin resistance, dyslipidemia, cardiovascular disease, NAFLD, and CKD through numerous mechanisms including, but not limited to (1) proinflammatory cytokine secretion, (2) endothelial dysfunction, (3) mitochondrial oxidative stress through the generation of reactive oxygen species, (4) reduced nitric oxide bioavailability, and (5) hepatocyte adenosine triphosphate depletion that enhances renal and hepatic de novo lipogenesis. Furthermore, a positive feedback loop exists whereby uric acid stimulates aldose reductase in the polyol pathway, promoting endogenous fructose production and hepatic triglyceride accumulation.[25,26] Mouse models unable to metabolize fructose are protected from renal dysfunction and lipid accumulation.[27] These interlinking pathways comprise synergistic mechanisms for both fructose-induced hepatic disease and uric acid-induced renal disease, respectively, contributing to the burden of NAFLD and CKD.

Oxidative Stress and Aging

Aging and oxidative stress with its associated dysfunction in mitochondria, the primary intracellular sites of oxygen consumption, are also key mediators in the pathogenesis of both NAFLD and CKD.[28] The aging process and increased visceral adiposity generates reactive oxygen species that diminish antioxidant capacity and adversely impact cellular signaling pathways, increasing insulin resistance, inflammation, and cell death.[28]

Nuclear erythroid related factor-2 (Nrf2), a transcription factor with high expression in the kidney and liver, upregulates the transcription of numerous antioxidant detoxifying enzymes.[29] In mice models involving wild-type and Nrf2-null mice that were fed a high-fat diet, wild-type mice possessed increased hepatic fat deposition without inflammation or fibrosis, whereas Nrf2-null mice developed substantially worse hepatic steatosis and inflammation.[29] In addition to exacerbating fat accumulation and upsetting fatty acid composition in the liver, Nrf2 deletion contributes to worsened oxidative stress, inflammation, and nephropathy, leading to lupuslike autoimmune nephritis.[30] Investigated in clinical trials, the Nrf2 activator, bardoxolone methyl, was associated with long-term renal function improvement in patients with coexisting advanced CKD and T2DM, but its impact on time to end-stage renal disease in CKD remain unelucidated.[31]

Oxidative stress and the accumulation of damaging reactive oxygen species also fundamentally comprises the free radical theory of aging, which is another mutual risk factor for NAFLD and CKD.[4] The aging process is associated with increased fetuin-A, diminished adiponectin, disruption of sinusoidal endothelial cells in the liver, and decreased urinary Klotho protein.[4] A serum glycoprotein secreted by the liver, fetuin-A binds to insulin receptor tyrosine kinase in skeletal muscles and hepatocytes to inhibit 5-AMP-activated protein kinase (AMPK) and induce free fatty acid–mediated expression of proinflammatory cytokines in adipocytes that ultimately promote insulin resistance.[32] Through overexpression of Wnt3a, fetuin-A lowers levels of adiponectin, an adipokine with antidiabetic and antiatherogenic effects.[33] Aging-related changes also include decreased urinary Klotho protein, one of the earliest biomarkers of CKD progression that is associated with vascular calcification, cardiac fibrosis, and cardiac hypertrophy in CKD.[34]

Oxidative stress and aging-related changes thus initiate inflammatory cascades involving players such as reactive oxygen species, fetuin-A, and adiponectin among adipocytes in the kidney and liver that significantly contribute to end-organ damage.

Intestinal Dysbiosis

The role of dysbiosis, or perturbation of the normal gut microbiota, and its interactions with immune and metabolic pathways has recently been implicated in the pathogenesis of NAFLD and CKD. Those bearing the burden of NAFLD and CKD demonstrate alterations in composition of the gut microbiome. For instance, patients with NAFLD possess decreased proportion of the Ruminococcaceae family compared with healthy controls, and those with NASH exhibited increased proportion of *Clostridium coccoides* compared with those with simple steatosis.[35,36] Patients with CKD frequently have increased levels of Enterobacteriaceae and reduced levels of Lactobacillaceae and Bifidobacteriaceae.[37] Alterations in intestinal bacteria populations affect proinflammatory and metabolic pathways that lead to the generation of harmful toxins that may damage the kidneys and liver.

When the gut microbiota metabolize dietary nutrients such as phenylalanine/tyrosine, tryptophan, and choline, they also, respectively, produce *p*-cresol, indole, and trimethylamine that then become the polar, ionically charged toxic uremic metabolites *p*-cresol sulfate, indole sulfate, and trimethylamine-N-oxide (TMAO), respectively.[4,24] The liver and kidneys may be damaged during the metabolism and generation of these molecules through oxidative and inflammatory pathways, and these end products also function as uremic toxins predisposed to causing further injury during renal excretion. For instance, proinflammatory indole sulfate is cleared by the proximal tubules and increases the risk of tubulointerstitial fibrosis, whereas TMAO is associated with worse long-term survival in CKD and promotes atherosclerosis and oxidative damage in the liver through foam cell production and upregulation of macrophage receptors.[38,39] Additional potentially toxic by-products include but are not limited to endotoxins (also known as lipopolysaccharides), hippuric acid, phenols, thiols, and ammonia.[4,40] As urea metabolites produced in the gastrointestinal lumen, ammonia and ammonium hydroxide impair intestinal epithelial tight junctions, increasing the transmigration of proinflammatory cytokines, luminal toxins, and lipopolysaccharides into the systemic and portal circulation.[40] In the setting of dysbiosis, gram-negative bacteria exhibit increased generation of lipopolysaccharides that further contributes to the vicious cycle of gastrointestinal barrier damage, disruption of intestinal epithelial tight junctions, and direct transfer of toxic lipopolysaccharides to the liver.[24] Upon reaching the liver, lipopolysaccharides activate Toll-like receptors on hepatocytes and Kupffer cells and initiate an inflammatory cascade that is associated with activation of fibrogenic cells and fibrosis.[41]

Two additional major categories of bacterial metabolites, short-chain fatty acids (SCFAs) and secondary bile acids, possess the capability to wreak havoc on normal organ function. Produced by anaerobic bacteria such as Lactobacilli and Bifidobacteria during fermentation of dietary fiber in the colon, SCFAs including acetate, butyrate, and propionate can impact hepatic glucose and fatty acid metabolism. For example, administration of propionate in mice models promotes the colonic L cell secretion of GLP-1 and incretins peptide YY that, respectively, stimulate insulin secretion and satiety.[42] Lower levels of SCFAs contribute to hepatic adiposity and insulin resistance in NAFLD.[24] On the other hand, primary bile acids have long been known to facilitate various metabolic pathways including lipid digestion, cholesterol metabolism, and energy homeostasis. Among the 1% to 5% of primary bile acids that are not reabsorbed via enterohepatic circulation, gut bacteria generate secondary bile acids, such as lithocholic acid, deoxycholic acid, and urodeoxycholic acid, in the ileum and colon. Because NAFLD is associated with changes in gut microbiome composition that are in turn associated with dysregulation of bile acid formation, the profiles of secondary bile acids are also adversely impacted.[4] Highly hydrophobic and toxic, secondary bile acids promote development and progression of NAFLD by (1) facilitating the transfer of toxic metabolites to the liver through interruption of intestinal epithelial tight junctions and (2) disrupting the mitochondrial membranes of hepatocytes due to its potent hydrophobicity.[24] Associated with high-fat diets, higher concentrations of secondary bile acids in the liver influence the development of cholestasis, inflammation, and carcinogenesis, although their effects in the kidneys remain under investigation.[24,43]

Dysbiosis thus contributes to the development of NAFLD and CKD through changes in intestinal bacterial populations, disruption of the gastrointestinal barrier, and the generation of proinflammatory toxins, bile acids, lipopolysaccharides, and SCFAs.

Platelet Activation

A growing body of evidence contends that platelet activation, regulated by oxidative stress and dyslipidemia, is a key inflammatory player interconnecting NAFLD and CKD.[4] Oxidative stress and the formation of reactive oxygen species significantly contributes to renal dysfunction, resulting in weakened antioxidant defenses such as urinary Klotho protein and diminished clearance of pro-oxidant metabolites including 8-oxo-7,8-dihydro-2'-deoxyguanosine, lipid hydroperoxides, malondialdehyde, protein carbonyls, asymmetric dimethylarginine, F2-isoprostanes, and advanced oxidation protein products.[34,44] Imbalances in reactive oxygen species formation and the cellular antioxidant system activate platelets to release dense granules and alpha granules that function as repositories for numerous inflammatory peptide and protein mediators. Examples of such inflammatory mediators are listed in **Table 1**.[45] The effects of oxidative stress on platelet activation are further compounded as urinary Klotho protein has been shown to modulate the effect of indole sulfate, a tryptophan metabolite and uremic toxin produced through intestinal bacteria, on platelet activation.[46]

Through inhibition of reactive oxygen species/p38MAPK signaling, urinary Klotho protein protects against indole sulfate-mediated thrombus formation and atherosclerosis in apoE-/- mice models with CKD.[46] Platelet hyperactivity and the platelet-derived release of serotonin and growth factors such as epidermal growth factor, platelet-derived growth factor, and tumor growth factor-beta 1 stimulate activation of hepatic stellate cells and fibrogenesis.[47] This imbalance between the increased

Table 1
Inflammatory peptide and protein mediators released through platelet activation

Location	Family	Molecule
Dense granules	Nucleotide	ATP
	Amino acid	Glutamate
	Phosphates	Polyphosphates
	Monoamine	Serotonin
α-Granules	Chemokines	PF4 or CXCL4
		β-Thromboglobulin (CXCL7 or NAP-2)
		RANTES or CCL5
		MIP-1α or CCL3
		MCP-3 or CCL7
		NAP-2 or CXCL7
		TARC or CCL17
		Interleukin-8 (CXCL8)
	Cytokines	CD40 ligand (CD40L)
		TNF-α
		IL-1α
		GRO-α or CXCL1
		ENA-78 or CXCL5
		SDF-1 or CXCL12
	Growth factors	PDGF
		TGF-β
		EGF

Imbalances between antioxidant levels and reactive oxygen species formation activate platelets to release dense and α-granules, which are repositories for numerous inflammatory peptide and protein mediators that include hormones, chemokines, cytokines, and growth factors.

Abbreviations: CXCL4, chemokine (CXC motif) ligand 4; ENA, epithelial cell-derived neutrophil-activating peptide-78; EGF, epidermal growth factor; GRO-α, growth-regulated oncogene-alpha; MCP-2, monocyte-chemotactic protein; MIP- α, macrophage inflammatory protein-1alpha; NAP-2, neutrophil activating peptide 2; IL-1α, interleukin 1 alpha; PDGF, platelet-derived growth factor; RANTES, regulated on activation, normal T cell expressed and secreted; PF4, platelet factor 4; SDF-1, stromal cell-derived factor 1; TARC, thymus- and activation-regulated chemokine; TGF-β, transforming growth factor-beta; TNF- α, tumor necrosis factor-alpha

production and attenuated dissolution of extracellular matrix disrupts the normal architecture of the liver and can result in advancement of liver disease to fibrosis, cirrhosis, and even hepatocellular carcinoma. In 2019, Malehmir and colleagues[48] demonstrated that platelet number, activation, and aggregation are amplified in NASH but not in steatosis or insulin resistance. By decreasing intrahepatic platelet accumulation and the frequency of platelet interactions with immune cells, dual antiplatelet therapy with either aspirin/clopidogrel or ticagrelor prevented NASH and the development of hepatocellular carcinoma in a murine hIL4rα/GP1bα transgenic mouse model of NASH.[48] Overall, platelet activation triggers molecular signaling cascades that cause damaging inflammation and inextricably link the development and progression of NAFLD and CKD.

PNPLA3 Polymorphism

In a 2008 genome-wide association scan of nonsynonymous sequence variations in an ethnically diverse study population (n = 9229) comprising Hispanic, African American, and European American individuals, Romeo and colleagues[49] showed that the genetic mutation, rs738409 C > G (p.Ile148Met), on the long arm of chromosome 22 in the patatinlike phospholipase domain-containing 3 gene (also known as PNPLA3, adiponutrin, or Ca^{2+}-independent phospholipase A2 epsilon [iPLA2ε]) was associated with susceptibility to NAFLD, independent of diabetes status, alcohol use, or BMI. This landmark study became the embers sparking enormous passion for the study of genetics and biology in NAFLD.

Since then, the loss-of-function PNPLA3 I148M mutation on the rs738409 site has been shown to be an independent risk factor for not only NAFLD but also the entire spectrum of severe liver disease through progression to steatohepatitis, fibrosis, cirrhosis, decompensation, hepatocellular carcinoma, and liver-related death.[50–52] The PNPLA3 I148M rs738409 gene polymorphism further underlies treatment response in NAFLD. Compared with those bearing the C-allele, patients with the G-allele of the PNPLA3 I148M rs738409 gene polymorphism demonstrated significantly increased reduction of hepatic adipose content, reduced insulin resistance, and weight loss in response to lifestyle modifications, dipeptidyl peptidase-4 inhibitors, and bariatric surgery.[53–55] On the other hand, patients with the C-allele of the PNPLA3 I148M rs738409 gene polymorphism demonstrated greater sensitivity to the beneficial pharmacologic effects of statins and omega-3 polyunsaturated fatty acids, when compared with those bearing the G-allele.[56–58] Recent emerging data also support the role of the PNPLA3 I148M rs738409 gene variant, particularly the G allele, in the development of CKD as evidenced by both lower eGFR and higher 2-hour proteinuria in adults and children with NAFLD, regardless of established renal risk factors and the histologic severity of NAFLD across different patient populations and ethnicities.[59]

The pathogenic mechanisms mediating the PNPLA3 I148M rs738409 gene polymorphism's impact on the development of hepatic and renal damage have yet to be completely understood. A 481-residue protein, PNPLA3 is highly expressed in the liver, more so in hepatic stellate cells than in hepatocytes, and resides in the endoplasmic reticulum and lipid droplet membrane.[60] Transcriptionally regulated by insulin, PNPLA3 has lipase activity in vitro against triglycerides in hepatocytes and retinyl esters in hepatic stellate cells. The I148M mutation results in loss of function with reduced secretion of very-low-density lipoproteins and retention of liver fat and vitamin A (retinol) in hepatocytes and hepatic stellate cells, respectively.[60] Owing to chronic inflammation, hepatic stellate cells transform from quiescent cells storing retinol to activated, highly proliferative, and contractile myofibroblastlike cells. During activation, hepatic stellate cells lose retinol through either secretion or oxidation into retinoic acid, which sensitizes early activated hepatic stellate cells to natural killer cell killing.[61] Meanwhile, fully activated hepatic stellate cells become resistant to natural killer cell killing, going on to indulge in the production of collagens leading to liver fibrosis.[61]

Alongside expression in the liver, *PNPLA3* mRNA is also highly expressed in the kidney, and the G allele of the PNPLA3 I148M rs738409 gene polymorphism may lead to lipid accumulation in the kidney.[59] Ectopic lipid buildup in the kidney can lead to insulin resistance, oxidative stress, and proinflammatory cytokines that impair the structure and function of podocytes, mesangial cells, and proximal tubular cells.[62] Owing to the burden of lipid accumulation, mesangial cells transform into foam cells that lose contractile function, and terminally differentiated podocytes become insulin resistant and undergo apoptosis without opportunity for renewal, thereby weakening the structural integrity of the capillary loop and leading to glomerular tuft stripping and glomerulosclerosis.[62] Podocyte loss then causes a maladaptive response in which the remaining podocytes undergo hypertrophy in an often futile attempt to compensate for the uncovering of the glomerular tuft, thus causing a secondary focal segmental glomerulosclerosis.[62] With glomerulosclerosis resulting in hyperfiltration and increased albuminuria, the proximal tubular cells absorb increasing amounts of albumin coated with nonesterified fatty acids that drive proximal tubular hypertrophy, insulin resistance, amplified renal gluconeogenesis, and eventually increased tubular atrophy and interstitial fibrosis.[62]

Fundamentally influencing the development of NAFLD and CKD while also modulating disease severity and treatment response, the PNPLA3 I148M mutation on the rs738409 site bears important clinical implications and warrants further investigation. Future research directions include investigating whether genotyping may clinically identify patients with NAFLD at higher risk of CKD, and whether a precise, personalized medical approach in NAFLD based on PNPLA3 rs738409 genotyping may be reasonable.

Common Therapeutic Options for Both Nonalcoholic Fatty Liver Disease and Chronic Kidney Disease

From the previous discussion, it is apparent that NAFLD and CKD are strongly interconnected with mutual metabolic risk factors. The presence of both diseases classifies certain pharmacologic treatment choices, such as glucagon-like peptide receptor (GLP-1) agonists and sodium glucose cotransporter 2 (SGLT2) inhibitors, as first-line therapies in coexisting NAFLD and CKD.

Glucagon-Like Peptide Receptor Agonists

An incretin-based therapy that reduces glucagon production, increases pancreatic secretion of insulin, delays gastric emptying, and promotes satiety, GLP-1 agonists are a promising treatment targeting both CKD an NAFLD. Aside from improving glycemic control, GLP-1 agonists are nephroprotective in actively inducing natriuresis through inhibition of proximal tubular Na^+/H^+ exchanger isoform 3 and decreased activation of the angiotensin II axis.[63] By decreasing reabsorption of sodium in the proximal tubule, GLP-1 agonists prevent glomerular hyperfiltration, reduce albuminuria, and exert anti-inflammatory, antioxidative, and antifibrotic protective effects against the development of CKD independent of improvement in glycemic control.[63] Yet, the effects of GLP-1 agonists in nondiabetic CKD remain unclear and requires future investigation. GLP-1 agonists also protect hepatocytes against fatty acid-related death through activation of autophagy that prevents dysfunctional endoplasmic reticulum-related apoptosis of hepatocytes.[64] Semaglutide and liraglutide are GLP-1 agonists that have been investigated for the treatment of NAFLD. In a double-blind phase 2 trial involving patients with biopsy-confirmed NASH and liver fibrosis F1 to F3, treatment with semaglutide resulted in significantly higher percentage of patients having resolution of NASH (0.1 mg group 40%, 0.2 mg group 36%, 0.4 mg group 59%, and placebo group 17%; $P < .001$ for 0.4 mg vs placebo).[65] According to a meta-analysis including 6 phase 3 randomized controlled trials from the Liraglutide Effect and Action in Diabetes (LEAD) program, treatment using 26 weeks of the GLP-1 agonist liraglutide 1.8 mg/d significantly improved liver enzymes and hepatic steatosis (assessed via liver-to-spleen attenuation ratio on computed tomographic scan) in patients with asymptomatic liver injury and type 2 diabetes in a dose-dependent manner.[66] However, reduction in mean ALT levels disappeared after correcting for reduction in weight and HbA_{1c}.[66] Another randomized control trial found that 12 weeks of liraglutide 1.8 mg/d reduced BMI and lipogenesis while increasing hepatic and adipose insulin sensitivity.[67] In the LEAN study, 39% of patients treated with 48 weeks of liraglutide 1.8 mg/d had histologic resolution of NASH based on end-of-treatment liver biopsy compared with 9% in the placebo control group.[68] Notably, reduction in weight and HbA_{1c} remained similar in those with liver histologic improvement compared with those without, suggesting that liraglutide's beneficial effects may be mediated through mechanisms other than weight loss and improved glycemic control.

Sodium Glucose Cotransporter 2 Inhibitors

Aside from GLP-1 agonists, SGLT2 inhibitors comprise another pharmacologic drug group that is promising in simultaneous treatment of both NAFLD and CKD. SGLT2 inhibitors may improve NAFLD through weight loss through increased fatty acid oxidation and lipolysis, insulin sensitization, increased angiotensin-converting enzyme-2 activation, and anti-inflammatory and anti-oxidative effects.[40] A systematic review revealed that GLT2 inhibitors improved liver enzyme levels, reduced hepatic steatosis, ameliorated fibrosis, and benefited metabolic parameters such as obesity, insulin resistance, glycemia, and lipid levels in T2DM with NAFLD.[69] Furthermore, by inhibiting the SGLT2 protein located in the proximal tubule, SGLT2 inhibitors increase urinary glucose excretion and reduce serum glucose levels. Similar to GLP-1 agonists, SGLT2 inhibitors also induce natriuresis through decreased SGLT2-mediated sodium reabsorption in the proximal tubule, thereby reducing afferent arteriolar vasoconstriction and glomerular hyperfiltration in CKD. Numerous randomized controlled trials have demonstrated that SGLT2 inhibitors reduced incident nephropathy, slowed declined in kidney function, and exhibited cardiovascular protection in diabetic patients.[70] In nondiabetic patients, SGLT2 inhibitors are a promising treatment choice as well. In the Dapagliflozin and Prevention of Adverse Outcomes in Chronic Kidney Disease trial involving 1398 patients with nondiabetic CKD, dapagliflozin exhibited a HR of 0.5 on the primary outcome, which was a composite of sustained eGFR decline of 50% or more, end-stage renal disease, or death from renal or cardiovascular causes.[70] In addition, the DIAMOND trial revealed that dapagliflozin transiently reduced eGFR but did not affect observed proteinuria in patients with nondiabetic CKD.[70]

SUMMARY

Recent compelling studies have substantiated a strong connection between increased prevalence and incidence of CKD and the increased prevalence and severity of NAFLD in those with or without coexisting cardiometabolic risk factors such as obesity, T2DM, or hypertension. Although it remains unclear whether CKD and NAFLD further share a causal relationship, numerous shared mechanisms including metabolic syndrome, fructose and uric acid accumulation, oxidative stress, intestinal dysbiosis, platelet activation, and genetic predispositions have been substantiated. Given this shared pathophysiology, the diagnosis of CKD thus warrants a thorough NAFLD risk assessment and further staging of fibrosis in the event of advanced liver disease. Likewise, it is reasonable to surveil patients with NAFLD for development of CKD. Identification of high-risk individuals with coexisting CKD and NAFLD may empower beneficial pharmacologic interventions such as GLP-1 agonists and SGLT2 inhibitors and amelioration of cardiometabolic disease burden.

CLINICS CARE POINTS

- The diagnosis of chronic kidney disease (CKD) warrants a thorough nonalcoholic fatty liver disease (NAFLD) risk assessment, and the reverse applies as well. Those with coexisting CKD and NAFLD may be considered for pharmacologic interventions with glucagon-like peptide-1 agonists or sodium-glucose transporter-2 inhibitors.

DISCLOSURE

M. Noureddin has been on the advisory board for 89BIO, Gilead, Intercept, Pfizer, Novartis, Novo Nordisk, Allergan, Blade, EchoSens, Fractyl, Terns, OWL, Siemens, Roche diagnostic, and Abbott; M. Noureddin has received research support from Allergan, BMS, Gilead, Galmed, Galectin, Genfit, Conatus, Enanta, Madrigal, Novartis, Shire, Viking, and Zydus; M. Noureddin is a minor shareholder or has stocks in Anaetos and Viking.

REFERENCES

1. Younossi Z, Anstee QM, Marietti M, et al. Global burden of NAFLD and NASH: trends, predictions, risk factors and prevention. Nat Rev Gastroenterol Hepatol 2018;15(1):11–20.
2. Loomba R, Sanyal AJ. The global NAFLD epidemic. Nat Rev Gastroenterol Hepatol 2013;10(11):686–90.
3. The top 10 causes of death. World Health Organization.
4. Byrne CD, Targher G. NAFLD as a driver of chronic kidney disease. J Hepatol 2020;72(4):785–801.
5. Targher G, Chonchol MB, Byrne CD. CKD and nonalcoholic fatty liver disease. Am J Kidney Dis 2014;64(4).
6. Xie Y, Bowe B, Mokdad AH, et al. Analysis of the Global Burden of Disease study highlights the global, regional, and national trends of chronic kidney disease epidemiology from 1990 to 2016. Kidney Int 2018;94(3):567–81.
7. Chalasani N, Younossi Z, Lavine JE, et al. The diagnosis and management of nonalcoholic fatty liver disease: Practice Guidance from the American association for the study of liver diseases. Hepatology 2017. https://doi.org/10.1002/hep.29367/suppinfo.
8. Park CC, Nguyen P, Hernandez C, et al. Magnetic resonance elastography vs transient elastography in detection of fibrosis and Noninvasive Measurement of steatosis in patients with biopsy-Proven nonalcoholic fatty liver disease. Gastroenterology 2017;152(3):598–607.e2.
9. Mikolasevic I, Orlic L, Franjic N, et al. Transient elastography (FibroScan(®)) with controlled attenuation parameter in the assessment of liver steatosis and fibrosis in patients with nonalcoholic fatty liver disease - where do we stand? World J Gastroenterol 2016;22(32):7236–51.
10. Imajo K, Kessoku T, Honda Y, et al. Magnetic resonance imaging more accurately classifies steatosis and fibrosis in patients with nonalcoholic fatty liver disease than transient elastography. Gastroenterology 2016;150(3):626–37.e7.
11. Newsome PN, Sasso M, Deeks JJ, et al. FibroScan-AST (FAST) score for the non-invasive identification of patients with non-alcoholic steatohepatitis with significant activity and fibrosis: a prospective derivation and global validation study. Lancet Gastroenterol Hepatol 2020;5(4):362–73.
12. Harrison SA, Ratziu V, Boursier J, et al. A blood-based biomarker panel (NIS4) for non-invasive diagnosis of non-alcoholic steatohepatitis and liver fibrosis: a prospective derivation and global validation study. Lancet Gastroenterol Hepatol 2020;5(11):970–85.
13. Kaswala DH, Lai M, Afdhal NH. Fibrosis assessment in nonalcoholic fatty liver disease (NAFLD) in 2016. Dig Dis Sci 2016;61(5):1356–64.
14. Kiapidou S, Liava C, Kalogirou M, et al. Chronic kidney disease in patients with non-alcoholic fatty liver disease: what the Hepatologist should know? Ann Hepatol 2020;19(2):134–44.

15. Musso G, Gambino R, Tabibian JH, et al. Association of non-alcoholic fatty liver disease with chronic kidney disease: a systematic review and meta-analysis. PLoS Med 2014;11(7). https://doi.org/10.1371/journal.pmed.1001680.
16. Mantovani A, Byrne CD, Bonora E, et al. Nonalcoholic fatty liver disease and risk of incident type 2 diabetes: a meta-analysis. Diabetes Care 2018;41(2):372.
17. Mantovani A, Zaza G, Byrne CD, et al. Nonalcoholic fatty liver disease increases risk of incident chronic kidney disease: a systematic review and meta-analysis. Metab Clin Exp 2018;79:64–76.
18. Sinn DH, Kang D, Jang HR, et al. Development of chronic kidney disease in patients with non-alcoholic fatty liver disease: a cohort study. J Hepatol 2017;67(6): 1274–80.
19. Targher G, Bertolini L, Rodella S, et al. Relationship between kidney function and liver histology in subjects with nonalcoholic steatohepatitis. Clin J Am Soc Nephrol. 2010;5(12):2166–71.
20. Yeung M-W, Wong GL-H, Choi KC, et al. Advanced liver fibrosis but not steatosis is independently associated with albuminuria in Chinese patients with type 2 diabetes. J Hepatol 2018;68(1). https://doi.org/10.1016/j.jhep.2017.09.020.
21. Kasapoglu B, Turkay C, Yalcın KS, et al. Increased microalbuminuria prevalence among patients with nonalcoholic fatty liver disease. Ren Fail 2016;38(1):15–9.
22. Cullaro G, Verna EC, Lee BP, et al. Chronic kidney disease in liver transplant Candidates: a rising burden impacting post–liver transplant outcomes. Liver Transplant 2020;26(4). https://doi.org/10.1002/lt.25694.
23. Hydes T, Buchanan R, Kennedy OJ, et al. Systematic review of the impact of non-alcoholic fatty liver disease on mortality and adverse clinical outcomes for individuals with chronic kidney disease. BMJ Open 2020;10(9):e040970.
24. Targher G, Byrne CD. Non-alcoholic fatty liver disease: an emerging driving force in chronic kidney disease. Nat Rev Nephrol 2017;13(5):297–310.
25. Musso G, Cassader M, Cohney S, et al. Emerging liver-kidney interactions in nonalcoholic fatty liver disease. Trends Mol Med 2015;21(10):645–62.
26. Kanbay M, Bulbul MC, Copur S, et al. Therapeutic implications of shared mechanisms in non-alcoholic fatty liver disease and chronic kidney disease. J Nephrol 2020. https://doi.org/10.1007/s40620-020-00751-y.
27. Fan CY, Wang MX, Ge CX, et al. Betaine supplementation protects against high-fructose-induced renal injury in rats. J Nutr Biochem 2014;25(3):353–62.
28. García-Ruiz C, Fernández-Checa JC. Mitochondrial oxidative stress and antioxidants balance in fatty liver disease. Hepatol Commun 2018;2(12):1425–39.
29. Wang C, Cui Y, Li C, et al. Nrf2 deletion causes "benign" simple steatosis to develop into nonalcoholic steatohepatitis in mice fed a high-fat diet. Lipids Health Dis 2013;12(1). https://doi.org/10.1186/1476-511X-12-165.
30. Ruiz S, Pergola PE, Zager RA, et al. Targeting the transcription factor Nrf2 to ameliorate oxidative stress and inflammation in chronic kidney disease. Kidney Int 2013;83(6):1029–41.
31. Pergola PE, Raskin P, Toto RD, et al. Bardoxolone methyl and kidney function in CKD with type 2 diabetes. N Engl J Med 2011;365(4):327–36.
32. Pal D, Dasgupta S, Kundu R, et al. Fetuin-A acts as an endogenous ligand of TLR4 to promote lipid-induced insulin resistance. Nat Med 2012;18(8):1279–85.
33. Agarwal S, Chattopadhyay M, Mukherjee S, et al. Fetuin-A downregulates adiponectin through Wnt-PPARγ pathway in lipid induced inflamed adipocyte. Biochim Biophys Acta - Mol Basis Dis 2017;1863(1):174–81.
34. Lu X, Hu MC. Klotho/FGF23 Axis in chronic kidney disease and cardiovascular disease. Kidney Dis 2017;3(1):15–23.

35. Mouzaki M, Comelli EM, Arendt BM, et al. Intestinal microbiota in patients with nonalcoholic fatty liver disease. Hepatology 2013;58(1):120–7.

36. Raman M, Ahmed I, Gillevet PM, et al. Fecal microbiome and volatile organic compound metabolome in obese humans with nonalcoholic fatty liver disease. Clin Gastroenterol Hepatol 2013;11(7):868–75.e3.

37. Sampaio-Maia B, Simões-Silva L, Pestana M, et al. Chapter three - the role of the gut microbiome on chronic kidney disease. In: Sariaslani Sima, Gadd Geoffrey, editors96. Online: Advances in Applied Microbiology; 2016. p. 65–94.

38. Nallu A, Sharma S, Ramezani A, et al. Gut microbiome in chronic kidney disease: challenges and opportunities. Translational Res 2017;179:24–37.

39. Wang Z, Klipfell E, Bennett BJ, et al. Gut flora metabolism of phosphatidylcholine promotes cardiovascular disease. Nature 2011;472(7341):57–63.

40. Musso G, Cassader M, Cohney S, et al. Fatty liver and chronic kidney disease: novel mechanistic insights and therapeutic opportunities. Diabetes Care 2016; 39(10):1830–45.

41. Vespasiani-Gentilucci U, Gallo P, Picardi A. The role of intestinal microbiota in the pathogenesis of NAFLD: starting points for intervention. Arch Med Sci 2018; 14(3):701–6.

42. Psichas A, Sleeth ML, Murphy KG, et al. The short chain fatty acid propionate stimulates GLP-1 and PYY secretion via free fatty acid receptor 2 in rodents. Int J Obes 2015;39(3):424–9.

43. Zeng H, Umar S, Rust B, et al. Secondary bile acids and short chain fatty acids in the colon: a Focus on colonic microbiome, cell proliferation, inflammation, and cancer. Int J Mol Sci 2019;20(5):1214.

44. Tucker PS, Dalbo VJ, Han T, et al. Clinical and research markers of oxidative stress in chronic kidney disease. Biomarkers 2013;18(2):103–15.

45. Arman M, Payne H, Ponomaryov T. Role of platelets in inflammation. In: Payne H, editor. The non-thrombotic role of platelets in health and disease. UK: IntechOpen; 2015. Ch. 3.

46. Yang K, Du C, Wang X, et al. Indoxyl sulfate induces platelet hyperactivity and contributes to chronic kidney disease–associated thrombosis in mice. Blood 2017;129(19):2667–79. https://doi.org/10.1182/blood-2016-10-744060.

47. Elpek GÖ. Cellular and molecular mechanisms in the pathogenesis of liver fibrosis: an update. World J Gastroenterol 2014;20(23):7260–76.

48. Malehmir M, Pfister D, Gallage S, et al. Platelet GPIbα is a mediator and potential interventional target for NASH and subsequent liver cancer. Nat Med 2019;25(4): 641–55.

49. Romeo S, Kozlitina J, Xing C, et al. Genetic variation in PNPLA3 confers susceptibility to nonalcoholic fatty liver disease. Nat Genet 2008;40(12):1461–5.

50. Lonardo A, Bellentani S, Argo CK, et al. Epidemiological modifiers of nonalcoholic fatty liver disease: Focus on high-risk groups. Dig Liver Dis 2015; 47(12):997–1006. https://doi.org/10.1016/j.dld.2015.08.004.

51. Marchesini G, Day CP, Dufour JF, et al. EASL-EASD-EASO Clinical Practice Guidelines for the management of non-alcoholic fatty liver disease. J Hepatol 2016;64(6):1388–402.

52. Grimaudo S, Pipitone RM, Pennisi G, et al. Association between PNPLA3 rs738409 C>G variant and liver-related outcomes in patients with nonalcoholic fatty liver disease. Clin Gastroenterol Hepatol 2020;18(4):935–44.e3. https://doi.org/10.1016/j.cgh.2019.08.011.

53. Shen J, Wong GL-H, Chan HL-Y, et al. PNPLA3 gene polymorphism and response to lifestyle modification in patients with nonalcoholic fatty liver disease. J Gastroenterol Hepatol 2015;30(1).
54. Palmer CNA, Maglio C, Pirazzi C, et al. Paradoxical lower serum triglyceride levels and higher type 2 diabetes mellitus susceptibility in obese individuals with the PNPLA3 148M variant. PLoS ONE 2012;7(6).
55. Kan H, Hyogo H, Ochi H, et al. Influence of the rs738409 polymorphism in patatin-like phospholipase 3 on the treatment efficacy of non-alcoholic fatty liver disease with type 2 diabetes mellitus. Hepatol Res 2016;46(3):E146–53.
56. Nobili V, Bedogni G, Donati B, et al. The I148M variant of PNPLA3 reduces the response to Docosahexaenoic acid in children with non-alcoholic fatty liver disease. J Med Food 2013;16(10). https://doi.org/10.1089/jmf.2013.0043.
57. Scorletti E, Bhatia L, McCormick KG, et al. Design and rationale of the WELCOME trial: a randomised, placebo controlled study to test the efficacy of purified long chain omega-3 fatty treatment in non-alcoholic fatty liver disease. Contemp Clin Trials 2014;37(2). https://doi.org/10.1016/j.cct.2014.02.002.
58. Dongiovanni P, Petta S, Mannisto V, et al. Statin use and non-alcoholic steatohepatitis in at risk individuals. J Hepatol 2015;63(3):705–12.
59. Mantovani A, Zusi C. PNPLA3 gene and kidney disease. Exploration Med 2020; 1(1):42–50.
60. Trépo E, Romeo S, Zucman-Rossi J, et al. PNPLA3 gene in liver diseases. J Hepatol 2016;65(2):399–412. https://doi.org/10.1016/j.jhep.2016.03.011.
61. Radaeva S, Wang L, Radaev S, et al. Retinoic acid signaling sensitizes hepatic stellate cells to NK cell killing via upregulation of NK cell activating ligand RAE1. Am J Physiol Gastrointest Liver Physiol 2007;293:809–16.
62. de Vries APJ, Ruggenenti P, Ruan XZ, et al. Review fatty kidney: emerging role of Ectopic lipid in obesity-related renal disease. Vol 2. 2014. Available at: www.thelancet.com/.
63. Skov J, Dejgaard A, Frøkiær J, et al. Glucagon-like peptide-1 (GLP-1): effect on kidney Hemodynamics and renin-angiotensin-aldosterone system in healthy men. J Clin Endocrinol Metab 2013;98(4):E664–71.
64. Sharma S, Mells JE, Fu PP, et al. GLP-1 analogs reduce hepatocyte steatosis and improve survival by enhancing the unfolded protein response and promoting macroautophagy. PLoS ONE 2011;6(9). https://doi.org/10.1371/journal.pone.0025269.
65. Newsome PN, Buchholtz K, Cusi K, et al. A placebo-controlled trial of Subcutaneous semaglutide in nonalcoholic steatohepatitis. New Engl J Med 2020;384(12):1113–24.
66. Armstrong MJ, Houlihan DD, Rowe IA, et al. Safety and efficacy of liraglutide in patients with type 2 diabetes and elevated liver enzymes: Individual patient data meta-analysis of the LEAD program. Aliment Pharmacol Ther 2013;37(2):234–42.
67. Armstrong MJ, Hull D, Guo K, et al. Glucagon-like peptide 1 decreases lipotoxicity in non-alcoholic steatohepatitis. J Hepatol 2016;64(2).
68. Armstrong MJ, Gaunt P, Aithal GP, et al. Liraglutide safety and efficacy in patients with non-alcoholic steatohepatitis (LEAN): a multicentre, double-blind, randomised, placebo-controlled phase 2 study. The Lancet 2016;387(10019):679–90.
69. Raj H, Durgia H, Palui R, et al. SGLT-2 inhibitors in non-alcoholic fatty liver disease patients with type 2 diabetes mellitus: a systematic review. World J Diabetes 2019;10(2):114–32.
70. Mima A. Sodium-glucose cotransporter 2 inhibitors in patients with non-diabetic chronic kidney disease. Adv Ther 2021;38(5):2201–12.

Polycystic Kidney/Liver Disease

Rebecca Roediger, MD[a],*, Douglas Dieterich, MD[a], Pramodh Chanumolu, MD[b], Priya Deshpande, MD[b]

KEYWORDS

- Polycystic liver disease • Polycystic renal disease
- Autosomal dominant polycystic kidney disease • End-stage kidney disease

KEY POINTS

- Autosomal dominant polycystic kidney disease presents in adulthood and leads to end-stage renal failure. The most common extrarenal manifestation of ADPKD is polycystic liver disease (PCLD), whereby liver cysts grow in size and number with age.
- Isolated PCLD is genetically distinct from PCLD in ADPKD but has a similar natural history of liver disease. PCLD presents with complications of hepatomegaly but liver function is preserved.
- The mainstay of medical management for ADPKD is tolvaptan, which slows cyst growth and decline of renal function. The only curative treatment of PCLD is transplantation. Renal transplantation can improve survival for ESKD patients with ADPKD.

INTRODUCTION

Polycystic kidney disease is cilia-related kidney disorder and a common cause of end-stage kidney disease (ESKD) both in children and adults. Autosomal dominant polycystic kidney disease (ADPKD), mainly presents in adults and whereas autosomal recessive polycystic kidney disease (ARPKD) is rarer but more severe and usually presents perinatally or in early childhood.

Polycystic liver is the most common extrarenal manifestation of ADPKD. Isolated PCLD is defined as polycystic liver without renal cysts.[1] In polycystic liver disease (PCLD), both from ADPKD and isolated PCLD, liver cysts grow both in number and size throughout the patient's life span and women having a higher cyst burden likely related to the influence of hormones.[1-3] We will focus this review on the diagnosis, genetics and current renal and liver management of ADPKD and isolated PCLD (iPCLD).

[a] Division of Liver Disease, Department of Medicine, Icahn School of Medicine, 1 Gustave L Levy Place, Box 1123, New York, NY 10029, USA; [b] Division of Nephrology, Department of Medicine, Icahn School of Medicine, 1 Gustave L Levy Place, Box 1123, New York, NY 10029, USA
* Corresponding author.
E-mail address: Rebecca.roediger@mssm.edu

Clin Liver Dis 26 (2022) 229–243
https://doi.org/10.1016/j.cld.2022.01.009
1089-3261/22/© 2022 Elsevier Inc. All rights reserved.

EPIDEMIOLOGY

ADPKD occurs in all races and has a prevalence of 1 in 400 and 1 in 1000 live births.[4] Approximately 5% of patients who initiate dialysis annually in the United States have end-stage kidney disease (ESKD) due to ADPKD. ESKD can occur in up to 75% of patients with ADPKD by 70 years.

Hepatic cysts are the most common extrarenal manifestation of ADPKD, with an MRI study finding hepatic cysts in 83% of patients with ADPKD.[5]

Isolated PCLD is much rarer and the prevalence is 1 to 10 cases per 1 million.[1,3] However, as most cases are asymptomatic, it is likely that the prevalence is higher and autopsy studies have seen a higher incidence.[6]

GENETICS

ADPKD is predominantly caused by mutations in one of the 2 genes: PKD1 and PKD2 which encode polycystin (PC1) and polycystin 2 (PC2), respectively. Mutations in PKD1 (chromosome 16p13.3) are responsible for almost 80% of cases of ADPKD, whereas ~15% of ADPKD cases are attributed to mutations in PKD2 (chromosome 4q22.1).[7]

Patients with a mutation in PKD1 have earlier-onset ESKD, lower glomerular filtration rate (GFR), and larger kidney volumes than patients with a mutation in PKD2. In elderly patients, mutations of PKD2 are responsible for a higher percentage of cases.[8,9] Compared with patients with PKD1, patients with PKD2 present later in life (median age at diagnosis, 56 vs 42), have longer renal survival (median survival to age 69 vs 53), and have fewer complications.[10] ADPKD is also fully penetrant; 100% of individuals who inherit a mutated PKD gene will develop renal cysts that can be detected sonographically by age 30. However, the severity of the disease, the age of onset of ESRD, and the spectrum of extrarenal manifestations vary between affected individuals, even within the same family.

About 5% to 10% of ADPKD cases may be caused by hepatocyte nuclear factor 1β (HNF1B), neutral α-glucosidase AB (GANAB), and DNAJB11. Patients with the GANAB mutation can present with an ADPKD or iPCLD phenotype.[14]

ADPKD can also result from mutations in genes that are primarily associated with iPCLD, including SEC63 and PRKCSH, which are involved in translocating PC1 and PC2 in the endoplasmic reticulum.[11–14]

Patients with ADPKD have a germline mutation in one allele of either PKD1 or PKD2 and at least another event, such as somatic inactivation of the remaining wild-type PKD1 or PKD2 allele or loss of heterozygosity, is required to initiate cyst formation.[15–17] (**Fig. 1**). The likelihood of cyst formation increases when the level of functional PC1 or PC2 drops below a critical threshold, thereby reducing a functional gene product (hypomorphic gene).[8,18]

Approximately 10% to 25% of patients do not have a family history of ADPKD. This may be attributed to *de novo* mutations, missing parental medical records, germline or somatic mosaicism, and mild disease from hypomorphic PKD1 mutations.

Isolated PCLD is genetically distinct from PCLD seen in ADPKD. For most cases of iPCLD a pathologic gene is not identified; however, mutations in PRKCSH, SEC63, and LRP5 account for more than 35% of cases.[14] A study performing whole-exome sequencing on patients with isolated polycystic disease estimates that there may be up to 15 causative genes for PCLD.[14]

PATHOPHYSIOLOGY

PC1 and PC2 are localized in the primary cilium, a hair-like structure that protrudes from the apical membrane of renal epithelial cells into the lumen of the nephron.[19,20]

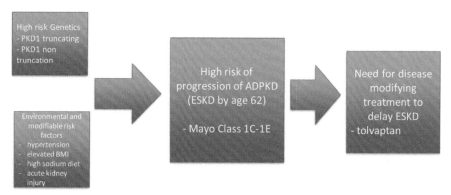

Fig. 1. Genetic and environmental risk factors contributing to progressive ADPKD. (*Adapted from* Chebiband Torres[23].)

The interaction of PC1 with PC2 is involved in the regulation of ion transport and indirectly affects Ca^{2+} signaling. Though the exact mechanism of cyst formation is unclear, it is thought that primary ciliary defects disrupt the normal orientation of tubular epithelial cells.[21–23] This process affects calcium flux and cAMP signaling resulting in fluid secretion and saccular dilation of tubules, which evolves into a cyst. Vasopressin, which is elevated in patients with ADPKD, interacts with the V2 receptor in the collecting ducts, increases cyclic AMP activity consequently cystogenesis.[24–26] As discussed later in discussion, inhibition of the V2 receptors by tolvaptan is a therapeutic target.

Histologically, liver cysts in ADPKD and iPCLD are indistinguishable. Both entities have cysts that arise from one of the 2 sites, either from biliary microhamartomas (von Meyenberg complexes) resulting from an overgrowth of biliary ductules or directly from peribiliary glands.[27] The cysts then become vascularized and grow from fluid secretion into the cyst and remodeling of the extracellular matrix.[3]

NATURAL HISTORY
Renal manifestations

ADPKD is a progressive disease in which renal cyst development occurs throughout life. The cysts start off as a few millimeters in length and can then exceed more than 40cm in length and weigh more than 8kg. Renal disease is also more severe in men than women. The clinical symptoms of ADPKD before renal insufficiency include early onset of hypertension, abdominal fullness and pain, hematuria, and urinary tract infections.

The earliest manifestation is a concentrating defect, and most patients have increased thirst, polyuria, and nocturia.[28] Hematuria can occur in between 35% and 50% of patients and follows a precipitating event, particularly a urinary tract infection or strenuous activity.[29] Hematuria results from a cyst rupture and self resolves after 5 to 7 days with conservative therapy. Gross hematuria typically occurs in patients with larger kidneys, hypertension, and higher plasma creatinine levels.[29] Gross hematuria before the age of 30 may portend poorer renal outcome.[30]

Nephrolithiasis is another cause of hematuria and occurs in 25% of patients with ADPKD. Uric acid stones are the predominant variety, followed by calcium oxalate.[31] Patients with ADPKD also had lower levels of urinary citrate, which is an inhibitor for stone formation.[32]

Renal cancers can present as hematuria and there have been conflicting reports on the incidence of renal cancers in ADPKD.[33,34] Diagnosis of malignancy is often delayed and requires a high level of suspicion.[35]

Acute flank or abdominal pain can occur with infections such as pyelonephritis and cyst infections and require prompt antimicrobial treatment.[36] Patients with severe chronic pain may need to be evaluated by pain management services for pain control. These patients are at a high risk of depression and need routine mental health screening as well.[37]

Hypertension can occur when the renal function is normal and carries a significant risk of progression to ESKD.[38] The activation of renin–angiotensin–aldosterone system is a major contributor to hypertension. However, derangements in mechanisms such as sympathetic activity and in endothelin and nitric oxide-mediated vascular tone may also contribute.[38]

Extrarenal manifestations

Patients with ADPKD can develop many extrarenal complications (**Table 1**). Given the scope of this review, we will focus on PCLD.

Liver manifestations

The natural history of iPCLD is similar to that in ADPKD. The liver cysts grow in size and number with age.[2] Compared with renal cysts, hepatic cysts appear later in life and grow more slowly in patients with ADPKD.[2] In ADPKD, the degree of renal disease only weakly correlates with the hepatic cyst burden[37] and there is no relationship between ADPKD genotype on the severity of PCLD.[39]

Polycystic livers are typically asymptomatic and diagnosed radiographically. Isolated PCLD is diagnosed later in life than liver involvement of ADPKD. Those with iPCLD have a larger number of and larger sized cysts at diagnosis than patients with ADPKD due to later presentation.[3,40]

Women have more severe diseases with more and larger size cysts and this may be related to female hormones, pregnancies, and contraceptive therapy.[2,40]

Liver function is preserved (despite cyst burden) and liver tests are normal with the exception of GGT (up to 1.4 times the upper limit of normal in 61% of patients with iPCLD) and alkaline phosphatase (mildly elevated in 21% of patients).[40] Elevations in these liver-specific laboratory values do not correlate with severity of disease.[40,41] The presence of symptoms is correlated with the presence of a known genetic mutation, younger age at diagnosis, and size of largest cyst, but is not correlated with the overall number of cysts.[40]

Table 1	
Extrarenal manifestations in ADPKD	
Liver	Mass effect from hepatomegaly → hepatic venous outflow obstruction, Budd Chiari, portal hypertension, biliary obstruction
	Liver cysts → Hemorrhage, infection, rupture
Brain	IAs → subarachnoid hemorrhage; carry the risk of high morbidity and mortality
Heart	Left ventricular hypertrophy
	Valvular abnormalities
GI tract	Diverticulosis
	Inguinal hernias

The enlarged liver can exert mass effect on adjacent organs leading to abdominal distention, dyspnea, early satiety, gastroesophageal reflux in about 20% of patients.[42] Mass effect can lead to hepatic venous outflow obstruction which was seen in 92% of patients who underwent transplant or resection.[43] There are case reports of Budd Chiari, portal hypertension, and biliary obstruction related to extrinsic compression (see **Table 1**).

The main cyst complications are hemorrhage, infection, and rupture. Cyst hemorrhage is highest risk in cysts with rapid growth or in the cases of abdominal trauma. Hemorrhage typically presents with abdominal pain and is diagnosed with contrasted imaging which can differentiate hemorrhagic cysts from cystadenocarcinoma or cystic adenoma.[41] Cyst infection occurs in 1% of patients and presents as fevers, malaise, and right upper quadrant pain. While rare it can lead to a mortality rate of 2% if not identified and treated. Diagnosis is made with a tagged white blood cell scan or with PET imaging as there are no diagnostic laboratories. Treatment is with systemic antibiotics and cyst drainage.[1,3,41] There are case reports of cyst rupture presenting as severe abdominal pain. This is diagnosed with perihepatic and pericystic free fluid seen on imaging and treatment is supportive.[1,41]

Other extrarenal manifestations that contribute significantly morbidity and mortality are intracranial aneurysms (IAs).[44] A family history of aneurysm carries the greatest risk.[44] Screening for IAs should be offered to patients with a family history of IAs or subarachnoid hemorrhage, personal history of ruptured aneurysm, if a patient has an occupation that may risk others' lives in the event of syncope, before surgery (if anticipated to have hypertension or hemodynamic instability) and to patients who want a negative result for reassurance.[44] The preferred screening method is the time of flight magnetic resonance angiography or computed tomography (CT) angiography.[45,46] Patients may need close follow-up with the neurosurgical team.

DIAGNOSIS

Before the onset of symptoms, the diagnosis of ADPKD can be made with abdominal imaging such as ultrasound, CT, or magnetic resonance imaging (MRI). As ultrasound is the cheapest modality, age-based criteria for diagnosing PKD 1 have been developed.[47] (**Table 2**).

MRI and CT scans are used to determine total kidney volume and assess the progression of disease. The total kidney volume is adjusted for height and age (hTKV). The Consortium of Radiologic Imaging Studies of Polycystic Kidney Disease (CRISP) study used MRI to assess the disease progression as determined by the baseline.[48] They concluded that a baseline hTKV of over 1500 mL predicted a decline in the GFR by about 4.33 ± 8.07 mL per year. Therefore, the higher the baseline hTKV predicts rapid disease progression.[48]

Table 2	
Kidney ultrasound confirmation of ADPKD diagnosis	
Age	**Cyst Burden**
15–29	Total of 3 cysts or more (either bilaterally or unilaterally)
30–45	Total of 3 cysts or more (either bilaterally or unilaterally)
40–59	$\geq$ 2 cysts in each kidney

Adapted from Pei Y, Watnick T, He N, et al. Somatic PKD2 Mutations in Individual Kidney and Liver Cysts Support a "Two-Hit" Model of Cystogenesis in Type 2 Autosomal Dominant Polycystic Kidney Disease. *J Am Soc Nephrol.* 1999;10(7):1524 to 1529. https://doi.org/10.1681/ASN.V1071524

Diagnosis of PCLD is made by abdominal ultrasound and CT; however, MRI is more sensitive and specific. Though there are no established radiographic criteria for diagnosis of PCLD, there must be 10 to 20 liver cysts in those without a known family history and at least 4 cysts in those with a family history. The differentiation between iPCLD and ADPKD is made by the number of renal cysts necessary to diagnose ADPKD.[27,42]

There are several classification systems to grade the severity of PCLD and guide treatment decisions (**Table 3**). Gigot's classification was designed to guide decisions for cyst fenestration.[49] Schnelldorfer classification uses imaging findings and symptoms to determine the optimal treatment modality.[50] Qian's classification grades the severity of liver involvement.[27]

MANAGEMENT

Identification of patients who are at a risk for progression and starting disease-modifying therapy is essential to the management of ADPKD. One approach is to use the 75th percentile of age when the overall ADPKD population would reach kidney failure. Per the Mayo ADPKD database, this is the age of 62. The age-adjusted hTKV, known as the Mayo imaging classification, predicts an individual patient's increase in kidney size and subsequent risk of kidney failure. Currently, this classification is the most individualized approach available.[51] (**Table 4**). The Mayo classification categorizes patients into 5 classes (1A, 1B, 1C, 1D, and 1E).[52] The patient's hTKV and age determine the class. The hTKV is obtained by measuring the coronal and sagittal height, depth, and width of the kidneys using a CT or MRI without contrast. These values are then entered into an ellipsoid equation and adjusted for height. Patients

Table 3
Classification systems for PCLD

Gigot[49]	Number of Cysts	Cyst Size	Remaining Areas of Normal Liver Parenchyma
Gigot Type 1	<10	Large	Large
Gigot Type 2	Multiple	(>10cm)	Large
Gigot Type 3	Multiple	Small, medium	Few
		Small, medium	

Schnelldorfer[50]	Symptoms	Cyst Characteristics	Remaining Areas of Normal liver Parenchyma	Venous Occlusion (Portal and Hepatic) of Preserved Parenchyma
Type A	Absent/mild	Any	Any	Any
Type B	Moderate/	Few but large	>2 sectors	Absent Present
Type C	severe	Any	>1 sector	
Type D	Severe	Any	<1 sector	
	Severe			

Qian[27]	Number of Cysts	Symptomatic Hepatomegaly
Grade 0	0	No
Grade 1	1–10	No
Grade 2	11–20	No
Grade 3	>20	No
Grade 4	>20	Yes

Table 4
Mayo classification of ADPKD, growth of cysts and yearly decline in estimated GFR

Mayo Classification	hTKV Growth Rate per Year	Estimated Slope of Estimated GFR (eGFR) Change per Year (mL/min/1.73 m^2)	Risk of Progression
1E	> 6%	- 4.78	High risk
1D	4.5%–6%	−3.48	High risk
1C	3%–4.5%	−2.63	High risk
1B	1.5%–3%	−1.33	Intermediate risk
1A	<1.5%	−0.23	Low risk

Adapted from Irazabal M V, Rangel LJ, Bergstralh EJ, et al. Imaging Classification of Autosomal Dominant Polycystic Kidney Disease: A Simple Model for Selecting Patients for Clinical Trials. J Am Soc Nephrol. 2015;26(1):160-172. https://doi.org/10.1681/ASN.2013101138.

with Class 1C, 1D, and 1E are in the high-risk category. The limitations of the Mayo classification include cost for CT or MRI and that non-White groups were not accurately represented.[51]

In addition to phenotypic characteristics, the genotype also plays a major role in determining progression. Truncating PKD1 mutations are associated with the severe form, which on average results in renal failure at the age of 56. The PKD1 nontruncating and PKD2 mutations are associated with kidney failure at average ages of 68 and 79, respectively.[8,53] Patients who are identified at high risk may benefit from medical management.

Medical Management of autosomal dominant polycystic kidney disease and polycystic liver disease

Tolvaptan

Tolvaptan is a vasopressin V2 receptor antagonist (see **Fig. 1**). The inhibition of the effect of vasopressin through an antagonist or through hydration can decrease cyst formation and protect kidney function.[54,55]

The Tolvaptan Efficacy and Safety in the Management of Autosomal Dominant Polycystic Kidney Disease and its Outcomes (TEMPO) 3:4 trial which was a 3-year, placebo-controlled, double-blind randomized control trial to evaluate the effects of tolvaptan on the trajectory of renal function.[56] Participants had a preserved GFR but total kidney volume over 750 mL. Over the 3-year study period, kidney volume increased by 2.8% increase in the tolvaptan group versus 5.5% in the placebo group (P < .001). The tolvaptan group also experienced a decreased rate of decline in GFR (−10 mL/min vs −6.8 mL/min; P < .001).[56]

The Replicating Evidence of Preserved Renal Function: an Investigation of Tolvaptan Safety and Efficacy in Later Stage ADPKD (REPRISE) trial was a double-blind, randomized withdrawal, placebo-controlled trial that evaluated 1370 patients with ADPKD with CKD stage 2 to early CKD stage 4 (estimated GFR between 25 and 65 mL/min) on the efficacy and safety of tolvaptan. The tolvaptan group had an annual decline in GFR by 2.34 mL/min/1.73 m^2, whereas the placebo group experienced a decline of 3.61 mL/min/1.73 m^2 (P < .001).[57] The Food and Drug Administration (FDA) then approved tolvaptan for the treatment of ADPKD with high risk of progression.[25]

Despite FDA approval, there are major barriers to starting a patient on tolvaptan: life-threatening hepatotoxicity and aquaresis. Cost can also be prohibitive. The most dangerous, albeit rare, effect of tolvaptan is hepatotoxicity. As a result, patients and prescribing nephrologists are involved in risk evaluation and mitigation strategies (REMS) to carefully monitor patients for adverse events.[51] In both TEMPO and REPRISE, interrupting or discontinuing tolvaptan resulted in the normalization of the transaminase levels.[51,56,57]

The aquaretic effects of tolvaptan influence adherence. Many patients feel thirsty while on tolvaptan and have a high intake of fluid and urine output..[51,58] In the event that the patient develops an illness (fever, diarrhea, volume depletion) or are unable to adequately hydrate due to travel or medical procedure, they are advised to temporarily stop tolvaptan ("sick day").[51,58] Patients on tolvaptan should be advised to restrict sodium and protein intake to prevent polyuria. Tolvaptan is also a substrate of cytochrome p450 and there may be interactions with medications that induce or inhibit this enzyme.

The effect of tolvaptan on liver volumes was not collected in these trials. Despite liver cyst epithelium not expressing vasopressin 2 receptors, there is one case report that found a significant reduction in liver volume during the treatment course with tolvaptan for ADPKD.[59]

ACEi and ARBs

The effects of blood pressure control in ADPKD were studied in the Halt Progression of Polycystic Kidney Disease (HALT-PKD) trial.[60] This study had two arms: rigorous versus standard blood pressure control and dual renin–angiotensin inhibition (RAASi, with lisinopril and telmisartan) versus lisinopril alone. The more rigorous blood pressure group (target BP 95/60–110/65 vs 120/70–130/80) was associated with slower increases in total kidney volume (without an overall change in estimated GFR), a greater decline in left ventricular mass index, and a decline in proteinuria.[60] There were no differences between the groups randomized to dual RAASi versus lisinopril.[60] In both early and late ADPKD (GFR 25–60mL/min), angiotensin converting enzyme inhibitors (ACEis)and angiotensin receptor blockers (ARBs) are considered first-line agents for hypertension management, but dual RAASi is not recommended.[37]

Approximately 50% of patients with ADPKD progress to ESKD and require renal replacement therapy (either through dialysis or transplantation).[61] In patients who require dialysis before transplant, either hemodialysis or peritoneal dialysis can be considered. Patients with ADPKD with ESKD have lower mortality as compared with patients with non-ADPKD likely because they are overall healthier given the genetic cause of kidney failure.

Somatostatin analogs

Somatostatin analogs are the main medical treatment of hepatomegaly in polycystic liver. Somatostatin inhibits cAMP in cystic cholangiocytes inhibiting fluid secretion into cysts as well as decreasing cholangiocyte proliferation.[62,63] Multiple randomized trials in humans have found a reduction in liver volume with the use of somatostatin analogs with minimal side effects such as loose stool or abdominal cramping. In a systematic review of the published somatostatin analog trials, there was no effect on patient quality of life despite a reduction in liver volumes. The treatment effect seems to be within the first year of use afterward the effect wears off and liver volumes revert. Similarly, if the drug is withdrawn, the liver volumes increase to pretreatment levels.[64]

Somatostatin agonists show some promise in decreasing renal cysts. The Octreotide-LAR in Later Stage Autosomal Dominant Polycystic Kidney Disease (ALADIN-2) was a randomized control study that found octreotide-LAR decreased the rate of kidney growth and progression to ESKD, particularly in patients with CKD stage 4.[65]

Ursodeoxycholic acid

Ursodeoxycholic acid (UDCA) is a hydrophilic bile acid that is a calcium agonist in cholangiocytes. UDCA inhibits liver cyst proliferation in animal models.[66] In a clinical trial comparing the effect of UDCA verses no treatment on liver volume in patients with polycystic livers found no difference after 24 weeks of ursodiol but in a post hoc subgroup analysis, there was a reduction in the growth of liver cyst in patients with ADPKD.[67]

Estrogen avoidance

Given the evidence that estrogen impacts the growth of liver cysts as women have more and larger cysts correlating also with the number of pregnancies and use of estrogen supplements, estrogen receptor antagonists are a theoretic target for decreasing the progression of polycystic livers. There is no data on estrogen antagonists on cyst development but it is recommended to avoid estrogen supplementation in patients with polycystic livers.[68]

Surgical management

There are multiple percutaneous and surgical treatment strategies aimed at addressing symptomatic large liver cysts[49,69–74] **(Table 5)**. They have the limitation of only addressing a single (or a few) large cysts. Though these procedures have short-term beneficial effects on symptoms, the remaining cysts continue to grow and symptoms recur in most of the patients requiring further interventions. In addition, the surgical options can lead to significant adhesions that make explantation difficult for liver transplantation.[75]

Transplantation

Renal transplantation of ESKD offers the best chances for survival but is not curative as the polycystic native kidneys can continue to cause symptoms. Native kidney nephrectomy is currently reserved for patients who have intractable pain, severe bleeding, recurrent cyst infections, or if the size of the native kidney(s) preclude proper placement of the allograft.[61] Living donor renal transplant is the preferential treatment of ESKD. Patients with transplanted ADPKD have excellent survival and graft survival rates.[61]

Liver transplantation is the only curative treatment of PCLD and is often performed with a simultaneous renal transplant in the setting of ADPKD. Other therapies, such as sclerotherapy and fenestration can offer a symptomatic benefit but only temporarily and in a subset of patients with large, symptomatic cysts in accessible areas. Liver transplantation has been found to have good long-term survival of 92% at 5 years.[75] As patients with polycystic livers have preserved hepatic function, they must have severe symptoms from hepatomegaly to qualify for or desire a transplant. They typically have low Model for end-stage liver disease (MELD) scores or in the cases of ADPKD may have elevated MELDs due to renal failure. As patients with PCLD have preserved synthetic function, The Organ Procurement and Transplant Network has provided guidance on MELD exception points for PCLD. Patients qualify for MELD exception points if they have diffuse hepatic involvement of cysts with severe symptoms and hepatic decompensation, GFR less than 20, hemodialysis, prior kidney transplant, or moderate to severe protein-calorie malnutrition.[76] With MELD exception points that continue to accrue, patients with PCLD get transplanted with more frequency than those with chronic liver disease despite having better hepatic function.[77] A study examining the quality of life for patients with PCLD posttransplant found a dramatic

Table 5
Percutaneous and surgical management options for symptomatic polycystic liver disease

Treatment Modality	Indication	Method	Efficacy	Adverse Outcomes
Aspiration and Sclerotherapy	Symptomatic cysts >5cm	Percutaneous aspiration of cyst and injection of sclerosant to prevent reaccumulation	Cyst volume reduction in 76%–100% of patients Symptom relief in 72%–100% of patients[69]	Abdominal pain Ethanol intoxication with long duration of ethanol sclerosant instillation
Transcatheter Embolization	Large, symptomatic cyst	Embolize hepatic artery branch feeding the cyst resulting in cystic epithelial cell death	Reduces liver volumes by 10%[70] Symptom relief in 86% of patients[71]	Fever Pain Center-dependent risk of liver failure leading to emergent resection or transplant (28%) or death (17%)[72]
Fenestration	Surgically accessible symptomatic cysts (anterior R lobe or L lateral segments)	Laparoscopic aspiration and excision of the cyst wall to prevent recurrence[49]	Symptom relief in 90% of patients[73]	11% with postoperative complications (Bile leak, Ascites, Pleural effusion, Infection)[73]
Hepatic Resection	Dense area of cysts with relative sparing of the rest of the parenchyma	Surgical resection of the cystic area	62% reduction in liver volume Symptom relief in 97% of patients[74]	Significant postoperative morbidity in 58% of patients (infection, pleural effusion, hemorrhage requiring repeat surgery, bile leak)[74]

improvement of quality of life with quality of life scores returning to the level of healthy age-matched controls.[78]

SUMMARY

In summary, ADPKD is a primary ciliary disorder that leads to the formation of renal cysts and is commonly associated with PCLD. Isolated PCLD can also be seen and has the same liver manifestations as ADPKD but has distinct genetic mutations. Radiographic and genetic sequencing techniques can identify patients who have a high risk of progression to ESKD. Somatostatin analogs can decrease the growth of cysts in the liver but the efficacy of this medication only lasts a year at the maximum. There are percutaneous and laparoscopic treatment options for symptomatic patients who have a few large cysts. Kidney and liver transplantation increases survival and improves the quality of life.

CLINICS CARE POINTS

- Polycystic kidney and liver disease is typically diagnosed radiographically.
- ADPKD can lead to end stage renal disease.
- Tolvaptan use in ADPKD can slow down the deterioration of renal function and growth of cysts.
- Liver function is typically preseverved in polycystic liver disease.
- The medication management for polycystic liver disease is limited. Somatostatin analogs can slow the growth of polycystic livers but the effect is short-lived.
- The only curative therapy for PCLD is liver transplantation.
- Renal transplantation can significantly improve survival in patients with ESKD due to ADPKD.

DISCLOSURE

No disclosures

REFERENCES

1. Kothadia JP, Kreitman K, Shah JM. Polycystic Liver Disease. [Updated 2021 May 19]. In: StatPearls [Internet]. Treasure Island (FL): StatPearls Publishing; 2021. Available from: https://www.ncbi.nlm.nih.gov/books/NBK549882/.
2. Gabow PA, Johnson AM, Kaehny WD, et al. Risk factors for the development of hepatic cysts in autosomal dominant polycystic kidney disease. Hepatology 1990;11(6):1033-7.
3. Qian Q. Isolated polycystic liver disease. Adv Chronic Kidney Dis 2010;17(2):181-9.
4. Garcia Iglesias C, Torres VE, Offord KP, et al. Epidemiology of adult polycystic kidney disease, Olmsted County, Minnesota: 1935-1980. Am J Kidney Dis 1983;2(6):630-9.
5. Bae KT, Zhu F, Chapman AB, et al. Magnetic resonance imaging evaluation of hepatic cysts in early autosomal-dominant polycystic kidney disease: the Consortium for Radiologic Imaging Studies of Polycystic Kidney Disease cohort. Clin J Am Soc Nephrol 2006;1(1):64-9.

6. Karhunen P, Tenhu M. Adult polycystic liver and kidney diseases are separate entities. Clin Genet 1986;30(1):29–37.

7. Cornec-Le Gall E, Torres VE, Harris PC. Genetic complexity of autosomal dominant polycystic kidney and liver diseases. J Am Soc Nephrol 2018;29(1):13–23.

8. Cornec-Le Gall E, Audrézet M-P, Chen J-M, et al. Type of PKD1 mutation influences renal outcome in ADPKD. J Am Soc Nephrol 2013;24(6):1006–13.

9. Heyer CM, Sundsbak JL, Abebe KZ, et al. Predicted mutation Strength of Non-truncating PKD1 mutations Aids genotype-phenotype Correlations in autosomal dominant polycystic kidney disease. J Am Soc Nephrol 2016;27(9):2872–84.

10. Torres VE, Harris PC. Autosomal dominant polycystic kidney disease: the last 3 years. Kidney Int 2009;76(2):149–68.

11. Porath B, Gainullin VG, Cornec-Le Gall E, et al. Mutations in GANAB, encoding the glucosidase IIα Subunit, cause autosomal-dominant polycystic kidney and liver disease. Am J Hum Genet 2016;98(6):1193–207.

12. Drenth JPH, te Morsche RHM, Smink R, et al. Germline mutations in PRKCSH are associated with autosomal dominant polycystic liver disease. Nat Genet 2003; 33(3):345–7.

13. Davila S, Furu L, Gharavi AG, et al. Mutations in SEC63 cause autosomal dominant polycystic liver disease. Nat Genet 2004;36(6):575–7.

14. Besse W, Dong K, Choi J, et al. Isolated polycystic liver disease genes define effectors of polycystin-1 function. J Clin Invest 2017;127(9):3558.

15. Watnick T, He N, Wang K, et al. Mutations of PKD1 in ADPKD2 cysts suggest a pathogenic effect of trans-heterozygous mutations. Nat Genet 2000;25(2):143–4.

16. Qian F, Watnick TJ, Onuchic LF, et al. The molecular basis of focal cyst formation in human autosomal dominant polycystic kidney disease type I. Cell 1996;87(6): 979–87.

17. Pei Y, Watnick T, He N, et al. Somatic PKD2 mutations in individual kidney and liver cysts Support a "Two-Hit" model of cystogenesis in type 2 autosomal dominant polycystic kidney disease. J Am Soc Nephrol 1999;10(7):1524–9.

18. Hopp K, Ward CJ, Hommerding CJ, et al. Functional polycystin-1 dosage governs autosomal dominant polycystic kidney disease severity. J Clin Invest 2012;122(11):4257–73.

19. Hughes J, Ward CJ, Peral B, et al. The polycystic kidney disease 1 (PKD1) gene encodes a novel protein with multiple cell recognition domains. Nat Genet 1995; 10(2):151–60.

20. Shen PS, Yang X, DeCaen PG, et al. The structure of the polycystic kidney disease channel PKD2 in Lipid Nanodiscs. Cell 2016;167(3):763–73.e11.

21. Lee K, Battini L, Gusella GL. Cilium, centrosome and cell cycle regulation in polycystic kidney disease. Biochim Biophys Acta - Mol Basis Dis 2011;1812(10): 1263–71.

22. Fischer E, Legue E, Doyen A, et al. Defective planar cell polarity in polycystic kidney disease. Nat Genet 2005;38(1):21–3.

23. Drummond IA. Polycystins, focal adhesions and extracellular matrix interactions. Biochim Biophys Acta - Mol Basis Dis 2011;1812(10):1322–6.

24. Belibi FA, Reif G, Wallace DP, et al. Cyclic AMP promotes growth and secretion in human polycystic kidney epithelial cells. Kidney Int 2004;66(3):964–73.

25. Torres VE. Pro: tolvaptan delays the progression of autosomal dominant polycystic kidney disease. Nephrol Dial Transpl 2019;34(1):30–4.

26. Yamaguchi T, Nagao S, Wallace DP, et al. Cyclic AMP activates B-Raf and ERK in cyst epithelial cells from autosomal-dominant polycystic kidneys. Kidney Int 2003;63(6):1983–94.

27. Qian Q, Li A, King BF, et al. Clinical profile of autosomal dominant polycystic liver disease. Hepatology 2003;37(1):164–71.
28. Gabow PA, Kaehny WD, Johnson AM, et al. The clinical utility of renal concentrating capacity in polycystic kidney disease. Kidney Int 1989;35(2):675–80.
29. Gabow PA, Duley I, Johnson AM. Clinical Profiles of Gross hematuria in autosomal dominant polycystic kidney disease. Am J Kidney Dis 1992;20(2):140–3.
30. Johnson AM, Gabow PA. Identification of patients with autosomal dominant polycystic kidney disease at highest risk for end-stage renal disease. J Am Soc Nephrol 1997;8(10):1560–7.
31. Torres VE, Wilson DM, Hattery RR, et al. Renal stone disease in autosomal dominant polycystic kidney disease. Am J Kidney Dis 1993;22(4):513–9.
32. Grampsas SA, Chandhoke PS, Fan J, et al. Anatomic and metabolic risk factors for nephrolithiasis in patients with autosomal dominant polycystic kidney disease. Am J Kidney Dis 2000;36(1):53–7.
33. Yu T-M, Chuang Y-W, Yu M-C, et al. Risk of cancer in patients with polycystic kidney disease: a propensity-score matched analysis of a nationwide, population-based cohort study. Lancet Oncol 2016;17(10):1419–25.
34. Wetmore JB, Calvet JP, Yu ASL, et al. Polycystic kidney disease and cancer after renal transplantation. J Am Soc Nephrol 2014;25(10):2335–41.
35. Keith DS, Torres VE, King BF, et al. Renal cell Carcinoma in autosomal dominant polycystic kidney disease. J Am Soc Nephrol 1994;4(9):1661–9.
36. Grantham JJ. Autosomal dominant polycystic kidney disease. N Engl J Med 2008;359(14):1477–85.
37. Torres VE, Chapman AB, Perrone RD, et al. The HALT polycystic kidney disease trials – analysis of baseline parameters. Kidney Int 2013;81(6):577–85.
38. Bergmann C, Guay-Woodford LM, Harris PC, et al. Polycystic kidney disease. Nat Rev Dis Prim 2018;4(1):50.
39. Chebib FT, Jung Y, Heyer CM, et al. Effect of genotype on the severity and volume progression of polycystic liver disease in autosomal dominant polycystic kidney disease. Nephrol Dial Transpl 2016;31(6):952–60.
40. Van Keimpema L, De Koning DB, Van Hoek B, et al. Patients with isolated polycystic liver disease referred to liver centres: clinical characterization of 137 cases. Liver Int 2011;31(1):92–8.
41. van Aerts RMM, van de Laarschot LFM, Banales JM, et al. Clinical management of polycystic liver disease. J Hepatol 2018;68(4):827–37.
42. Abu-Wasel B, Walsh C, Keough V, et al. Pathophysiology, epidemiology, classification and treatment options for polycystic liver diseases. World J Gastroenterol 2013;19(35):5775–86.
43. Barbier L, Ronot M, Béatrice A, et al. Polycystic liver disease: hepatic venous outflow obstruction lesions of the noncystic parenchyma have major consequences. Hepatology 2018;68(2):652–62.
44. Perrone RD, Malek A, Watnick T. Vascular complications in autosomal dominant polycystic kidney disease. Nat Rev Nephrol 2015;11(10):589–98.
45. Chapman AB, Rubinstein D, Hughes R, et al. Intracranial aneurysms in autosomal dominant polycystic kidney disease. N Engl J Med 1992;327(13):916–20.
46. Gibbs GF, Huston J, Qian Q, et al. Follow-up of intracranial aneurysms in autosomal-dominant polycystic kidney disease. Kidney Int 2004;65(5):1621–7.
47. Pei Y, Obaji J, Dupuis A, et al. Unified criteria for Ultrasonographic diagnosis of ADPKD. J Am Soc Nephrol 2009;20(1):205–12.
48. Grantham JJ, Torres VE, Chapman AB, et al. Volume progression in polycystic kidney disease. N Engl J Med 2006;354(20):2122–30.

49. Gigot JF, Jadoul P, Que F, et al. Adult polycystic liver disease: is fenestration the most adequate operation for long-term management? Ann Surg 1997;225(3): 286–94.

50. Schnelldorfer T, Torres VE, Zakaria S, et al. Polycystic liver disease: a critical appraisal of hepatic resection, cyst fenestration, and liver transplantation. Ann Surg 2009;250(1):112–8.

51. Chebib FT, Torres VE. Assessing risk of rapid progression in autosomal dominant polycystic kidney disease and special Considerations for disease-modifying therapy. Am J Kidney Dis 2021;78(2):282–92.

52. Irazabal MV, Rangel LJ, Bergstralh EJ, et al. Imaging classification of autosomal dominant polycystic kidney disease: a simple model for Selecting patients for clinical trials. J Am Soc Nephrol 2015;26(1):160–72.

53. Cornec-Le Gall E, Audrézet M-P, Renaudineau E, et al. PKD2-Related autosomal dominant polycystic kidney disease: prevalence, clinical presentation, mutation spectrum, and Prognosis. Am J Kidney Dis 2017;70(4):476–85.

54. Gattone VH, Wang X, Harris PC, et al. Inhibition of renal cystic disease development and progression by a vasopressin V2 receptor antagonist. Nat Med 2003; 9(10):1323–6.

55. Hopp K, Wang X, Ye H, et al. Effects of hydration in rats and mice with polycystic kidney disease. Am J Physiol - Ren Physiol 2015;308(3):F261–6.

56. Torres VE, Chapman AB, Devuyst O, et al. Tolvaptan in patients with autosomal dominant polycystic kidney disease. N Engl J Med 2012;367(25):2407–18.

57. Torres VE, Chapman AB, Devuyst O, et al. Tolvaptan in later-stage autosomal dominant polycystic kidney disease. N Engl J Med 2017;377(20):1930–42.

58. Devuyst O, Chapman AB, Shoaf SE, et al. Tolerability of aquaretic-related symptoms following tolvaptan for autosomal dominant polycystic kidney disease: results from TEMPO 3:4. Kidney Int Rep 2017;2(6):1132–40.

59. Mizuno H, Hoshino J, Suwabe T, et al. Tolvaptan for the treatment of enlarged polycystic liver disease. Case Rep Nephrol Dial 2017;7(2):108–11.

60. Schrier RW, Abebe KZ, Perrone RD, et al. Blood pressure in early autosomal dominant polycystic kidney disease. N Engl J Med 2014;371(24):2255–66.

61. Kanaan N, Devuyst O, Pirson Y. Renal transplantation in autosomal dominant polycystic kidney disease. Nat Rev Nephrol 2014;10(8):455–65.

62. Masyuk T, Masyuk A, LaRusso N. Therapeutic targets in polycystic liver disease. Curr Drug Targets 2018;18(8):950–7.

63. Masyuk TV, Masyuk AI, Torres VE, et al. Octreotide inhibits hepatic cystogenesis in a Rodent model of polycystic liver disease by reducing cholangiocyte Adenosine 3′,5′-cyclic Monophosphate. Gastroenterology 2007;132(3):1104–16.

64. Khan S, Dennison A, Garcea G. Medical therapy for polycystic liver disease. Ann R Coll Surg Engl 2016;98(1):18–23.

65. Perico N, Ruggenenti P, Perna A, et al. Octreotide-LAR in later-stage autosomal dominant polycystic kidney disease (ALADIN 2): a randomized, double-blind, placebo-controlled, multicenter trial. PLoS Med 2019;16(4). https://doi.org/10.1371/JOURNAL.PMED.1002777.

66. Munoz-Garrido P, Marin JJG, Perugorria MJ, et al. Ursodeoxycholic acid inhibits hepatic cystogenesis in experimental models of polycystic liver disease. J Hepatol 2015;63(4):952–61.

67. D'Agnolo HMA, Kievit W, Takkenberg RB, et al. Ursodeoxycholic acid in advanced polycystic liver disease: a phase 2 multicenter randomized controlled trial. J Hepatol 2016;65(3):601–7.

68. Pirson Y. Extrarenal manifestations of autosomal dominant polycystic kidney disease. Adv Chronic Kidney Dis 2010;17(2):173–80.
69. Wijnands TFM, Görtjes APM, Gevers TJG, et al. Efficacy and safety of aspiration sclerotherapy of simple hepatic cysts: a systematic review. Am J Roentgenol 2017;208(1):201–7.
70. Hoshino J, Ubara Y, Suwabe T, et al. Intravascular embolization therapy in patients with enlarged polycystic liver. Am J Kidney Dis 2014;63(6):937–44.
71. Zhang JL, Yuan K, Wang MQ, et al. Transarterial embolization for treatment of symptomatic polycystic liver disease: more than 2-year follow-up. Chin Med J (Engl) 2017;130(16):1938–44.
72. Yang J, Ryu H, Han M, et al. Comparison of volume-reductive therapies for massive polycystic liver disease in autosomal dominant polycystic kidney disease. Hepatol Res 2016;46(2):183–91.
73. Bernts LHP, Echternach SG, Kievit W, et al. Clinical response after laparoscopic fenestration of symptomatic hepatic cysts: a systematic review and meta-analysis. Surg Endosc 2019;33(3):691–704.
74. Que F, Nagorney DM, Gross JB, et al. Liver resection and cyst fenestration in the treatment of severe polycystic liver disease. Gastroenterology 1995;108:487–94.
75. Van Keimpema L, Nevens F, Adam R, et al. Excellent survival after liver transplantation for isolated polycystic liver disease: an European Liver Transplant Registry study. Transpl Int 2011;24(12):1239–45.
76. U.S. Department of Health & Human Services. Guidance to liver transplant Programs and the National liver review board for: Adult MELD exception review. Organ Procurement and transplant Network 2021. Available at: https://optn. transplant.hrsa.gov/media/3939/20200804_nlrb_adult_other_guidance.pdf. Accessed August 19, 2021.
77. Doshi SD, Bittermann T, Schiano TD, et al. Waitlisted candidates with polycystic liver disease are more likely to be transplanted than those with chronic liver failure. Transplantation 2017;101(8):1838–44. Waitlisted.
78. Kirchner GI, Rifai K, Cantz T, et al. Outcome and quality of life in patients with polycystic liver disease after liver or Combined liver-kidney transplantation. Liver Transpl 2006;122:1268–77.

Kidney Replacement Therapy in Patients with Acute Liver Failure and End-Stage Cirrhosis Awaiting Liver Transplantation

Karthik Kovvuru, MD[a,b,*], Juan Carlos Q. Velez, MD[a,b]

KEYWORDS

- Kidney Replacement Therapy • Liver Failure • End-stage cirrhosis • Cirrhosis
- Dialysis • Liver Transplantation • Peritoneal Dialysis • Ascites
- Renal Replacement Therapy

KEY POINTS

- Kidney replacement therapy for isolated liver failure has been used for cerebral edema, severe acidosis, volume and electrolyte management. Survival benefit has been limited to case reports and series.
- Hemodialysis complemented with intermittent paracentesis remains the modality of choice in stable patients.
- Peritoneal dialysis has been successfully used in patients with compensated cirrhosis.
- Albumin dialysis could be a life saving procedure for a carefully selected subgroup of patients in liver faiure.

INTRODUCTION

Kidney dysfunction in patients with liver failure increases mortality by 7-fold and challenges health care providers with very complex clinical scenarios. This increased mortality has prompted inclusion of kidney dysfunction into the model for end-stage liver disease scoring system for organ transplantation allocation.[1] With increased prevalence of chronic kidney disease (CKD) and improved overall medical care for cirrhosis, the prevalence of CKD in patients with cirrhosis has increased. In hospitalized patients with cirrhosis, the prevalence of CKD, defined as estimated glomerular filtration rate

[a] Department of Nephrology, Ochsner Health, New Orleans, LA, USA; [b] The University of Queensland/Ochsner Clinical School, Brisbane, Queensland, Australia
* Corresponding author. Division of Nephrology, Department of Medicine, Ochsner Clinic Foundation, 1514 Jefferson Hwy, Clinic Tower 5th Floor, New Orleans, LA 70121.
E-mail address: Karthikreddy.999@gmail.com

Clin Liver Dis 26 (2022) 245–253
https://doi.org/10.1016/j.cld.2022.01.003
1089-3261/22/© 2022 Elsevier Inc. All rights reserved.

less than 60 mL/min/1.73 m^2 for greater than 3 months, is reported to be around 47%.[2] Acute kidney injury (AKI) is also very common in patients with liver failure, and its prevalence increases in severe cases. Although the overall incidence of AKI in hospitalized patients with cirrhosis is 20%,[1] the incidence of AKI that requires kidney replacement therapy (KRT) in liver disease is less clear. Studies have reported 4% to 6% incidence of cirrhosis in patients with end-stage kidney disease (ESKD) on maintenance KRT.[3] Providing KRT in this subset of patients presents unique challenges.

INDICATIONS FOR KIDNEY REPLACEMENT THERAPY IN PATIENTS WITH LIVER FAILURE

Indications for KRT in patients with acute or acute-on-chronic liver failure can be broadly categorized into KRT for kidney failure and KRT as part of supportive management for liver failure. KRT for kidney failure is indicated in patients with acute liver failure, compensated cirrhosis, and decompensated cirrhosis awaiting transplantation. KRT for patients with decompensated cirrhosis not candidate for liver transplantation should be approached on an individual basis.[4]

KRT for isolated liver failure (in the absence of kidney failure) has been used for patients with cerebral edema secondary to hepatic encephalopathy, for patients with severe acidosis secondary to liver failure, and for volume or electrolyte management that failed medical therapy (**Table 1**). Liver failure leads to accumulation of toxins that can be broadly grouped into water soluble and protein bound. KRT removes small water-soluble toxins, free plasma amino acids, and ammonia. This removal is typically only modest. Thus, continuous therapies do not impact plasma concentrations unless liver function is concurrently improving. Despite multiple case reports and case series reporting some benefit with KRT in liver failure, there is no randomized controlled study that proved improved survival with this approach.[5]

CHOOSING MODALITY OF KIDNEY REPLACEMENT THERAPY IN LIVER FAILURE

Low arterial blood pressure in patients with liver failure plays a significant role in selecting modality. The pathophysiology for low arterial blood pressure in chronic liver failure stems from portal hypertension, which induces progressive splanchnic and systemic vasodilation via nitric oxide and other vasoactive substances secondary to endothelial stretching and stress.[6] In patients with decompensated cirrhosis and acute liver failure, arterial blood pressure may also drop owing to distributive shock stemming from liver failure itself. Consequently, any further drop in blood pressure during dialysis can significantly affect cerebral perfusion pressures. Patients with acute or decompensated liver failure usually have an intact blood-brain barrier and are at risk of cerebral edema and increased intracranial pressure owing to an accumulation of toxins. Removing osmoles more rapidly from plasma than that from the brain itself could lead to movement of water

Table 1 Indications for kidney replacement therapy in patients with liver failure	
1	Kidney failure that failed medical management
2	Liver failure + Hepatic encephalopathy with cerebral edema Metabolic acidosis[a] Severe electrolyte abnormalities[a] Volume overload[a]

[a] Failed medical management.

back into the brain, exacerbating cerebral edema.[7] Studies have demonstrated that in patients with fulminant hepatic failure, changes in intracranial pressure occur during KRT either because of a drop in cerebral perfusion pressure from intradialytic hypotension or because of a rapid drop in serum osmolality. This risk can be mitigated by choosing a modality that offers better hemodynamic stability and slower osmolar shifts. Peritoneal dialysis (PD) could offer these benefits. However, starting PD for AKI is limited by availability and associated with increased risk of peritonitis,[8] leakage of ascites, protein loss, and compromised respiratory dynamics.[9] Intermittent hemodialysis (iHD) is known to cause increased intracranial pressure, making it a poor choice.[10] Thus, continuous kidney replacement therapy (CKRT) should be considered treatment of choice, as it offers the least cerebral and hemodynamic instability.[5]

Patients on CKRT who recover liver function without needing liver transplant can be transitioned to peritoneal or iHD until kidneys recover. Patients who receive liver transplantation cannot be transitioned to PD, as it would introduce a risk for postoperative site infection. On the other hand, PD has been successfully used for patients who developed ESKD many years after liver transplant[11] (**Fig. 1**).

CONTINUOUS KIDNEY REPLACEMENT THERAPY

As discussed above, CKRT remains the safest modality of choice for patients with hemodynamic instability and hepatic encephalopathy. Depending on availability, it can be delivered by slow low efficient dialysis (SLED) or continuous venovenous hemodiafiltration/hemodialysis/hemofiltration. SLED can be managed as CKRT or as prolonged intermittent KRT. Studies have not conclusively proven benefit of one over the other.[12]

All current continuous venovenous hemodiafiltration solutions have a sodium concentration of 140 mEq/L, and patients with liver failure are frequently hyponatremic.[13] Thus, dysnatremia protocols should be implemented to prevent rapid correction of

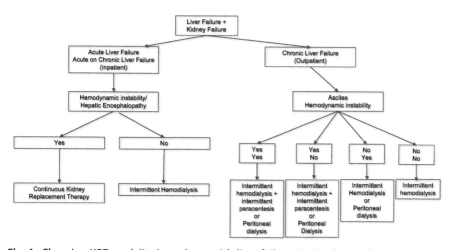

Fig. 1. Choosing KRT modality in patients with liver failure: Optimal modality of choice depends primarily on the presence of hepatic encephalopathy and hemodynamic instability. In the inpatient setting, CKRT would be the preferred choice if any of those are present; iHD would be reasonable in their absence. In the outpatient setting, iHD is the commonly used modality. Midodrine can be considered for patients with borderline hemodynamics. CKRT and iHD may need to be augmented with intermittent paracentesis. PD is less commonly used but offers the benefit of not needing additional paracentesis.

sodium. SLED offers a unique advantage in this aspect, as the dialysate sodium can be set as low as 130 mEq/L.

Filter clotting may represent a barrier for effective CKRT, and patients with liver failure are susceptible to this. Prescription adjustments, such us anticoagulant-free CKRT circuit relying on higher blood flow, low filtration fraction, and predilution replacement fluid administration, can be tried to decrease the clotting risk. Anticoagulants are probably required if filter clots occur, after ruling out catheter issues. Counterintuitively, patients with advanced liver failure can be more prothrombotic than coagulopathic.[14,15] The effect of heparin may be unpredictable owing to reduced levels of antithrombin and heparin cofactor II. Thus, some patients with liver failure may paradoxically require higher doses of heparin, whereas others are at high risk of bleeding owing to inherent coagulopathy.[16]

Regional citrate anticoagulation has caveats in liver failure. Under standard conditions, the infused citrate is partly cleared as a calcium citrate complex in the effluent (30%–70%), and the rest is metabolized by liver and muscle into bicarbonate. Because of the lack of hepatic clearance in patients with liver failure, the half-life of citrate is increased, leading to a higher risk of citrate accumulation and toxicity (12%) **(Fig. 2)**.[17] If citrate anticoagulation is to be used, it can be considered to start at lower

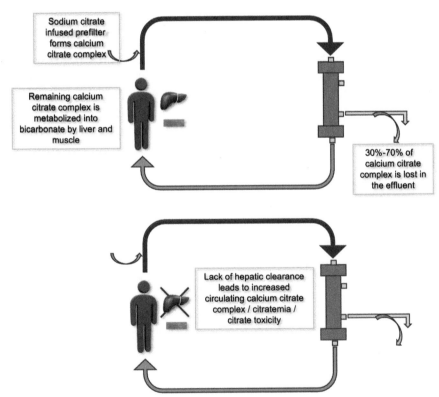

Fig. 2. Citrate metabolism. Depending on the effluent rate, 30% to 70% of the infused citrate is lost in the effluent as a calcium citrate complex. The rest of the citrate is metabolized to bicarbonate by liver and muscle. In patients with liver failure, hepatic clearance of citrate is impaired leading to high risk of citrate toxicity. This risk can be mitigated by using lower blood flow rate along with lowest dose of citrate needed to maintain a therapeutic postfilter calcium and by increasing the effluent rate if needed to augment citrate removal.

(50%–60%) than the usual dose and titrate it by 10% to the lowest dose to maintain therapeutic postfilter ionized calcium while frequently monitoring systemic calcium levels and citrate toxicity. If the patient starts to develop citrate toxicity with the minimum dose of citrate needed to maintain therapeutic postfilter ionized calcium, the effluent dose can be increased to augment citrate loss.[18]

HEMODIALYSIS

Most patients are transitioned from CKRT to iHD owing to challenges with PD during acute illness and lack of resources. Hemodynamic instability, anticoagulation, and inability to remove ascitic fluid are the main challenges for hemodialysis in patients with liver failure. Oral midodrine, low dialysate temperature, and intravenous albumin prime could potentially help prevent hypotension to some extent.[19,20] Bleeding at the site of catheter insertion and prolonged bleeding after needle removal may occur. Ascites fluid in a patient with cirrhosis behaves as a separate compartment, and hemodialysis alone cannot effectively remove it. Some patients would continue to need intermittent paracentesis despite being on hemodialysis.[21,22]

PERITONEAL DIALYSIS

PD has been successfully used in patients who have compensated cirrhosis. It also offers an additional advantage of draining the ascitic fluid and provision of caloric load.[3]

There is an understandable concern for an increased risk of peritonitis in patients with cirrhosis owing to their malnourished state and potentially weak immune system. However, published data have been mixed. An early, small series of 5 patients reported a higher incidence of peritonitis with a rate of 1 episode per 9 patient-months (average rate of 1 episode per 24 patient-months) with predominantly gram-negative organisms.[23] The largest study that looked into peritonitis risk is a retrospective study that compared peritonitis rates between cirrhotic (n = 25) and noncirrhotic (n = 36) patients with hepatitis B virus infection on PD. There was no significant difference in the peritonitis rate, peritonitis-free survival, or time to first peritonitis. Rates of gram-negative and gram-positive infection were also similar.[24]

Increased loss of protein via PD fluid represents another concern in this patient population. PD proponents theorize that the increase in intra-abdominal pressure during fills might effectively oppose the portal pressure and decrease the ascites fluid formation and protein losses. They also suggest that the dialysate might serve as an additional source of calories.[25] Several retrospective longitudinal studies have shown that peritoneal fluid protein losses could be initially high, but they decrease over time.[23,26,27] Patients with cirrhosis on PD did not have any issues with metabolism of lactate in PD fluid.[27] For patients listed for liver transplantation, there has been debate about increased risk of peritonitis, protein loss, and portal vein thrombosis, which could preclude a patient from getting a transplant. However, there are no conclusive data to support this notion. In a recent report of 12 patients on PD with combined kidney failure and cirrhosis, 3 patients underwent successful simultaneous liver kidney transplant, 4 patients remained active on transplant wait list, and 5 patients were deemed not to be transplant candidates because of comorbid conditions.[28]

INTRAOPERATIVE DIALYSIS DURING LIVER TRANSPLANTATION

Some liver transplant centers practice periliver transplant KRT (**Table 2**).[29] The benefit of perioperative KRT compared with conservative care is unclear because of a lack of prospective controlled studies.[30]

Table 2	
Rationale for intraoperative kidney replacement therapy during liver transplantation	
1	Metabolic acidosis in the anhepatic phase
2	Hyperkalemia during reperfusion
3	Hyponatremia before transplant and abrupt correction during reperfusion
4	Management of large-volume shifts

Hyponatremia is relatively common in patients with decompensated or end-stage cirrhosis. In early decades of liver transplantation, many centers reported encephalopathy and death owing to central pontine myelinosis.[31,32] This was likely due to rapid correction of serum sodium during the transplant surgery from low 120 mEq/L to 140 mEq/L because of the sodium content in blood and other products given during transplant surgery. CKRT has been used to prevent this overcorrection.[33,34] CKRT has also been used to maintain other electrolyte and acid-base balance during and in the immediate postoperative period.[35] Liver transplant abruptly changes the hemodynamics from high portal pressures with low systemic vascular resistance to normal portal pressure and normal/low systemic vascular resistance. This abrupt change can precipitate acute right-sided heart failure, prompting need of CKRT intraoperatively to help correct volume if needed to prevent right-sided heart failure.[5]

The liver may need to be resected first in some very severe cases of acute liver failure, leaving the patient anhepatic while awaiting transplant, and CKRT has been used to sustain acid-base status.[5] More recently, MARS (Molecular Adsorbent Recirculation System, Gambro, Sweden) has been used for this indication.[36]

ALBUMIN DIALYSIS

Artificial liver support systems have been in use for more than a decade. However, their availability and use have been limited because of cost, lack of clear guidelines, training, and expertise. Bioartificial systems were initially investigated until the invention of high-flux artificial polysulfone membrane (which can separate protein-bound substances from protein-containing liquids like plasma) in the early 1990s. This method has been traditionally called albumin dialysis.[37] Single-pass albumin dialysis, MARS, and Prometheus (Fractionated Plasma Separation and Adsorption System; Fresenius Medical Care, Germany) are the currently available modalities. Each of these has their own benefits and disadvantages.[38] MARS has been the most widely studied and has been used in various clinical settings, including acute liver failure, acute-on-chronic liver failure, as a bridge for liver transplantation, for removal of albumin bound drugs, liver graft failure, and intractable cholestatic pruritus.[39]

The Food and Drug Administration has currently approved MARS for only 2 indications: (1) drug overdose and poisoning (drug or chemical should be dialyzable and bound by charcoal and/or ion exchange resin); (2) treatment of hepatic encephalopathy owing to decompensation of chronic liver disease (not as a bridge to liver transplantation). Availability of MARS is limited to very few hospitals in the United States, and it has been used infrequently. MARS has been shown to potentially improve mortality in patients with acute liver failure[40] and is yet to be proven to be efficacious in acute-on-chronic liver failure.[41] The reported adverse events are very limited.[42] Although further studies are needed to standardize the treatment protocols and improve the treatment efficacy, this modality has a potential in the management of selected patients with liver failure who are otherwise at very high risk for mortality.[36]

SUMMARY

Providing dialysis to patients with liver failure is challenging primarily because of their tenuous hemodynamics and refractory ascites. With better machinery and increased availability, CKRT has been successfully delivered to acutely ill patients in liver failure over the past few decades. IHD continues to remain the modality of choice outside the intensive care unit and on occasion needs to be complemented with paracentesis. PD has not been widely used, but the recent literature is showing promising outcomes barring for publication bias. Albumin dialysis could be a lifesaving procedure for a carefully selected subgroup of patients with liver failure.

CLINICS CARE POINTS

- Continuous kidney replacement therapy offers the least cerebral and hemodynamic instability.
- Risk of Citrate toxicity can be minimized by starting the citrate at 50-60% lower than the usual dose and titrating closely.
- Continuous kidney replacement therapy has been used intraoperatively during liver transplant to prevent rapid correction of sodium, control hyperkalemia and acidosis.

DISCLOSURE

J.C.Q. Velez has participated in consulting engagements with Mallinckrodt, Bayer, and Travere and in speaking bureau for Otsuka.

REFERENCES

1. Fede G, D'Amico G, Arvaniti V, et al. Renal failure and cirrhosis: a systematic review of mortality and prognosis. J Hepatol 2012;56(4):810–8.
2. Wong F, Reddy KR, O'Leary JG, et al. Impact of chronic kidney disease on outcomes in cirrhosis. Liver Transpl 2019;25(6):870–80.
3. Rajora N, De Gregorio L, Saxena R. Peritoneal dialysis use in patients with ascites: a review. Am J Kidney Dis 2021;78(5):728–35.
4. Velez JCQ. Patients with hepatorenal syndrome should be dialyzed? PRO Kidney360 2021;2(3):406–9.
5. Davenport A. Continuous renal replacement therapies in patients with liver disease. Semin Dial 2009;22(2):169–72.
6. Vora RS, Subramanian RM. Hypotension in cirrhosis. Clin Liver Dis (Hoboken) 2019;13(6):149–53.
7. Arieff AI, Massry SG, Barrientos A, et al. Brain water and electrolyte metabolism in uremia: effects of slow and rapid hemodialysis. Kidney Int 1973;4(3):177–87.
8. Chionh CY, Soni SS, Finkelstein FO, et al. Use of peritoneal dialysis in AKI: a systematic review. Clin J Am Soc Nephrol 2013;8(10):1649–60.
9. Almeida CP, Ponce D, de Marchi AC, et al. Effect of peritoneal dialysis on respiratory mechanics in acute kidney injury patients. Perit Dial Int 2014;34(5):544–9.
10. Davenport A, Will EJ, Davison AM. Early changes in intracranial pressure during haemofiltration treatment in patients with grade 4 hepatic encephalopathy and acute oliguric renal failure. Nephrol Dial Transplant 1990;5(3):192–8.
11. Saiprasertkit N, Nihei CH, Bargman JM. Peritoneal dialysis in orthotopic liver transplantation recipients. Perit Dial Int 2018;38(1):44–8.

12. Shirazian A, Peralta-Cuervo AF, Aguilera-Pena MP, et al. Sustained low-efficiency dialysis is associated with worsening cerebral edema and outcomes in intracerebral hemorrhage. Neurocrit Care 2021;35(1):221–31.
13. Rosner MH, Connor MJ Jr. Management of severe hyponatremia with continuous renal replacement therapies. Clin J Am Soc Nephrol 2018;13(5):787–9.
14. Kohli R, Shingina A, New S, et al. Thromboelastography parameters are associated with cirrhosis severity. Dig Dis Sci 2019;64(9):2661–70.
15. Harrison MF. The misunderstood coagulopathy of liver disease: a review for the acute setting. West J Emerg Med 2018;19(5):863–71.
16. Davenport A. Continuous renal replacement therapy for liver disease. Hemodial Int 2003;7(4):348–52.
17. Zhang W, Bai M, Yu Y, et al. Safety and efficacy of regional citrate anticoagulation for continuous renal replacement therapy in liver failure patients: a systematic review and meta-analysis. Crit Care 2019;23(1):22.
18. Mariano F, Morselli M, Bergamo D, et al. Blood and ultrafiltrate dosage of citrate as a useful and routine tool during continuous venovenous haemodiafiltration in septic shock patients. Nephrol Dial Transplant 2011;26(12):3882–8.
19. Hryciw N, Joannidis M, Hiremath S, et al. Intravenous albumin for mitigating hypotension and augmenting ultrafiltration during kidney replacement therapy. Clin J Am Soc Nephrol 2021;16(5):820–8.
20. Palmer BF, Henrich WL. Recent advances in the prevention and management of intradialytic hypotension. J Am Soc Nephrol 2008;19(1):8–11.
21. Ing TS, Daugirdas JT, Popli S, et al. Treatment of refractory hemodialysis ascites with maintenance peritoneal dialysis. Clin Nephrol 1981;15(4):198–202.
22. Selgas R, Bajo MA, Del Peso G, et al. Peritoneal dialysis in the comprehensive management of end-stage renal disease patients with liver cirrhosis and ascites: practical aspects and review of the literature. Perit Dial Int 2008;28(2):118–22.
23. Bajo MA, Selgas R, Jimenez C, et al. CAPD for treatment of ESRD patients with ascites secondary to liver cirrhosis. Adv Perit Dial 1994;10:73–6.
24. Chow KM, Szeto CC, Wu AK, et al. Continuous ambulatory peritoneal dialysis in patients with hepatitis B liver disease. Perit Dial Int 2006;26(2):213–7.
25. Khan S, Rosner MH. Peritoneal dialysis for patients with end-stage renal disease and liver cirrhosis. Perit Dial Int 2018;38(6):397–401.
26. Huang ST, Chuang YW, Cheng CH, et al. Outcome of peritoneal dialysis in cirrhotic patients with end-stage renal disease: a 24-years' experience in Taiwan. Clin Nephrol 2011;76(4):306–13.
27. De Vecchi AF, Colucci P, Salerno F, et al. Outcome of peritoneal dialysis in cirrhotic patients with chronic renal failure. Am J Kidney Dis 2002;40(1):161–8.
28. Jones RE, Liang Y, MacConmara M, et al. Peritoneal dialysis is feasible as a bridge to combined liver-kidney transplant. Perit Dial Int 2018;38(1):63–5.
29. Sedra AH, Strum E. The role of intraoperative hemodialysis in liver transplant patients. Curr Opin Organ Transpl 2011;16(3):323–5.
30. Cheng XS, Tan JC, Kim WR. Management of renal failure in end-stage liver disease: a critical appraisal. Liver Transpl 2016;22(12):1710–9.
31. Adams DH, Ponsford S, Gunson B, et al. Neurological complications following liver transplantation. Lancet 1987;1(8539):949–51.
32. Lee EM, Kang JK, Yun SC, et al. Risk factors for central pontine and extrapontine myelinolysis following orthotopic liver transplantation. Eur Neurol 2009;62(6):362–8.
33. Davenport A. Is there a role for continuous renal replacement therapies in patients with liver and renal failure? Kidney Int Suppl 1999;(72):S62–6.

34. Nagai S, Moonka D, Patel A. Novel intraoperative management in the model for end-stage liver disease-sodium era: continuous venovenous hemofiltration for severe hyponatremia in liver transplantation. Liver Transpl 2018;24(2):304–7.
35. Kim HY, Lee JE, Ko JS, et al. Intraoperative management of liver transplant recipients having severe renal dysfunction: results of 42 cases. Ann Surg Treat Res 2018;95(1):45–53.
36. Hanish SI, Stein DM, Scalea JR, et al. Molecular adsorbent recirculating system effectively replaces hepatic function in severe acute liver failure. Ann Surg 2017; 266(4):677–84.
37. Stange J, Ramlow W, Mitzner S, et al. Dialysis against a recycled albumin solution enables the removal of albumin-bound toxins. Artif Organs 1993;17(9):809–13.
38. Krisper P, Stadlbauer V, Stauber RE. Clearing of toxic substances: are there differences between the available liver support devices? Liver Int 2011;31(Suppl 3):5–8.
39. Stadlbauer V, Jalan R. Acute liver failure: liver support therapies. Curr Opin Crit Care 2007;13(2):215–21.
40. He G-L, Feng L, Duan C-Y, et al. Meta-analysis of survival with the molecular adsorbent recirculating system for liver failure. Int J Clin Exp Med 2015;8(10): 17046–54.
41. Shen Y, Wang XL, Wang B, et al. Survival benefits with artificial liver support system for acute-on-chronic liver failure: a time series-based meta-analysis. Medicine (Baltimore) 2016;95(3):e2506.
42. Faybik P, Bacher A, Kozek-Langenecker SA, et al. Molecular adsorbent recirculating system and hemostasis in patients at high risk of bleeding: an observational study. Crit Care 2006;10(1):R24.

Peritransplant Renal Dysfunction in Liver Transplant Candidates

Rajiv Heda, MD[a], Alexander J. Kovalic, MD[b],
Sanjaya K. Satapathy, MBBS, MD, DM, MS[c,d],*

KEYWORDS

- Liver transplantation • Chronic kidney disease • Acute kidney injury
- Hepatorenal syndrome • Novel biomarkers

KEY POINTS

- The most common manifestations of acute kidney injury (AKI) in patients with cirrhosis include prerenal AKI, hepatorenal syndrome type of AKI (HRS-AKI), and acute tubular necrosis (ATN).
- HRS-AKI, a potentially life-threatening condition, may result in rapid deterioration of the kidney function in patients with decompensated cirrhosis is diagnosed after excluding other potential etiologies of kidney injury and after 48 hours of aggressive volume expansion.
- Urinary neutrophil gelatinase-associated lipocalin, or uNGAL, is a novel biomarker that is elevated in HRS-AKI (specifically type 1 HRS), and can help distinguish HRS-AKI from prerenal AKI.
- Identifying patients at risk for posttransplant renal failure is important to help tailor posttransplant immunosuppression to avoid worsening renal function and overall mortality.

INTRODUCTION

Renal dysfunction among patients with cirrhosis is an important prognostic indicator and a major determinant for liver transplant candidacy. Patients with cirrhosis, especially those with decompensated cirrhosis, are at heightened risk for developing acute kidney injury (AKI). The pathophysiology of this increased risk is thought to be related

[a] Department of Internal Medicine, Tulane University School of Medicine, New Orleans, LA 70112, USA; [b] Department of Internal Medicine, Division of Gastroenterology and Hepatology, Donald and Barbara Zucker School of Medicine at Hofstra/Northwell, Northwell Health, Manhasset, NY 11030, USA; [c] Department of Medicine, Division of Hepatology, Sandra Atlas Bass Center for Liver Diseases and Transplantation, Manhasset, NY 11030, USA; [d] Donald and Barbara Zucker School of Medicine at Hofstra/Northwell Health, 400 Community Drive, Manhasset, NY 11030, USA
* Corresponding author. Barbara and Zucker School of Medicine/Northwell Health, 400 Community Drive, Manhasset, NY 11030.
E-mail address: ssatapat@northwell.edu

Clin Liver Dis 26 (2022) 255–268
https://doi.org/10.1016/j.cld.2022.01.010
1089-3261/22/© 2022 Elsevier Inc. All rights reserved.

liver.theclinics.com

Abbreviations	
RAAS	renin-angiotensin-aldosterone system

to the splanchnic vasodilation and decreased effective intra-arterial volume that markedly increases the activation of the renin-angiotensin-aldosterone system (RAAS), both of which provide a heightened vulnerability for developing renal failure. The most common manifestations of AKI in patients with cirrhosis include prerenal AKI, hepatorenal syndrome type of AKI (HRS-AKI), and acute tubular necrosis (ATN) (**Table 1**). Prerenal AKI, a common presentation in decompensated cirrhosis patients, is typically more representative of a benign disorder and responds well to plasma volume expansion. On the other hand, ATN requires more specific renal support and is associated with substantial mortality. HRS-AKI could lead to devastating consequences and is characterized by a dysregulated inflammatory response.

The primary aim of this review will be to discuss the diagnostic criteria, characterize the pathophysiology, and discuss management of renal dysfunction among patients with cirrhosis awaiting liver transplantation (LT) and in the peritransplantation phase.

PATHOPHYSIOLOGY

Renal dysfunction in cirrhosis has multiple potential etiologies. Medications, volume status, contrast agents, infection, intrinsic renal disease, and urinary obstruction can all contribute to renal function among patients with or without cirrhosis. The etiology of renal dysfunction can be solely attributed to progressive worsening of liver disease, typically triggered by the presence of underlying portal hypertension. The crucial result lies within the decreased effective intra-arterial volume due to splanchnic vasodilation. Among compensated cirrhosis, there is a compensatory increase in cardiac output and plasma volume to restore the effective intra-arterial blood volume (**Fig. 1**). However, progression of cirrhosis leads to worsening of portal hypertension, which further culminates in increased splanchnic vasodilation. Although similar compensatory mechanisms are in motion, there reaches a clinical threshold among patients with decompensated cirrhosis where an increase in cardiac output and plasma volume cannot sufficiently increase intra-arterial volume.[1] The rampant activation of the RAAS results in sodium reabsorption, water retention, and ascites formation, all of which contribute to decreasing effective intra-arterial volume, thus creating a maladaptive positive feedback mechanism resulting in further RAAS activation. Ultimately, this leads to vasoconstriction, impaired cardiac output, and worsening renal failure.

Clinical Significance of Renal Dysfunction Among Patients with Cirrhosis

The onset of renal dysfunction has significant implications in the clinical course and survival of patients with cirrhosis. Compared to patients without cirrhosis, one study identified a 7-fold increase in mortality among cirrhotics, and also showed a 50% mortality rate within 1 month of onset of renal dysfunction.[2] The importance of renal function in cirrhotic patients is reflected in the inclusion of serum creatinine in the Model for End-Stage Liver Disease (MELD) scoring system, a tool used to predict 90-day mortality and aid in prioritizing higher acuity liver transplant candidates. Furthermore, in cirrhotic patients undergoing liver transplant evaluation, patients with pretransplant CKD stage 3 (or estimated glomerular filtration rate [GFR] <30 mL/min) and AKI were associated with reduced posttransplant survival at 1 year.[3] Although pretransplant renal dysfunction plays a major role in transplant candidacy, identifying patients at higher risk for renal failure posttransplant is critical because of the associated increased mortality and risk for

Table 1
Clinical and laboratory characteristics differentiating ATN, prerenal AKI, and HRS-AKI among patients with cirrhosis

	ATN	Prerenal AKI	HRS-AKI
Progression of serum creatinine	Serum creatinine increase of at least 0.3 mg/dL or 50% increase within 48 h	Serum creatinine increase of at least 0.3 mg/dL or 50% increase within 48 h	Often more gradual time course, but AKI development as early as 2 weeks in type 1 HRS
Urinary casts	Granular or epithelial casts	None	None
FeNa (%)	>2%	<2%	<2%
Urinary sodium (mEq/L)	>20	<20	<20
Proteinuria	May be present	No	No
Biomarkers:			
Cystatin C	>1.12 mg/L	0.57–1.12 mg/L[a]	<0.57 mg/L
uNGAL	239–2242 µg/g Creatinine[b]	20–59 µg/g Creatinine[b]	83–263 µg/g Creatinine
Response to intravascular volume repletion (albumin and/or IVF) and diuretic holiday	Dependent on underlying etiology	Yes	No

Abbreviations: AKI, acute kidney injury; ATN, acute tubular necrosis; FeNa, fractional urinary sodium excretion; HRS, hepatorenal syndrome; IVF, intravenous fluids; uNGAL, urinary neutrophil gelatinase-associated lipocalin.

[a] Normal reference range[55]; Cystatin C can also be low in prerenal AKI.

[b] Ranges based 2012 study; HRS-AKI range listed for patients without active infection.[25]

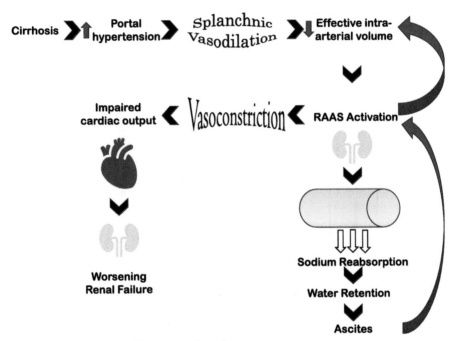

Fig. 1. Pathophysiology of hepatorenal syndrome.

major adverse cardiovascular events as compared with patients without renal dysfunction in the posttransplant period.[4–6]

Of note, pretransplant renal dysfunction is an independent predictor of posttransplant renal dysfunction (defined as serum creatinine > 1.2 mg/dL and/or GFR < 70 mL/min/1.73 m²). Furthermore, patients who developed severe renal failure (defined as median GFR < 30 mL/min/1.73 m² for a minimum of 6 months) were more likely to have diabetes mellitus, coronary artery disease, or primary graft nonfunction and were associated with lower survival.[7]

A retrospective analysis further stratified posttransplant acute renal failure (defined as a 50% rise in serum creatinine) into early (within 1 week) and late (second through fourth week). Significant risk factors for early posttransplant acute renal failure were identified as a serum albumin less than 3.2 g/dL, preoperative acute renal failure, treatment with dopamine more than 6 days, and graft dysfunction. However, for late-onset acute renal failure, only surgical reoperation and bacterial infection were identified as significant risk factors.[8]

DEVELOPMENT AND MANAGEMENT OF ACUTE RENAL DYSFUNCTION IN THE LIVER TRANSPLANT CANDIDATE

The criteria proposed for diagnosing AKI in cirrhotic patients are an increase in serum creatinine of ≥0.3 mg/dL or an increase in serum creatinine of 50% or more from baseline within less than 48 hours. Patients with AKI in the setting of cirrhosis should be evaluated earlier for LT, because of increased mortality risk. Urine output is intentionally excluded in this proposal, as refractory ascites will typically lead to a urine output less than 0.5 cc/kg/h, even in the absence of kidney injury.[9]

Hepatorenal syndrome (HRS) is associated with increased mortality and is a reversible cause of renal failure. As such, these patients should be evaluated for transplant early in the course of renal dysfunction while attempting to restore renal function with standard medical therapies, which is often ineffective. When contrasted with the much more stringent definition of HRS (**Box 1**), AKI is a more inclusive term and can help better characterize an at-risk population, especially when prioritizing patients for LT. AKI in cirrhosis is common in the setting of reduced effective arterial blood volume either due to aggressive diuresis or impending HRS. A prolonged course of decreased effective intra-arterial blood volume can lead to ischemia and subsequent ATN.[10] Furthermore, risk factors for renal dysfunction in hospitalized cirrhotic patients include ascites, spontaneous bacterial peritonitis, and treatment with intravenous aminoglycosides.[11] Therefore, medication-induced causes and infection should be considered in the diagnostic work-up. It is important to note that NSAIDs still cause a notable number of hospitalizations due to renal failure in cirrhotic patients despite discouraging use by several major guidelines.[12,13]

Although a diagnosis of HRS may be entertained, it is important to recall that several other diagnoses must first be ruled out before the definitive diagnosis of HRS. Infection, ATN, hypovolemia due to diuretic use, gastrointestinal bleeding, intrinsic renal disease, and urinary obstruction can all affect renal function and must be ruled out before arriving at the diagnosis of type 1 HRS.[12] Of note, when renal failure due to bacterial infection has been identified, the most common sources are peritoneal (i.e. spontaneous bacterial peritonitis) followed by respiratory then urinary tract. Similarly, gram-positive, gram-negative, then less commonly fungal micro-organisms were the common etiologies of infection as a cause of renal dysfunction.[12] The pathophysiology linking infection with renal dysfunction is thought to be due to the release of vasoactive cytokines disrupting a circulatory system that is already compromised by the presence of cirrhosis.

Type 1 HRS

The International Club of Ascites and the American Association for the Study of Liver Diseases have outlined criteria for HRS (see **Box 1**). HRS occurs due to splanchnic

---

Box 1
Diagnostic criteria for hepatorenal syndrome

Advanced hepatic failure and portal hypertension in the setting of acute or chronic liver disease

Acute kidney injury (defined as increase in serum creatinine by 0.3 mg/dL within 48 hours or 50% increase in serum creatinine from baseline within past 7 days)

Exclusion of other causes of acute kidney injury:
- Shock (septic, cardiogenic, distributive)
- Current or prior treatment with nephrotoxic agents.
- Obstructive uropathy

Absence of parenchymal kidney disease as indicated by proteinuria less than 500 mg/d

Absence of microhematuria (ie, <50 red blood cells per high power field) and/or normal renal ultrasonography

No improvement of serum creatinine after 48 hours of diuretic withdrawal and volume expansion with albumin (1 g/kg of body weight per day up to a maximum of 100 g/d)

Abbreviation: INR, international normalized ratio.

Data from Biggins SW, Angeli P, Garcia-Tsao G, et al. Diagnosis, Evaluation, and Management of Ascites, Spontaneous Bacterial Peritonitis and Hepatorenal Syndrome: 2021 Practice Guidance by the American Association for the Study of Liver Diseases. *Hepatology.* Aug 2021;74(2):1014-1048. doi:10.1002/hep.31884.

vasodilation from increased production of nitric oxide, which causes decreased systemic blood flow leading to activation of the RAAS, and subsequent intrarenal vasoconstriction. Regarding the measurement of intrarenal vasoconstriction, a resistive index measured by duplex ultrasonography of the kidneys of greater than 0.7 is associated with HRS in cirrhotic patients when compared to cirrhotic patients with a resistive index less than 0.7.[14] In fact, it was previously thought that LT was the only cure for type 1 HRS. However, with the identification of risk factors for HRS and subsequent treatments to prevent HRS, the need for LT may be evaded.[9] For instance, a major risk factor for HRS is spontaneous bacterial peritonitis; early recognition of this infection can lead to prevention of type 1 HRS by early (within 6 hours) administration of albumin, which has been shown to play a role as a vasoconstrictor by binding to vasodilators in addition to also playing a role in volume expansion.[15,16] However, even after the diagnosis of type 1 HRS has been made, it is possible to reverse the renal dysfunction with the administration of vasopressors such as terlipressin, which has been shown to be an effective treatment by the CONFIRM study, a 2021 phase 3 trial. However, these patients did not have significant improvement in 90-day mortality.[17] Therefore, although renal function may be preserved, these patients often succumb to other complications of cirrhosis, requiring liver transplant evaluation. Although terlipressin and administration of other effective vasopressors (ie, norepinephrine) generally require monitoring in the intensive care unit, treatment with octreotide, midodrine, and albumin has demonstrated potential beneficial effects in patients with type 1 HRS not being managed in an intensive care setting.[18] Although it is a common cause of AKI in cirrhotic patients, the criteria used for HRS diagnosis often underestimate the true prevalence and severity of HRS as cirrhotic patients often have sarcopenia with lower muscle mass, and therefore, low baseline serum creatinine values that do not accurately reflect renal function. These factors should be taken into consideration and clinicians should be vigilant to identify early HRS with close monitoring of renal function in hospitalized patients with cirrhosis.

NOVEL MODALITIES FOR THE ASSESSMENT OF UNDERLYING RENAL FUNCTION AMONG CIRRHOTICS

Serum creatinine can be an elusive marker for accurately assessing renal function in all patients with cirrhosis. Although it depends on the etiology of cirrhosis and progression of disease, serum creatinine levels can be decreased in the setting of sarcopenia and impaired synthetic function. This phenomenon can lead to an overestimation of GFR.[19] Furthermore, creatinine assays can potentially be impaired in the presence of elevated bilirubin, which is frequently observed among patients with cirrhosis.[19] Noninvasive means of predicting renal dysfunction through calculation of resistive index by renal ultrasound with doppler has also been studied; in fact, patients with normal serum creatinine pretransplant with resistive index greater than 0.7 are at high risk for posttransplant renal dysfunction and need for hemodialysis.[14,20]

Novel biomarkers reflective of more accurate calculation of renal function have recently been described. Cystatin C is a low molecular weight protein not altered by muscle mass, gender, or bilirubin has become a useful addition to serum creatinine in accurately determining GFR.[21] A combination of serum creatinine and cystatin C is more accurate in determining GFR than serum creatinine alone.[22] Cystatin C is also less cumbersome than measuring the clearance of inulin or iohexol, which are gold-standard methods of assessing GFR.[23] Finally, a recent systematic review and meta-analysis validated the overestimation of GFR using serum creatinine, and while cystatin C did not overestimate GFR, it demonstrated an overestimation in the setting of ascites or renal dysfunction.[24]

Another novel biomarker is urinary neutrophil gelatinase-associated lipocalin (uNGAL). uNGAL has been demonstrated to accurately aid in the diagnosis of renal dysfunction, most notably type I HRS, among cirrhotics. One study found that uNGAL was significantly increased among type I HRS as compared with ATN, CKD, and pre-renal azotemia.[25] Although, it is suggested that urinary tract infections be ruled out first before interpreting these results because this can increase uNGAL excretion. Other studies have validated that uNGAL levels are lower among patients with prerenal AKI or azotemia, and seemingly the most elevated in ATN, however, there can be over-lap among these clinical scenarios.[26,27] Overall, uNGAL and cystatin C have proven to be powerful tools in the assessment of renal dysfunction among patients with cirrhosis, especially for type I HRS.[28]

EVALUATING CIRRHOTIC PATIENTS WITH RENAL DYSFUNCTION FOR SLKT

Several studies including reports based on Organ Procurement and Transplantation Network (OPTN) data suggest a survival benefit from simultaneous liver-kidney trans-plantation (SLKT).[29] The controversy surrounding SLKT is driven by scarcity of organs and potential unwanted kidney transplantation in patients who may recover their renal function. Since the introduction of the model for end-stage disease (MELD) score in 2002, there has been an increased use of SLKT. Although there is little controversy with regards to the current allocation policy for SLKT among patients with end-stage renal disease (ESRD) with cirrhosis and among patients with cirrhosis and chronic kidney dis-ease the policy remains controversial among patients with cirrhosis and AKI, mainly because of the inability to accurately differentiate the cause of AKI, especially HRS versus intrarenal etiology. There is immense interest in the utility of urine biomarkers of tubular injury and/or clinical models to accurately stratify AKI etiology and to predict renal recov-ery after LT as the basis to best utilize the scarce donor kidney pool.

Patients with NASH-related cirrhosis are at increased risk for renal failure. Singal and colleagues found an increase in SLKT among NASH patients, which increased from 6.3% in 2002 to 2003 to 19.2% in 2010 to 2011.[30] They further observed a higher incidence of kidney graft loss among the NASH patients as compared with other eti-ologies of liver disease. Satapathy and colleagues have shown that LT recipients with more preserved renal function had lower mortality risk but similar liver allograft loss risk after transplantation; however, SLKT recipients had similar mortality and liver allo-graft loss risk but superior kidney transplant-free survival compared with recipients with severe renal dysfunction independent of demographics, comorbidities, and donor-related data.[31] Yu and colleagues have examined the impact of pre-LT obesity on SLK outcomes using the OPTN registry from October 1987 to June 2016, the au-thors identified 7205 SLK transplants and divided them into groups based on their body mass index (BMI).[32] Of these, 1677 patients were overweight/obese (OW, BMI 30–39 kg/m^2) and 183 were morbidly obese (MO, BMI $\geq$40 kg/m^2). Twenty-nine percent of patients had NASH in the MO group versus 16.4% and 4.7% in the OW and normal weight (NW) groups, respectively. The 1-, 3-, and 5-year overall patient survival, in addition to kidney and liver graft survival were comparable between the 3 groups. Multivariate analysis identified donor age, diabetes mellitus, and delayed kidney transplant function as risk factors for poor patient and both liver and kidney graft survival.[32] These studies highlight that consideration should be given to the inherent disease process for each patient, as this may specifically impact posttrans-plant outcomes.

INTRAOPERATIVE CARE IN PATIENTS WITH RENAL DYSFUNCTION

LT for patients with renal dysfunction is frequently complicated by major fluid shifts, acidosis, and electrolyte and coagulation abnormalities. Nadim and colleagues have shown outcomes of intraoperative hemodialysis as compared to continuous renal replacement therapy (RRT) in dialysis-free outcomes post-LT.[33] The 90-day patient and dialysis-free survival rates were 90% and 99%, respectively. One-year patient survival rates based on the pretransplant renal replacement status as compared to the MELD status were not statistically different. In another study, Zimmerman and colleagues compared 3 groups of patients: patients with pre-LT renal dysfunction who underwent intraoperative RRT (78%), patients with pre-LT renal dysfunction who did not receive intraoperative RRT (88%), and patients without evidence of pre-transplant renal dysfunction.[34] In this study, similar postoperative survival was demonstrated at 17.7-month follow-up. Baek and colleagues further examined the outcomes of patients with the need for an intraoperative requirement for RRT.[35] Compared with the nondialytic conservative treatment group, the intraoperative continuous RRT group escaped volume overload and unnecessary changes in serum sodium concentration $\geq$10 mmol/L during surgery in addition to superior patient survival, graft survival, recovery of renal function, and postoperative complications.[35]

In addition to evaluating the need for RRT requirement intraoperatively, surgical and anesthesia techniques also play significant roles in preserving renal function in patients undergoing LT. The cava-preserving piggyback (PB) technique involves only partial clamping of inferior vena cava during the anhepatic phase of transplantation may prevent hemodynamic instability as compared to the classic cava replacement (CR).[36,37] In a large retrospective study from China, the utilization of intraoperative venovenous bypass was associated with a significantly lower incidence of posttransplant AKI in patients with compromised pretransplant renal function.[38]

RENAL DYSFUNCTION AND CONSIDERATIONS IN THE PERIOPERATIVE PERIOD

Identifying which patients are at higher risk for renal dysfunction posttransplant can lead to guided management, such as the use of nephrotoxin-sparing immunosuppression regimens, frequent laboratory monitoring, and closer follow-up. Specifically, monitoring of renal function at 1-year posttransplant is highly predictive of long-term renal dysfunction.[39] For instance, 65% of patients 1-year posttransplant with renal dysfunction (defined as GFR <40) continued to have renal dysfunction at the 3-year posttransplant mark; when compared to the entire cohort, only 20% developed a GFR less than 40 at 3-year follow-up posttransplant.[39] Studies also suggest that incidence of renal dysfunction and progression to ESRD will increase as patients continue to live longer due to strict selection of transplant candidates, improved experience in LT, and use of nephrotoxic immunosuppression.[40–42] Lastly, the progression of renal disease in the setting of liver transplant candidacy has led to an increase in simultaneous liver-kidney transplant.[43]

Calcineurin inhibitors (CNIs) such as cyclosporine and tacrolimus are the mainstay for immunosuppressive therapy in addition to the treatment of autoimmune disorders and primary renal diseases.[43] Although inhibition of calcineurin enzymatic activity causes disrupted T-cell signaling and hampering of the immune system, CNIs also promote nephrotoxicity through various mechanisms. For instance, increased vasoconstriction of arterioles with CNI use is accomplished by the activation of the RAAS as well as increased sympathetic tone (through increased norepinephrine release), increased vascular tone (through increased endothelin-1), and decreased vasodilatory production of prostaglandins.[44] Renal dysfunction due to the aforementioned renal vasoconstriction is thought to be dose-dependent and reversible with CNI withdrawal; however, with continued use, hyalinization and tubulointerstitial fibrosis can lead to structural damage and subsequent chronic nephrotoxicity.[45,46] An important predictor for nephrotoxicity from CNIs are serum creatinine and eGFR at 1-year follow-up posttransplant.[39]

There have been several techniques for immunosuppressive therapy with a focus on the underlying renal function, many referred to as renal sparing regimens. Substitution of CNI with mycophenolate mofetil monotherapy has been shown to reduce nephrotoxicity but unfortunately comes with a higher risk of transplant rejection.[5] Other regimens include the initiation of the mechanistic target of rapamycin [mTOR] inhibitor, everolimus, either as monotherapy or in combination with low dose tacrolimus. A meta-analysis studying mTOR inhibitors (ie, sirolimus, everolimus) as a nephroprotective alternative to CNIs included 4 randomized control trials, totaling nearly 900 patients. When everolimus was initiated 4 weeks posttransplant, when compared with controls, significant improvement in renal function was noted 12 months posttransplant. Although a significant increase in infections was noted, no change in biopsy-proven acute rejection was appreciated.[47] No long-term improvement in renal function was observed.

Basiliximab

Basiliximab is a monoclonal antibody and interleukin-2 receptor antagonist. Depending on the individual liver transplant center, basiliximab may be used instead of CNIs for the induction of immunosuppression. Basiliximab is still implemented in conjunction with corticosteroids and mycophenolate mofetil, with CNIs possibly introduced pending improvement of renal function post-LT. This renal sparing immunosuppressive strategy, with basiliximab and delayed introduction of tacrolimus, has been shown to improve renal function and outcomes.[48,49] A recent network meta-analysis has identified a benefit with respect to mortality and graft failure among patients receiving basiliximab for immunosuppression induction; however, this needs to be a focus of future clinical studies.[50] Anti-human T-lymphocyte globulin (ATG) is an alternative to interleukin-2-receptor antagonistic for induction therapy but potentially has higher hematologic and infectious adverse event rates which has been widely reported in renal transplantation literature. However, induction with a lower dose of ATG in patients with pretransplant renal dysfunction is a possible strategy for preserving posttransplant renal function.[57]

Fenoldopam

Fenoldopam, a selective dopamine-1 receptor agonist, has vasodilatory and antihypertensive properties and is useful in treating several conditions, including renovascular hypertension. Its role in preventing renal dysfunction has been extensively studied. In addition to the favorable hemodynamic profile, fenoldopam has also been shown to counteract the vasoconstrictive effects of cyclosporine, a nephrotoxic medication commonly used for post-LT immunosuppression, and therefore, improve creatinine clearance.[51] A meta-analysis of 471 patients (6 trials) showed that fenoldopam treatment in the perioperative period leads to less incidence of AKI in patients receiving major surgery.[52] In patients specifically undergoing LT, the use of fenoldopam lead to significantly lower BUN, serum creatinine, and requirement of furosemide when compared with dopamine.[53]

Atrial Natriuretic Peptide

Atrial natriuretic peptide (ANP) is endogenously released in response to hypervolemia (detected as right atrial stretch). Its diuretic effects at the level of the glomerulus help to neutralize hypervolemia. The use of exogenous ANP in patients undergoing cardiothoracic surgery is well-studied.[54] However, ANP has also been shown to significantly improve creatinine clearance and the need for postoperative hemodialysis in patients undergoing living-donor LT when compared with controls.

Although the diuretic effects of ANP seem to be beneficial in the posttransplant period, their effects in cirrhotic patients not undergoing LT, however, have shown to be harmful, and use of ANP should therefore be reserved to patients in the posttransplant period as an experimental measure.[54]

SUMMARY

The onset of renal dysfunction is a critical event among patients with cirrhosis that portends to a poor prognosis. As patients develop decompensated cirrhosis, the compensatory mechanisms combating decreased effective intra-arterial volume are thwarted. The ensuing activation of the RAAS creates further sodium reabsorption, water retention, and vasoconstriction that eventually leads to HRS. However, it is important to note that several other clinical conditions must be ruled out before diagnosing HRS, including hypovolemia, infection, ATN, intrinsic renal disease, or urinary obstruction. Novel biomarkers, such as cystatin C and uNGAL, may be able to aid in future management strategies, allowing for more accurate and earlier detection of renal failure, and potentially may help distinguish their underlying etiologies. Renal dysfunction in the pretransplant period has significant implications on intraoperative surgical strategy and the need for RRT for the preservation of kidney function during the post-LT period. In addition, the status of the kidney in the pre-LT period also dictates the choice of immunosuppression in the post-LT period with the use of renoprotective immunosuppression regimens. Assessment of the presence and severity of renal dysfunction also helps in stratifying the need for SLKT versus LT alone in this patient population.

CLINICS CARE POINTS

- Differentiating HRS -AKI from other forms of AKI is key to improving survival in decompensated cirrhosis as early institutions of the therapy may lead to potential reversal of the AKI.

- Treatment of HRS-AKI may include octreotide, midodrine, and albumin in the non-ICU setting or vasopressors such as norepinephrine or terlipressin or vasopressin with IV albumin in the ICU setting.

- Immunosuppression modification should be considered in patients with high risk for graft dysfunction in the posttransplant period by including renal sparing regimens such as later introduction of CNIs by using lymphocyte non-depleting monoclonal antibody agents (e.g. Basilixumumab) or lymphocyte depleting (e.g. Anti-thymocyteglobulin) or use of reduced dose of CNIs in combination with mycophenylate mofetil (MMF) and by substituting CNIs with m-TORs when appropriate.

AUTHOR CONTRIBUTIONS

S.K. Satapathy conceptualized the manuscript; R. Heda and A.J. Kovalic wrote the initial draft; and S.K. Satapathy contributed significantly by providing major intellectual inputs and revising the initial draft of the manuscript. All authors then participated in additional intellectual input, critical revision, and approval of the manuscript under supervision of S.K. Satapathy.

DISCLOSURE

The authors have nothing to disclose.

REFERENCES

1. Ginès P, Schrier RW. Renal failure in cirrhosis. N Engl J Med 2009;361(13): 1279–90.
2. Fede G, D'Amico G, Arvaniti V, et al. Renal failure and cirrhosis: a systematic review of mortality and prognosis. J Hepatol 2012;56(4):810–8.
3. Chauhan K, Azzi Y, Faddoul G, et al. Pre-liver transplant renal dysfunction and association with post-transplant end-stage renal disease: a single-center examination of updated UNOS recommendations. Clin Transplant 2018;32(12):e13428.
4. Ojo AO, Held PJ, Port FK, et al. Chronic renal failure after transplantation of a non-renal organ. N Engl J Med 2003;349(10):931–40.
5. Saliba F, Fischer L, de Simone P, et al. Association between renal dysfunction and major adverse cardiac events after liver transplantation: evidence from an international randomized trial of everolimus-based immunosuppression. Ann Transplant 2018;23:751–7.
6. Shenoy S, Hardinger KL, Crippin J, et al. Sirolimus conversion in liver transplant recipients with renal dysfunction: a prospective, randomized, single-center trial. Transplantation 2007;83(10):1389–92.
7. Pawarode A, Fine DM, Thuluvath PJ. Independent risk factors and natural history of renal dysfunction in liver transplant recipients. Liver Transpl 2003;9(7):741–7.
8. Cabezuelo JB, Ramírez P, Ríos A, et al. Risk factors of acute renal failure after liver transplantation. Kidney Int 2006;69(6):1073–80.
9. Wong F, Nadim MK, Kellum JA, et al. Working party proposal for a revised classification system of renal dysfunction in patients with cirrhosis. Gut 2011;60(5): 702–9.
10. Gleisner AL, Jung H, Lentine KL, et al. Renal dysfunction in liver transplant candidates: evaluation, classification and management in contemporary practice. J Nephrol Ther 2012;(Suppl 4). https://doi.org/10.4172/2161-0959.S4-006. SI Kidney Transplantation.
11. Hampel H, Bynum GD, Zamora E, et al. Risk factors for the development of renal dysfunction in hospitalized patients with cirrhosis. Am J Gastroenterol 2001;96(7): 2206–10.
12. Martín-Llahí M, Guevara M, Torre A, et al. Prognostic importance of the cause of renal failure in patients with cirrhosis. Gastroenterology 2011;140(2):488–96.e4.
13. Moore KP, Wong F, Gines P, et al. The management of ascites in cirrhosis: report on the consensus conference of the International Ascites Club. Hepatol 2003; 38(1):258–66.
14. Platt JF, Ellis JH, Rubin JM, et al. Renal duplex Doppler ultrasonography: a noninvasive predictor of kidney dysfunction and hepatorenal failure in liver disease. Hepatology 1994;20(2):362–9.
15. Fernández J, Navasa M, Garcia-Pagan JC, et al. Effect of intravenous albumin on systemic and hepatic hemodynamics and vasoactive neurohormonal systems in patients with cirrhosis and spontaneous bacterial peritonitis. J Hepatol 2004; 41(3):384–90.

16. Salerno F, Gerbes A, Ginès P, et al. Diagnosis, prevention and treatment of hepatorenal syndrome in cirrhosis. Postgrad Med J 2008;84(998):662–70.
17. Wong F, Pappas SC, Curry MP, et al. Terlipressin plus albumin for the treatment of type 1 hepatorenal syndrome. N Engl J Med 2021;384(9):818–28.
18. Skagen C, Einstein M, Lucey MR, et al. Combination treatment with octreotide, midodrine, and albumin improves survival in patients with type 1 and type 2 hepatorenal syndrome. J Clin Gastroenterol 2009;43(7):680–5.
19. Heda R, Yazawa M, Shi M, et al. Non-alcoholic fatty liver and chronic kidney disease: retrospect, introspect, and prospect. World J Gastroenterol 2021;27(17): 1864–82.
20. Platt JF, Marn CS, Baliga PK, et al. Renal dysfunction in hepatic disease: early identification with renal duplex Doppler US in patients who undergo liver transplantation. Radiology 1992;183(3):801–6.
21. Gerbes AL, Gülberg V, Bilzer M, et al. Evaluation of serum cystatin C concentration as a marker of renal function in patients with cirrhosis of the liver. Gut 2002; 50(1):106–10.
22. Mindikoglu AL, Dowling TC, Weir MR, et al. Performance of chronic kidney disease epidemiology collaboration creatinine-cystatin C equation for estimating kidney function in cirrhosis. Hepatol 2014;59(4):1532–42.
23. Sampaio MS, Martin P, Bunnapradist S. Renal dysfunction in end-stage liver disease and post-liver transplant. Clin Liver Dis 2014;18(3):543–60.
24. Singapura P, Ma TW, Sarmast N, et al. Estimating glomerular filtration rate in cirrhosis using creatinine-based and cystatin C-based equations: systematic review and meta-analysis. Liver Transpl 2021;27:1538–52.
25. Fagundes C, Pépin MN, Guevara M, et al. Urinary neutrophil gelatinase-associated lipocalin as biomarker in the differential diagnosis of impairment of kidney function in cirrhosis. J Hepatol 2012;57(2):267–73.
26. Verna EC, Brown RS, Farrand E, et al. Urinary neutrophil gelatinase-associated lipocalin predicts mortality and identifies acute kidney injury in cirrhosis. Dig Dis Sci 2012;57(9):2362–70.
27. Belcher JM, Sanyal AJ, Peixoto AJ, et al. Kidney biomarkers and differential diagnosis of patients with cirrhosis and acute kidney injury. Hepatol Aug 2014;60(2): 622–32.
28. Gomaa SH, Shamseya MM, Madkour MA. Clinical utility of urinary neutrophil gelatinase-associated lipocalin and serum cystatin C in a cohort of liver cirrhosis patients with renal dysfunction: a challenge in the diagnosis of hepatorenal syndrome. Eur J Gastroenterol Hepatol 2019;31(6):692–702.
29. Singal AK, Ong S, Satapathy SK, et al. Simultaneous liver kidney transplantation. Transplant Int 2019;32(4):343–52.
30. Singal AK, Hasanin M, Kaif M, et al. Nonalcoholic steatohepatitis is the most rapidly growing indication for simultaneous liver kidney transplantation in the United States. Transplant 2016;100(3):607–12.
31. Molnar MZ, Joglekar K, Jiang Y, et al. Association of pretransplant renal function with liver graft and patient survival after liver transplantation in patients with nonalcoholic steatohepatitis. Liver Transplant 2019;25(3):399–410.
32. Yu JW, Gupta G, Kang L, et al. Obesity does not significantly impact outcomes following simultaneous liver kidney transplantation: review of the UNOS database - a retrospective study. Transplant Int 2019;32(2):206–17.
33. Nadim MK, Annanthapanyasut W, Matsuoka L, et al. Intraoperative hemodialysis during liver transplantation: a decade of experience. Liver Transplant 2014;20(7): 756–64.

34. Zimmerman MA, Selim M, Kim J, et al. Outcome analysis of continuous intraoperative renal replacement therapy in the highest acuity liver transplant recipients: a single-center experience. Surgery 2017;161(5):1279–86.

35. Baek SD, Jang M, Kim W, et al. Benefits of intraoperative continuous renal replacement therapy during liver transplantation in patients with renal dysfunction. Transplant Proc 2017;49(6):1344–50.

36. Cabezuelo JB, Ramirez P, Acosta F, et al. Does the standard vs piggyback surgical technique affect the development of early acute renal failure after orthotopic liver transplantation? Transplant Proc 2003;35(5):1913–4.

37. Barbas AS, Levy J, Mulvihill MS, et al. Liver transplantation without venovenous bypass: does surgical approach matter? Transplant Direct 2018;4(5):e348.

38. Sun K, Hong F, Wang Y, et al. Venovenous bypass is associated with a lower incidence of acute kidney injury after liver transplantation in patients with compromised pretransplant renal function. Anesth Analg 2017;125(5):1463–70.

39. Cohen AJ, Stegall MD, Rosen CB, et al. Chronic renal dysfunction late after liver transplantation. Liver Transpl 2002;8(10):916–21.

40. Fisher NC, Nightingale PG, Gunson BK, et al. Chronic renal failure following liver transplantation: a retrospective analysis. Transplantation 1998;66(1):59–66.

41. Gonwa TA, Mai ML, Melton LB, et al. End-stage renal disease (ESRD) after orthotopic liver transplantation (OLTX) using calcineurin-based immunotherapy: risk of development and treatment. Transplantation 2001;72(12):1934–9.

42. Lynn M, Abreo K, Zibari G, et al. End-stage renal disease in liver transplants. Clin Transplant 2001;15(Suppl 6):66–9.

43. Davis CL, Gonwa TA, Wilkinson AH. Pathophysiology of renal disease associated with liver disorders: implications for liver transplantation. Part I. Liver Transplant 2002;8(2):91–109.

44. Campistol JM, Sacks SH. Mechanisms of nephrotoxicity. Transplantation 2000; 69(12 Suppl):Ss5–10.

45. Olyaei AJ, de Mattos AM, Bennett WM. Immunosuppressant-induced nephropathy: pathophysiology, incidence and management. Drug Saf 1999;21(6):471–88.

46. Ong AC, Fine LG. Loss of glomerular function and tubulointerstitial fibrosis: cause or effect? Kidney Int 1994;45(2):345–51.

47. Lin M, Mittal S, Sahebjam F, et al. Everolimus with early withdrawal or reduced-dose calcineurin inhibitors improves renal function in liver transplant recipients: a systematic review and meta-analysis. Clin Transplant 2017;31(2). https://doi.org/10.1111/ctr.12872.

48. Lange NW, Salerno DM, Sammons CM, et al. Delayed calcineurin inhibitor introduction and renal outcomes in liver transplant recipients receiving basiliximab induction. Clin Transplant 2018;32(12):e13415.

49. Boyd A, Brown A, Patel J, et al. Basiliximab with delayed tacrolimus improves short-term renal outcomes post-liver transplantation-a real-world experience. Transplant Proc 2021;53(5):1541–7.

50. Best LM, Leung J, Freeman SC, et al. Induction immunosuppression in adults undergoing liver transplantation: a network meta-analysis. Cochrane Database Syst Rev 2020;1(1):Cd013203.

51. Biancofiore G, Della Rocca G, Bindi L, et al. Use of fenoldopam to control renal dysfunction early after liver transplantation. Liver Transplant 2004;10(8):986–92.

52. Gillies MA, Kakar V, Parker RJ, et al. Fenoldopam to prevent acute kidney injury after major surgery-a systematic review and meta-analysis. Crit Care 2015; 19:449.

53. Rocca GD, Pompei L, Costa MG, et al. Fenoldopam mesylate and renal function in patients undergoing liver transplantation: a randomized, controlled pilot trial. Anesth Analg 2004;99(6):1604–9.
54. Swärd K, Valsson F, Odencrants P, et al. Recombinant human atrial natriuretic peptide in ischemic acute renal failure: a randomized placebo-controlled trial. Crit Care Med 2004;32(6):1310–5.
55. Köttgen A, Selvin E, Stevens LA, et al. Serum cystatin C in the United States: the third national health and nutrition examination survey (NHANES III). Am J Kidney Dis 2008;51(3):385–94.
57. Dopazo, C., Charco, R., Caralt, M., Pando, E., Lázaro, J. L., Gómez-Gavara, C., Castells, L., & Bilbao, I. (2018). Low Total Dose of Anti-Human T-Lymphocyte Globulin (ATG) Guarantees a Good Glomerular Filtration Rate after Liver Transplant in Recipients with Pretransplant Renal Dysfunction. *Can J Gastroenterol Hepatol 2018*.

Pros and Cons of the Safety Net Rule for Prioritization of Liver Transplant Recipients Who Receive Liver Alone Transplant but Develop End-Stage Renal Disease

Mark W. Russo, MD, MPH[a],*, Vincent Casingal, MD[b]

KEYWORDS

- Kidney • Cirrhosis • Candidate • Criteria • Equity

KEY POINTS

- The number of liver transplant candidates presenting with end-stage renal disease (ESRD) is increasing partly because MELD-sodium score includes creatinine.
- In August 2017, standardized criteria for simultaneous liver-kidney transplant (SLKT) were implemented and includes a safety net rule for liver transplant alone (LTA) recipients who do not meet criteria for SLKT but do not recover renal function 60 to 365 days after liver transplant.
- A benefit of the safety net rule is that it provides a priority allocation pathway for kidney transplant for LTA recipients with ESRD that did not qualify for SLKT and do not recover renal function.
- A risk of the safety net pathway is that LTA recipients who develop ESRD are at high risk for morbidity and mortality and may become too sick while waiting for kidney transplant.

INTRODUCTION

Before 2002, fewer patients underwent simultaneous liver-kidney transplant (SLKT) because unlike MELD, UNOS criteria did not incorporate creatinine into organ allocation. During 2000, 135 candidates underwent SLKT.[1] After the introduction of MELD in 2002 followed by MELD-sodium for liver allocation, the number of SLKTs increased to 730 in 2016 or more than a 5-fold increase.[1] In addition to the transition to MELD score

a Division of Hepatology, Atrium Health Wake Forest Baptist, Atrium Health-Carolinas Medical Center, 6th Floor MMP 1025 Morehead Medical Drive, Charlotte, NC 28204, USA; b Transplant Surgery, Atrium Health Wake Forest Baptist, Atrium Health-Carolinas Medical Center, 6th Floor MMP 1025 Morehead Medical Drive, Charlotte, NC 28204, USA
* Corresponding author.
E-mail address: mark.russo@atriumhealth.org

Clin Liver Dis 26 (2022) 269–281
https://doi.org/10.1016/j.cld.2022.01.005
liver.theclinics.com
1089-3261/22/© 2022 Elsevier Inc. All rights reserved.

for organ allocation, other potential factors that may be associated with the increase in SLKTs are the increasing prevalence of comorbidities associated with kidney disease, such as diabetes as well as variability in patient selection for SLKT among transplant centers with the proportion of patients undergoing SLKT ranging from 0% to 43.7%.[2] Some transplant centers may have had a lower threshold to perform SLKT because there was not an established priority allocation pathway for kidney transplant for LTA recipients who developed ESRD.

SAFETY NET RULE

Before the implementation of the SLKT and safety net policies in 2017, the decision to perform SLKT was largely left up to the discretion of the transplant center.[3] Centers may have had a lower threshold to perform SLKT in candidates with renal injury because morbidity and mortality are high in liver transplant recipients on dialysis and average waitlist time for a liver transplant recipient awaiting kidney transplant was 470 days .[4,5] A lower threshold to perform SLKT may have been due to the lack of a policy to rescue LTA recipients who did not recover renal function. A consequence of lack of a safety net rule was that 40% of SLKTs were performed in patients who were not on dialysis with pretransplant creatinine less than 2.5 mg/dL and some of these patients may have had recovery of renal function with LTA.[6]

A result of unregulated kidney allocation to SLKT recipients is that organ availability would decrease and waiting times would increase for candidates awaiting kidney transplant alone (KTA). Furthermore, as mentioned, some SLKT recipients may have had recovery of renal function after LTA. To address the concern for lack of prioritization for kidney transplant in LTA recipients who develop kidney failure, criteria were developed for kidney transplant after liver transplant (KALT) that increased priority for KALT, referred to as the 'safety net' rule (**Box 1**). The SLKT policy and safety net rule are intimately connected and will be discussed in this context. In this article, the pros and cons of the safety net policy for LTA recipients who do not recover renal function are debated.

PROS
Not all Liver Transplant Candidates with Kidney Injury Need a Kidney Transplant

Before implementation of defined SLKT eligibility, any patient could be listed for an SLKT without constraints. The rate of listing for SLKT was increasing and given the severe organ shortage, the transplant community advocated for a standardized approach. Although most agreed that end-stage liver disease (ESLD) patients with end-stage renal disease (ESRD) or longstanding chronic kidney disease (CKD) met criteria, there were many patients with acute kidney injury that could recover renal

---

Box. 1
Kidney after liver transplant "safety net" criteria

Liver transplant recipient receives priority for kidney transplant if the following criteria are met:
- The candidate is registered on the kidney waiting list before the 1-year anniversary of the most recent liver transplant
- The candidate is at least 60 days but not more than 365 days for the liver transplant date

And one of the following criteria is met:
- Candidate's calculated creatinine clearance or glomerular filtration rate (GFR) ≤20 mL/min
- Candidate is on dialysis

function after LTA.[5] Recipient age, pretransplant hemodialysis, elevated serum creatinine, hepatitis C, and diabetes mellitus are risk factors for the development of ESRD after liver transplant,[7] but many of these patients recover renal function. For those who do not recover renal function after LTA, the safety net provides increased priority for KALT. Waitlist mortality for LTA recipients awaiting kidney transplant is not compromised.[8] Thus, despite the risk of prolonged renal failure after LTA, the safety net rule provides priority for kidney transplant without placing the recipient at undo risk for waitlist mortality (**Box 2**).

Equity and Utility

As of August 2021, there were over 90,000 patients waiting for a kidney transplant, and 11,000 waiting for a liver transplant.[1] In 2016, 19,060 KTA were performed and 730 SLKTs were performed or 3.8% of kidney transplants were performed as SLKTs.[1] Kidneys were transplanted in SLKT recipients instead of KTA candidates and some of the SLKT recipients may have recovered renal function. Thus, a policy addressing equity and utility was needed because KTA candidates could have derived greater benefits.

Equity, equal opportunity, and access to organ transplant should also be considered when allocating kidneys.[8–10] The safety net policy addresses the equity and utility of kidney transplantation (**Table 1; Box.3**). Although individuals awaiting liver transplant are allocated organs based on medical urgency (MELD-Na score), kidney transplant candidates derive their allocation points from matching and waiting time or time on dialysis. The current wait times are typically much longer for KTA candidates than LTA candidates. Although kidney and liver transplant candidates are difficult to compare as it relates to medical urgency, *equity* should be considered as it relates to access to organs. In an ideal setting, a kidney would be available for a liver transplant candidate with renal failure; however, in reality, kidney transplant candidates may be disadvantaged if SLKTs are prioritized over KTA.

The difference in equity between KTA and SLKT was magnified when evaluating allocation of kidneys before 2017 SLKT and safety net rules. Compared with SLKT recipients, KTA recipients were more likely to receive a lower quality kidney graft, as measured by kidney donor profile index (KDPI). Before 2017, SLKTs were allocated regardless of KDPI, and therefore SLKT recipients had greater access to "younger" organs. In multiorgan transplant, the average KDPI ranges from 18% to 36% compared with 46% for KTA recipients.[6,8] This disparity was addressed in the safety net policy that preserved access, while allowing lower KDPI kidneys to be allocated to pediatric, low estimated posttransplant survival (EPTS) score, and other multiorgan candidates (**Fig. 1**). The KALT safety net rule allows for more stringent criteria to be applied for SLKT, while improving equity.

An important component of the SLKT and safety net policies is to incorporate utility or medical benefit and avoid unnecessary or futile kidney transplants. Before

---

Box. 2
Pros of the safety net rules

Allows for standardized criteria for SLKT while providing a priority pathway for LTA recipients who do not recover adequate renal function

Addresses equity and utility of kidney allocation

Reduces the number of unnecessary kidney transplants

Survival outcomes postpolicy implementation similar to prepolicy implementation

Table 1
Ethical issues in transplantation: equity and utility

Equity	Utility
Equal opportunity, imminently lifesaving, first come first served.	*Nonmaleficence*—medical benefit, quality of benefit, avoiding futile transplants
SLKT patients tend to be sicker, despite similar degree of single organ dysfunction SLKT vs KTA (medical urgency)	The degree of medical benefit tends to be less for 1 recipient vs 2 recipients.
Higher quality organs used in multiorgan transplant remove limits access for single organ transplant	SLKT patients tend to benefit from the most "immediate" life-saving measures associated with LTA.
When a multiorgan transplant patient receives an organ that is "beneficial, but not required"—takes that organ from a single organ transplant, who loses that opportunity.	*Beneficence*—maximize the net overall benefit to the transplant community as a whole is increased when organs are allocated only as needed, and without futility

implementation of the policy, there was reason to believe that a sizable number of SLKT recipients would have recovered renal function had they undergone LTA. In fact, in 95% of LTA recipients who met SLKT criteria, the mean estimated glomerular filtratation rate (eGFR) increased from 23 mL/min preoperatively to 48 mL/min 1-year post-LTA.[11] The current policies, although more restrictive for SLKT, reduce the number of futile kidney transplants while allowing for a priority allocation pathway for LTA recipients who do not have return of kidney function.

Other approaches to address utility for kidney allocation are to estimate life-years gained after organ transplantation as a metric or EPTS score.[12] A candidate's EPTS score represents the percentage of kidney candidates in the nation with a longer expected posttransplant survival time EPTS score is based on: (1) candidate time on dialysis, (2) current diagnosis of diabetes, (3) history of any prior solid organ transplant, and (4) candidate's age. Patients receiving a kidney under the safety net will be eligible for allocation sequence B, C, and D (KDPI>20%). This compromise is a balance of equity and utility, preserving KDPI less than 20% for pediatric patients, and those with an EPTS score less than 20%. The safety net policy optimizes utility by improving access of the kidney donor pool to patients with the potential to achieve the longest survival.

Excellent Survival After Implementation of the Safety Net Policy

A risk of patients with chronic renal failure undergoing LTA is increased morbidity and mortality associated with renal failure and subsequent poor outcomes after KALT. On average, 5% of liver transplant recipients are placed on chronic dialysis, placed on the kidney transplant waiting list, or received a living donor kidney transplant within a year

Box. 3
Cons to KALT safety net rule

Morbidity and mortality in liver transplant recipients on dialysis

Lack of data on long-term kidney graft survival compared with SLKT

Lack of immunologic protection

Potential for racial, ethnic, and gender disparities

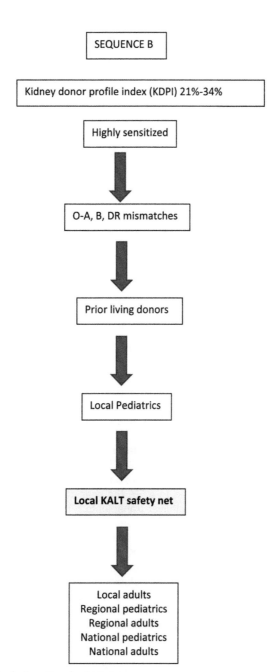

Fig. 1. Sequence of allocation for kidneys.

of transplant.[11] Although there has been an increase in patients on hemodialysis listed for LTA in the safety net era, there is no difference in posttransplant survival compared to patients not on hemodialysis.[13–15] Patients who receive a KALT have similar patient and graft survival as patients receiving KTA (**Fig. 2**).[13] One-year survival is similar between LTA and safety net recipients (93.4% and 96.4%, respectively, $P = .234$).[14]

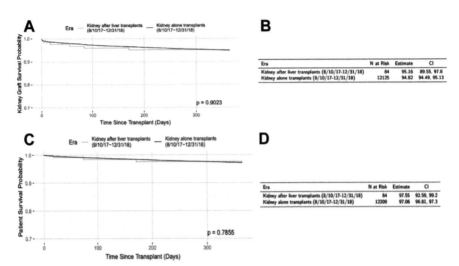

Fig. 2. (*A*) Graft survival for kidney after liver transplant and kidney alone transplants. (*B*) Probabilify of graft survival for kidney after liver transplant and kidney alone transplants. (*C*) Patient survival for kidney after liver transplant and kidney alone transplants. (*D*) Probability of patient survival for kidney after liver transplant and kidney alone transplant.

These data support the notion that the safety net rule does not compromise outcomes in KALT recipients.

As liver transplant is a sensitizing event, both from an organ and blood transfusion perspective, there is concern that many patients will have limited access to safety net organs. In those patients listed for KALT, the median CPRA = 0%, and a third of patients listed were transplanted within 6 months suggesting that LTA and associated blood products are not sensitizing events.[14]

Implementation of the SLKT policy and safety net rules was intended to provide equity for the availability of kidneys between SLKT and KTA candidates resulting in a decrease in SLKTs. Before the policies, SLKTs comprised 5.5% of all deceased donor kidney transplants and this declined to 4.5% the year after implementation.[4] SLKTs declined from 10.2% to 9.0% of all liver transplants.[4] These data support that the goal of the safety net rule to reduce SLKTs was initially achieved.

Although the number of SLKTs initially started to decrease after SLKT and safety net rules were implemented, the number of SLKTs subsequently increased. A factor to consider is the evolving behavior of transplant center listing practices and the changing landscape of patient characteristics, including an increase in age and comorbid conditions of those listed for SLKT.[15] Patients who otherwise may have been too old or too sick for SLKT several years ago may now be considered suitable candidates. This evolution is a success of proper patient selection and advancement in perioperative care and not a failure of the safety net rule. Despite more SLKTs in older patients and those with more comorbidities, fewer patients with GFR greater than 30 mL/min have undergone SLKT postpolicy (11.8% vs 8.8%).[16]

CONS
The Safety Net Rule Has Not Reduced SLKTs or Kidney Transplants in Liver Transplant Recipients

The SLKT and KALT policies were anticipated to reduce the number of SLKTs by 19%.[6] Despite an initial decline in SLKTs after policy implementation, the number

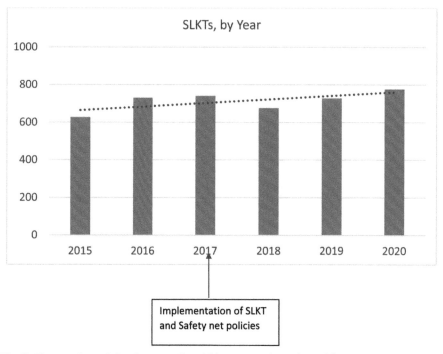

Fig. 3. The number of simultaneous liver kidney transplants (SLKTs) by year.

of SLKTs has increased to above prepolicy numbers (**Fig. 3**). Although the number of SLKTs decreased from 730 in 2016 to 676 SLKTs in 2018 after implementation of the SLKT and KALT policies, the number of SLKTs has increased to 728 in 2019.[1,17,18] In fact, the number of SLKTs is higher postpolicy than prepolicy (see **Fig. 3**). In addition, the number of KALTs increased from an average of 1.4 prepolicy to 7.3 per month postpolicy[17] (**Fig. 4**). Listing for KALT within a year of transplant has increased from 2.9% prepolicy to 8.8% postpolicy and KALTs have increased from 0.7% to 4% per year.[16] Thus, the policy has not maintained the intended goal of reducing the number of SLKTs or KALTs in order to increase organ availability to KTA candidates.

Increased Mortality in Liver Transplant Recipients with Renal Dysfunction

Liver transplant recipients who do not recover renal function have lower survival compared with recipients with preserved renal function.[19,20] LTA recipients with an measured glomerular filtraation rate (mGFR) less than 30 mL/min/1.72 m^2 were associated with a 2.67-fold increased risk of mortality and an mGFR less than 15 mL/min/1.73 m^2 had a 5-fold increased risk of death.[21] LTA recipients have a 77% increased risk of death if they require renal replacement therapy after transplant.[19] One year patient survival was 75% for LTA recipients requiring renal replacement therapy compared with 88% in SLKT recipients.[19] Liver transplant recipients who had a serum creatinine greater than 2.5 mg/dL or underwent dialysis before liver transplant had lower 1-year patient survival compared with the SLKT group (79.5% and 84.5%, respectively, $P < .001$).[22] In a study of liver transplant recipients requiring dialysis, the median time from initiation of dialysis to death was 1.5 years and 1-year mortality was 20% in LTA recipients on chronic dialysis.[20]

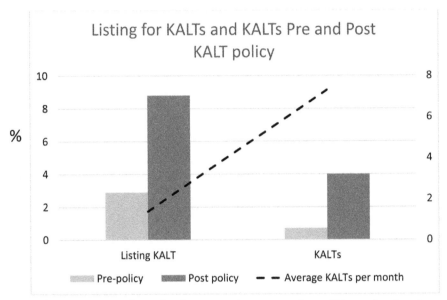

Fig. 4. The number of kidney after liver transplants pre and post kidney after liver transplant (KALT) policy.

The data demonstrate LTA recipients with renal dysfunction have worse outcomes compared with LTA recipients with preserved renal function. Thus, renal failure is associated with significant mortality in LTA recipients, and they may not have the luxury of waiting for KALT.

Although a criticism of the lack of SLKT and safety net criteria was variability among transplant centers in determining eligibility for SLKT, renal recovery in liver transplant recipients may not occur as expected. Renal injury may not be from hepatorenal syndrome and recipients may have intrinsic kidney disease. Liver transplant recipients may have glomerulonephritis, hypertensive nephrosclerosis, tubulointerstitial disease, or early liver allograft dysfunction that causes kidney failure.[23,24]

Under the current criteria, if a liver transplant candidate does not meet the criteria for a kidney transplant, then the candidate undergoes LTA and if renal recovery does not return, the recipient is listed for kidney transplant under the safety net rules. Unlike prepolicy when there was no additional waiting time for a kidney transplant in SLKT candidates while under the safety net policy, the median wait time for KALT in the postpolicy era is 109 days.[25] Unfortunately, waitlist mortality remains high at 15%.[13] Prepolicy SLKT recipients were not exposed to waiting time morbidity and mortality associated with KALT. Candidates who would have previously qualified for SLKT but do not meet the criteria for SLKT postpolicy are exposed to increased morbidity and mortality while waiting for KALT under the safety net rules.

Long Term Outcomes of KALT may be Inferior to SLKT and KTA

Under the safety net rule, long-term survival should be equivalent or better in KALT recipients compared with historical rates in SLKT recipients. Kidney graft survival is lower in KALT recipients compared with KTA and SLKT recipients. Among 368 LTA recipients who underwent KALT within 1 year of transplant, 1-year kidney graft failure was 8.4% compared with 5.3% to 8.9% for SLKT recipients.[26,27] Reasons for better outcomes with SLKT include better donor quality and lower KDPI in SLKT recipients compared with KALT, mean KDPI 38% and 50%, respectively.[28]

The safety net rule may not improve the utility of kidney organs. KALT recipients have worse outcomes than KTA recipients. Results from analysis of the UNOS database from 1988 to 2015 comparing adult KALT recipients to KTA recipients who received a kidney from the same donor (N = 745 one kidney went to KALT and the other kidney to KTA) reported inferior graft survival in the KALT compared with KTA group in the subgroup with KDPI 21% to 85%.[29] KTA recipients with a KDPI 21% to 85% had superior graft survival compared with the KALT group (1-year graft survival 92.3% and 88.9%, respectively, $P = .0068$).[29] In a subgroup analysis, KALT recipients who waited less than 1 year had lower patient and graft survival compared with recipients of KTA who waited more than 1 year. The safety net policy shifts more patients to KALT, and because outcomes are inferior in KALT compared with KTA, utility is compromised postsafety net rules.

An important con to current policy of KALT is that there is a greater decline in GFR and graft loss with KALT compared with SLKT.[30] The apparent decline in kidney function and graft loss may be partly attributed to an increase in subclinical inflammation and cellular alloreactivity in the KALT group compared with the SLKT group. A proposed mechanism for the preservation of GFR and reduced graft loss seen with SLKT is that cellular alloreactivity against the kidney is less common in SLKT.[30] This is attributed to early infiltration of the liver by dendritic cell precursors and T cells that are associated with a decreased incidence of kidney allograft rejection. Liver antigen-presenting cells are inferior stimulators of effectors T cells.[30–32]

Immunologic Disadvantages of KALT versus SLKT

SLKT confers immune protection from rejection of the renal allograft that does not occur with KALT. Proposed mechanisms for immunoprotection include neutralization of existing alloantibodies and cytotoxic T lymphocytes in the systemic circulation and removal of preformed lymphocytotoxic antibodies by the transplanted liver.[33–36] Data that support clearance of preformed antibodies by the liver after SLKT is demonstrated in patients who have a positive crossmatch before SLKT and have a negative crossmatch after SLKT.[34] Other proposed mechanisms associated with SLKT include hematopoietic chimerism and the production of HLA-G molecules with tolerogenic properties.[34]

KALT is not associated with the same immunologic advantages of SLKT, especially in patients with high levels of donor-specific antibodies (DSAs), and long-term graft survival is lower with KALT. Although 1-year kidney graft survival is similar in SLKT and early KALT (30–365 days of LT) recipients, 5- and 10-year censored kidney transplant survival is lower in early KALT compared with SLKT recipients (81% and 49% and 90% and 83%, respectively).[28] The improved long-term graft survival in the SLKT group compared with the KALT group can be partly attributed to immunoprotection by the liver graft.

Recipients of SLKT are protected against decline in renal function and acute or chronic rejection compared with KTA recipients. In a study of SLKT and KTA recipients with high levels of DSAs (>2000 mean fluorescence intensity) at the time of transplant and 5 years after transplant, mean GFR was stable in the SLKT group but declined by 44% in the KTA group.[30] More recipients in the KTA group reached a combined clinical endpoint of graft failure and decline in kidney function. In patients who were DSA+, antibody-mediated rejection was also lower in the SLKT

DSA+ group compared with the KTA DSA+ group (7.1% and 46.4%, respectively).[30] Furthermore, no SLKT recipient developed histologic findings of chronic glomerulopathy compared to KTA DSA+ recipients who developed chronic glomerulopathy in 37% and 53.6% of recipients 2 and 5 years posttransplant, respectively (P = .01 for both time points). Outcomes for SLKT DSA- and KTA DSA-recipients were similar except the mean eGFR declined by 15% in the KTA DSA-group but remained stable in the SLK DSA-group (P = .002). In multivariable analysis, SLKT was associated with an 89% reduction in antibody-mediated rejection or chronic transplant glomerulopathy (odds ratio [OR] = 0.11 95% confidence interval [CI] 0.03–0.32, P = .0002), T-cell mediated rejection or subclinical inflammation (OR = 0.13 95% CI 0.06–0.27, P < .0001), and decline in kidney graft function (OR = 0.22, 95% CI 0.06–0.59, P < .0001).[30]

Disparities in KALT Safety Net Rule

Although no significant differences were seen in the proportion of SLKTs between African-Americans, Hispanics, and Whites prepolicy and postpolicy, Hispanic patients were sicker and had higher median MELD scores at SLKT.[4,36] A lower proportion of early KALTs occurred in African-Americans relative to SLKTs (7% vs 16%; P = .04).[28] The proportion of SLKT recipients who were Black before and after policy implementation was 15.3% and 14.3%, respectively, and although this difference was not statistically significant, longer follow-up is needed to determine if a downward trend continues.[4] Gender disparities exist as well. The proportion of female KAL registrations and KALTs was lower in women compared with men (41% and 34% versus 59% and 65%, respectively).[13]

Limitations of Studies Demonstrating a Benefit of KALT Safety Net Policy

Studies comparing outcomes in transplant recipients, SLKT, KALT, KTA, before and after implementation of OPTN policy in 2017 have not captured important outcomes, such as mortality in LTA recipients who are not listed for KALT because they become too sick. To fully capture risks associated with the safety net policy, the mortality rate needs to be captured for LTA recipients who prepolicy would have undergone SLKT, but postpolicy develop ESRD that qualify for the safety net but are not listed because they are too sick. There are limited data on outcomes in LTA recipients who develop rapid kidney dysfunction early posttransplant, before 60 days, but are not subsequently listed for a kidney transplant. Also, morbidity, quality of life, and costs in the KALT group have not been reported in studies. Organ acquisition is costly and KALT is associated with higher charges compared with SLKT[37] (Table 2).

Table 2 Charges associated with organ procurement	
	Procurement ($)
Liver Transplant	104,200
Kidney Transplant	113,900
Liver Kidney Transplant	187,000
Kidney After Liver Transplant	218,000

https://milliman-cdn.azureedge.net/-/media/milliman/pdfs/articles/2020-us-organ-tissue-transplants.ashx

DISCLOSURE

The authors have nothing to disclose.

CLINICS CARE POINTS

- The safety net rule for KALT allows a pathway for prioritization of LTA recipients for KALT who previously may have undergone SLKT.
- After implementation of the SLKT criteria and safety net rule, initially fewer SLKTs were performed, and patient and graft survival were similar before and after implementation.
- Long-term patient and graft survival will need to be monitored to determine if KALT is associated with similar graft survival to SLKT because of the immunoprotective effect the liver has on the kidney graft after SLKT.

REFERENCES

1. Available at: https://optn.transplant.hrsa.gov/data/view-data-reports/national-data/#. Accessed August 5, 2021.
2. Eason JD, Gonwa TA, Davis CL, et al. Proceedings of consensus conference on simultaneous liver kidney transplantation (SLK). Am J Transplant 2008;8: 2243–51.
3. Luo X, Massie AB, Haugen CE, et al. Baseline and center-level variation in simultaneous liver- kidney listing in the United States. Transplantation 2018;102:609.
4. Altshuler PJ, Shah AP, Frank AM, et al. Simultaneous liver kidney allocation policy and the safety net: an early examination of utilization and outcomes in the United States. Transpl Int 2021;34:1052–64.
5. Hughes DL, Sharma P. Simultaneous liver-kidney transplant following standardized medical eligibility criteria and creation of the safety net: less appears to be more. Liver Transpl 2021;27(8):1089–91. https://doi.org/10.1002/lt.26182.
6. Formica RN Jr. Simultaneous liver-kidney allocation: let's not make perfect the enemy of good. Am J Transplant 2016;16:2765.
7. Israni AK, Xiong H, Liu J, et al. Predicting end-stage renal disease after liver transplant. Am J Transplant 2012;13:782–92.
8. Nagai S, Suzuki Y, Kitajima T, et al. Paradigm change in liver transplant practice after the implementation of the liver-kidney allocation policy. Liver Transplant 2021;27(11):1563–76. https://doi.org/10.1002/LT.26107.
9. Available at: https://optn.transplant.hrsa.gov/media/2500/ethics_whitepaper_201806.pdf. Accessed July 22, 2021.
10. Available at: https://optn.transplant.hrsa.gov/media/2801/ethics_publiccomment_20190122.pdf. Accessed August 16, 2021.
11. Jiang DD, Roayaie K, Woodland D, et al. Survival and renal function after liver transplantation alone in patients meeting the new United Network for Organ Sharing simultaneous liver-kidney criteria. Clin Transpl 2020;34:e14020.
12. Cheng XS, Kim WR, Tan JC, et al. Comparing simultaneous liver-kidney transplant strategies: a modified cost-effectiveness analysis. Transplantation 2018;102: e219–28.
13. Booker S, Wilk AR. OPTN Simultaneous Liver Kidney (SLK) Allocation Policy Two Year Monitoring Report. DHHS Contract No. 250-2019-00001c.
14. Cannon RM, Goldberg DS, Eckhoff DE, et al. Early outcomes with the liver-kidney safety net. Transplantation 2021;105:1261–72.

15. Culllaro G, Sharma P, Jo J, et al. Temporal trends and evolving outcomes after simultaneous liver-kidney transplant (SLKT): results from the United States SLKT Consortium. Liver Transpl 2021;27(11):1613–22.

16. Samoylova ML, Wegermann K, Shaw BI, et al. The impact of the 2017 kidney allocation policy change on simultaneous liver-kidney utilization and outcomes. Liver Transpl 2021;27:1106–15.

17. Wiseman AC. Simultaneous liver-kidney transplant: long-term management (steroid withdrawal and safter net patients). Clin Liv Dis 2019;13:176–9.

18. Bari K, Sharma P. Optimizing the selection of patients for simultaneous liver-kidney transplant. Clin Liver Dis 2021;25(1):89–102.

19. Gonwa TA, McBride MA, Anderson K, et al. Continued influence of preoperative renal function on outcome of orthotopic liver transplant (OLTX) in the US: where will MELD lead us? Am J Transpl 2006;6:2651–9.

20. Al Riyami D, Alam A, Badovinac K, et al. Decreased survival in liver transplant patients requiring chronic dialysis: a Canadian experience. Transplantation 2008;85:1277–80.

21. Allen AM, Kim WR, Thernau TM, et al. Chronic kidney disease and associated mortality after liver transplantation – a time-dependent analysis using measured glomerular filtration rate. J Hepatol 2014;61:286–92.

22. Fong TL, Khemichian S, Shah T, et al. Combined liver-kidney transplantation is preferable to liver transplant alone for cirrhotic patients with renal failure. Transplantation 2012;94:411–6.

23. Gonwa TA, McBride MA, Mai ML, et al. Kidney transplantation after previous liver transplantation: analysis of the organ procurement transplant network database. Transplantation 2011;92:31–5.

24. Wadei HM, Keaveny AP, Taner B, et al. Post-liver early allograft dysfunction modifies the effect of pre-liver transplant renal dysfunction on post-liver transplant survival. Liver Transpl 2021;27(9):1291–301.

25. Wilk AR, Booker SE, Stewart DE, et al. Developing simultaneous liver-kidney transplant medical eligibility criteria while providing a safety net: a two-year review of the OPTN's allocation policy 2021. Am J Transplant 2021;21(11):3593–607.

26. Cullaro G, Verna EC, Emond JC, et al. Early kidney allograft failure after simultaneous liver-kidney transplantation (SLKT): evidence for utilization of the Safety Net? Transplantation 2021;105:816–23.

27. Agopian VG. Liver transplantation in patients with pretransplant renal dysfunction: a "safety net" is in place, but who should walk the tightrope? Transplantation 2021;105:709–10.

28. Jay CL, Washburn WK, Rogers J, et al. Difference in survival in early kidney after liver transplantation compared with simultaneous liver-kidney transplantation: evaluating the potential of the "safety net". J Am Coll Surg 2020;230:463–73.

29. Eerhart MJ, Reyes JA, Leverson GE, et al. Kidney after liver transplantation marched-pair analysis: are kidneys allocated to appropriate patients to maximize their survival? Transplantation 2020;104:804–12.

30. Taner T, Heimbach JK, Rosen CB, et al. Decreased chronic cellular and antibody-mediated injury in the kidney following simultaneous liver-kidney transplantation. Kidney Int 2016;89:909–17.

31. Ingelsten M, Karlsson-Parra A, Granqvist AB, et al. Postischemicinflammatory response in an auxiliary liver graft predicts renal graftoutcome in sensitized patients. Transplantation 2011;91:888–94.

32. Thomson AW, Geller DA, Gandhi C, et al. Hepatic antigen-presenting cells and regulation of liver transplant outcome. Immunol Res 2011;50:221–7.
33. Simpson N, Cho YW, Cicciarelli JC, et al. Comparison of renal allograft outcomes in combined liver-kidney transplantation versus subsequent kidney transplantation in liver transplant recipients: analysis of UNOS database. Transplantation 2006;82:1298.
34. Fung J, Makowka L, Tzakis A, et al. Combined liver-kidney transplantation: analysis of patients with preformed lymphocytoxic antibodies. Transpl Proc 1988;20: 88–91.
35. Creput C, Durrbach A, Menier C, et al. Human leukocyte antigen-G (HLA-G) expression in biliary epithelial cells is associated with allograft acceptance in liver-kidney transplantation. J Hepatol 2003;39:587–94.
36. Goyes D, Nsubuga JP, Medina-Morales E, et al. New OPTN simultaneous liver-kidney transplant (SLKT) policy improves racial and ethnic disparities. J Clin Med 2020;9:3901.
37. Available at: https://milliman-cdn.azureedge.net/-/media/milliman/pdfs/articles/2020-us-organ-tissue-transplants.ashx. Accessed July 31, 2021.

Kidney Allocation Issues in Liver Transplantation Candidates with Chronic Kidney Disease and Severe Kidney Liver Injury

Daniel Lia, MD, MS, Elliot I. Grodstein, MD*

KEYWORDS

- Liver transplant • Simultaneous liver-kidney transplant • Chronic kidney disease

KEY POINTS

- MELD (Model for End-Stage Liver Disease)-based allocation favors patients with renal impairment
- Lack of guidelines for simultaneous liver-kidney transplant
- Shortage of kidneys available for transplant

MODEL FOR END-STAGE LIVER DISEASE AND KIDNEY DISEASE

Cirrhosis is often accompanied by kidney dysfunction. Both acute kidney injury (AKI) and chronic kidney disease (CKD) are common in the patient with end-stage liver disease (ESLD) awaiting liver transplantation.[1–34] Problems surrounding the management of these patients were amplified in 2002, when the liver allocation system changed to a MELD (Model for End-Stage Liver Disease)-based scoring system (**Fig. 1**). The MELD score, although very helpful in predicting mortality risk from liver dysfunction, puts a relatively heavy weight on a patient's serum creatinine level. Although intentioned to save the lives of the highest MELD patients, this shift in allocation protocol prioritized liver transplant candidates with some degree of renal disease or failure. Since implementation of the MELD score, the proportion of patients undergoing liver transplant who receive simultaneous kidney transplant has drastically increased. With an extreme shortage of available organs for kidney-alone transplantation, the addition of liver-kidney recipients has put added stress on the kidney allocation system.

Transplant Surgery Fellowship, Donald and Barbara Zucker School of Medicine at Hofstra/Northwell, 400 Community Drive, Manhasset, NY 11765, USA
* Corresponding author.
E-mail address: egrodstein@northwell.edu

Clin Liver Dis 26 (2022) 283–289
https://doi.org/10.1016/j.cld.2022.01.004
1089-3261/22/© 2022 Elsevier Inc. All rights reserved.

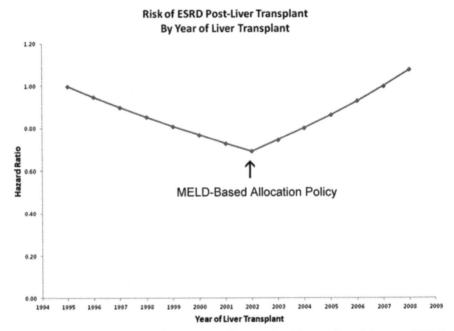

Risk of ESRD Post-Liver Transplant
By Year of Liver Transplant

MELD-Based Allocation Policy

Hazard Ratio

Year of Liver Transplant

Fig. 1. Increasing Risk of ESRD after MELD Implementation (Sharma P, et al. Impact of MELD-based allocation on end-stage renal disease after liver transplantation. Am J Transplant 2011 Nov;11(11):2372-8.)

BACKGROUND

Kidney dysfunction is a serious problem in liver transplant recipients, occurring in more than half of patients with decompensated cirrhosis; it contributes to an increased morbidity and mortality pretransplant, and if uncorrected it is a risk factor for poor outcome posttransplant. The need for dialysis in the first year after liver transplantation results in a 5% decrease in 1-year survival compared with having a liver transplant with normal postoperative renal function (**Fig. 2**). This simple statistics has led many transplant programs to err on the side of transplanting kidneys with livers.

The highest burden of kidney disease is from AKI, typically induced by hemodynamic changes associated with advanced cirrhosis. Many patients with ESLD are sarcopenic, leading to artificially low creatinine levels and underestimations of glomerular filtration rate (GFR). Considering this, relatively small changes in serum creatinine levels can indicate large changes in GFR. A serum creatinine level elevation of 0.3 mg/dL within 48 hours above baseline has been used to define AKI in the cirrhotic setting. Often, these patients do not require concomitant kidney transplantation. Kidney dysfunction can sometimes correct with diuretic withdrawal and volume expansion, vasoconstricting agents, or other therapies.

In addition to AKI, there is a strong correlation of ESLD and CKD. As the incidence of diabetes has increased over the past decades, more patients are being transplanted with nonalcoholic fatty liver disease. Of this cohort, many patients have concomitant diabetic nephropathy. There are other disease-specific associations between liver and kidney disease. Hepatitis C infection is associated with glomerulonephritis and cryoglobulinemia, which may continue after viral eradication. Alcoholic liver disease is associated with IgA nephropathy.

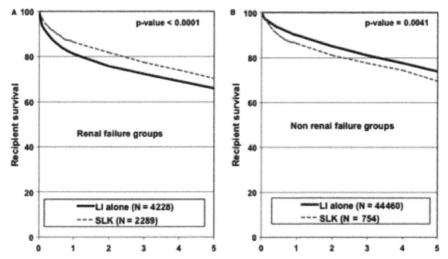

Fig. 2. Increasing Risk of ESRD after MELD Implementation (American J Transplantation, Volume: 16, Issue: 3, Pages 756-788, First published 2016, DOI: (10.1111at.13831).)

THE PROBLEM

To design an allocation system that accommodates simultaneous liver and kidney transplantation without unnecessarily transplanting kidneys, there must be metrics to prognosticate renal recovery in patients with ESLD. Clearly, patients who would recover kidney function after liver transplant would not need a kidney transplant.

In 2008, a consensus conference evaluated allocation of kidneys to liver transplant candidates with kidney dysfunction. Agreed-upon criteria to predict nonrecovery of native kidney function after liver transplant included the following:

- CKD with GFR less than 30
- CKD on kidney biopsy
- AKI with SCr level greater than 2 and dialysis more than 8 weeks
- Comorbid conditions (hyoertension, diabetes mellitus, age >65 years)
- Metabolic kidney disease

At that time, however, the decision to list a patient for simultaneous liver-kidney transplant remained up to the transplant center itself. Problematically, despite having consensus, none of the agreed-upon predictors of nonrecovery were very highly predictive. If anything, they were more suggestive. Plenty of patients, for instance, with comorbid conditions, would indeed recover renal function after liver transplantation. Owing to the nonmandatory nature of the criteria, simultaneous liver-kidney transplantation practices continued to vary from center to center (**Fig. 3**).

THE FINAL RULE AND KIDNEY TRANSPLANT FOR END-STAGE RENAL DISEASE

The Final Rule is a national policy that dictates the goals of organ allocation policy by the Organ Procurement and Transplantation Network. The rule states that the allocation policy must be based on sound medical judgment to achieve the best use of organs and avoid futile transplants. Furthermore, it dictates that allocation policy must be based on standardized criteria. Patients on the kidney transplant waiting list were dissatisfied that kidneys were being unnecessarily transplanted into liver recipients. Policy makers thought this was a violation of The Final Rule.

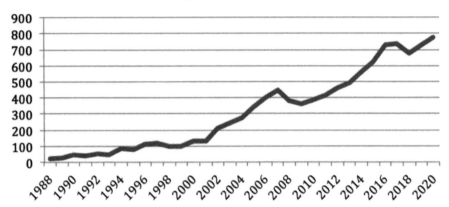

Fig. 3. Increasing Risk of ESRD after MELD Implementation (OPTN Transplant information Database.)

The kidney transplant waiting list is not a good place to be for patients without ESLD. Because of the deceased donor kidney shortage, patients with end-stage renal disease (ESRD) are frequently denied the opportunity for transplant. Annually, approximately 5000 people die while waiting for a kidney and an additional 3700 become too sick to undergo transplantation. A wasted kidney represents a lost opportunity to save one of these patients.

Furthermore, many of the kidneys used for simultaneous liver-kidney transplants are from the best kidney donors. About 50% of these kidneys would have otherwise been prioritized for pediatric recipients had they not been given to liver recipients. If the outcomes are scrutinized, renal allografts do better when transplanted into patients with ESRD than when transplanted as simultaneous liver-kidney transplants into patients with ESLD. One-year graft survival is about 5% worse in this setting. Taking kidneys away from children and putting them into adults with liver disease who had worse kidney outcomes exacerbated the calls for a need to change policy.

The Safety Net

Because renal recovery is difficult to accurately predict, there will always be a group of patients who are denied the opportunity for simultaneous liver-kidney transplant, but never regain renal function. As previously mentioned, these patients fare far worse than similar patients who would have received a kidney transplant. In fact, even if listed for an isolated kidney transplant after a liver transplant, they have a higher rate of wait-list death than other patients with ESRD awaiting transplantation.

The development of a safety net for these patients is an important element of allocation policy. The safety net allows practitioners to confidently list patients with kidney disease who do not meet criteria for simultaneous liver-kidney transplantation; it removes the penalty of guessing incorrectly that a patient would regain renal function.

In policy at the time of the writing of this article, if a recipient continues to have a GFR less than 20 mL/min or is on dialysis between 60 and 365 days after liver transplantation, they will gain priority on the kidney transplant waiting list. Although these

If the candidate's transplant nephrologist confirms a diagnosis of:	Then the transplant program must report to the OPTN and document in the candidate's medical record:
Chronic kidney disease (CKD) with a measured or calculated glomerular filtration rate (GFR) less than or equal to 60 mL/min for greater than 90 consecutive days	At least *one* of the following: That the candidate has begun regularly administered dialysis as an end-stage renal disease (ESRD) patient in a hospital based, independent non-hospital based, or home setting. At the time of registration on the kidney waiting list, that the candidate's most recent measured or calculated creatinine clearance (CrCl) or GFR is less than or equal to 30 mL/min. On a date after registration on the kidney waiting list, that the candidate's measured or calculated CrCl or GFR is less than or equal to 30 mL/min.
Sustained acute kidney injury	At least *one* of the following, or a combination of *both* of the following, for the last 6 weeks: That the candidate has been on dialysis at least once every 7 days. That the candidate has a measured or calculated CrCl or GFR less than or equal to 25 mL/min at least once every 7 days. If the candidate's eligibility is not confirmed at least once every seven days for the last 6 weeks, the candidate is not eligible to receive a liver and a kidney from the same donor.
Metabolic disease	A diagnosis of at least *one* of the following: Hyperoxaluria Atypical hemolytic uremic syndrome (HUS) from mutations in factor H or factor I Familial non-neuropathic systemic amyloidosis Methylmalonic aciduria

Fig. 4. Increasing Risk of ESRD after MELD Implementation

recipients have relative priority on the kidney-alone waiting list, they are not prioritized above pediatric patients. Furthermore, the safety net does not allow for the highest quality deceased donor grafts to be allocated to prior liver recipients.

Allocation Policy

The lack of standardized practice toward simultaneous liver-kidney transplant violated The Final Rule. Correspondingly, discussions began to develop a universal allocation policy. Ultimately it was implemented in 2017 (**Fig. 4**).

CLINICS CARE POINTS

- Renal failure in liver transplant recipients became more common after implementation of MELD-based allocation
- Requirement of dialysis post-liver transplant decreases 1 year patient survival
- Both chronic kidney disease and prolonged acute-kidney injury predict non-recovery of native kidney function after liver transplantation

DISCLOSURE

The authors of this work have no commercial or financial conflicts of interest to report. There are no sources of funding to report.

REFERENCES

1. O'Leary JG, Levitsky J, Wong F, et al. Protecting the kidney in liver transplant candidates: practice-based Recommendations from the American Society of transplantation liver and Intestine Community of practice. Am J Transplant 2016; 16(9):2516–31.
2. Wong F, O'Leary JG, Reddy KR, et al. New consensus definition of acute kidney injury accurately predicts 30-day mortality in patients with cirrhosis and infection. Gastroenterology 2013;145(1280–8):e1.
3. Fernandez J, Navasa M, Planas R, et al. Primary prophylaxis of spontaneous bacterial peritonitis delays hepatorenal syndrome and improves survival in cirrhosis. Gastroenterology 2007;133:818–24.
4. European Association for the Study of the Liver. EASL clinical practice guidelines on the management of ascites, spontaneous bacterial peritonitis, and hepatorenal syndrome in cirrhosis. J Hepatol 2010;53:397–417.
5. Wiest R, Krag A, Gerbes A. Spontaneous bacterial peritonitis: Recent guidelines and beyond. Gut 2012;61:297–310.
6. Salerno F, Navickis RJ, Wilkes MM. Albumin infusion improves outcomes of patients with spontaneous bacterial peritonitis: a meta-analysis of randomized trials. Clin Gastroenterol Hepatol 2013;11:123–30.
7. Sort P, Navasa M, Arroyo V, et al. Effect of intravenous albumin on renal impairment and mortality in patients with cirrhosis and spontaneous bacterial peritonitis. N Engl J Med 1999;341:403–9.
8. Bendtsen F, Krag A, Moller S. Treatment of acute variceal bleeding. Dig Liver Dis 2008;40:328–36.
9. Garcia-Tsao G, Sanyal AJ, Grace ND, et al. Practice guidelines Committee of the American association for the study of liver D; practice Parameters Committee of the American College of G.. Prevention and management of gastroesophageal varices and variceal hemorrhage in cirrhosis. Hepatology 2007;46:922–38.
10. Bernardi M, Caraceni P, Navickis RJ, et al. Albumin infusion in patients undergoing large-volume paracentesis: a meta-analysis of randomized trials. Hepatology 2012;55:1172–81.
11. Nadim MK, Sung RS, Davis CL, et al. Simultaneous liver-kidney transplantation summit: Current state and future directions. Am J Transplant 2012;12:2901–8.
12. Naesens M, Kuypers DR, Sarwal M. Calcineurin inhibitor nephro- toxicity. Clin J Am Soc Nephrol 2009;4(2):481–508.
13. Formica RN, Aeder M, Boyle G, et al. Simultaneous liver-kidney allocation policy: a proposal to Optimize Appropriate Utilization of Scarce Resources. Am J Transplant 2016;16(3):758–66.
14. Ruebner RL, Reese PP, Denburg MR, et al. Risk factors for end-stage kidney disease after pediatric liver transplantation. Am J Transplant 2012;12(12):3398–405.
15. Ruebner R, Goldberg D, Abt PL, et al. Risk of end-stage renal disease among liver transplant recipients with pretransplant renal dysfunction. Am J Transplant 2012;12(11):2958–65.
16. Wadei HM, Geiger XJ, Cortese C, et al. Kidney allocation to liver transplant candidates with renal failure of undetermined etiology: role of percutaneous renal biopsy. Am J Transplant 2008;8(12):2618–26.

17. Sharma P, Schaubel DE, Guidinger MK, et al. Impact of MELD-based allocation on end-stage renal disease after liver transplantation. Am J Transplant 2011; 11(11):2372–8.
18. Wadei HM, Lee DD, Croome KP, et al. Early allograft dysfunction after liver transplantation is associated with Short- and Long-term kidney function impairment. Am J Transplant 2016;16(3):850–9.
19. Levitsky J, Salomon DR, Abecassis M, et al. Clinical and plasma proteomic markers correlating with chronic kidney disease after liver transplantation. Am J Transplant 2011;11(9):1972–8.
20. Goldaracena N, Marquez M, Selzner N, et al. Living vs. deceased donor liver transplantation provides comparable recovery of renal function in patients with hepatorenal syndrome: a matched case-control study. Am J Transplant 2014; 14(12):2788–95.
21. Davis CL, Feng S, Sung R, et al. Simultaneous liver-kidney trans- plantation: evaluation to decision making. Am J Transplant 2007;7:1702–9.
22. Dellon ES, Galanko JA, Medapalli RK, et al. Impact of dialysis and older age on survival after liver transplantation. Am J Transplant 2006;6:2183–90.
23. Gonwa TA. Continued influence of preoperative renal function on outcome of orthotopic liver transplant (OLTX) in the US: where will MELD lead us? Am J Transplant 2006;6:2651–9.
24. Kiberd B, Skedgel C, Alwayn I, et al. Simultaneous liver kidney transplantation: a medical decision analysis. Transplantation 2011;91:121–7.
25. Levitsky J, O'Leary JG, Asrani S, et al. Protecting the kidney in liver transplant recipients. Am J Transplant 2016;16(9):2532–44.
26. Locke JE, Warren DS, Singer AL, et al. Declining outcomes in simultaneous liver-kidney transplantation in the MELD era: Ineffective usage of renal allografts. Transplantation 2008;85:935–42.
27. Marik PE, Wood K, Starzl TE. The course of type 1 hepato-renal syndrome post liver transplantation. Nephrol Dial Transplant 2006;21:478–82.
28. Martin-Llahi M, Guevara M, Torre A, et al. Prognostic importance of the cause of renal failure in patients with cirrhosis. Gastroenterology 2011;140(488–96):e4.
29. Ojo AO, Held PJ, Port FK, et al. Chronic renal failure after trans- plantation of a nonrenal organ. N Engl J Med 2003;349:931–40.
30. Pawarode A, Fine DM, Thuluvath PJ. Independent risk factors and natural history of renal dysfunction in liver transplant recipients. Liver Transpl 2003;9:741–7.
31. Ruiz R, Kunitake H, Wilkinson AH, et al. Long-term analysis of combined liver and kidney transplantation at a single center. Arch Surg 2006;141:735–41.
32. Sanchez EQ, Gonwa TA, Levy MF, et al. Preoperative and perioperative predictors of the need for renal replacement therapy after orthotopic liver transplantation. Transplantation 2004;78:1048–54.
33. Wong F, Nadim MK, Kellum JA, et al. Working Party proposal for a revised classification system of renal dysfunction in patients with cirrhosis. Gut 2011;60: 702–9.
34. Francoz C, Glotz D, Moreau R, et al. The evaluation of renal function and disease in patients with cirrhosis. J Hepatol 2010;52(4):605–13.

The Use of Hepatitis C Virus–Positive Organs in Hepatitis C Virus–Negative Recipients

Christian Kuntzen, MD*, Zohaib Bagha, MD

KEYWORDS

- Hepatitis C • HCV • Liver transplant • Donor • Recipient • Positive • Negative
- Fibrosing cholestatic hepatitis

KEY POINTS

- There is a significant shortage of solid organs available for transplant worldwide. The success of new direct-acting antiviral regimens and, in the United States, the increase in drug-related deaths owing to the opioid pandemic encourage the use of hepatitis C virus (HCV)-positive organs.
- Several studies have reported outcomes of transplant of HCV-viremic livers and kidneys into HCV-negative recipients, with excellent results of posttransplant treatment. However, the adoption of this approach still varies among transplant centers.
- The rates of hepatitis C- or treatment-related complications after transplant of an HCV-positive liver into an HCV-negative recipient, including fibrosing cholestatic hepatitis, are low. Mortality and inability to take oral medications after liver transplant have to be considered.
- Optimal timing after transplant, possible treatment regimens, treatment duration, and long-term outcomes need further evaluation.

INTRODUCTION

In the United States, there were 106,917 candidates waiting for an organ transplant as of November 30, 2021: 90,518 for a kidney, 11,619 for a liver, 3506 for a heart, and 1054 for a lung transplant (Organ Procurement and Transplantation Network, http://optn.transplant.hrsa.gov, accessed December 30, 2021). Despite increasing awareness and rates of organ transplantation, the demand greatly exceeds the supply, and in 2020, 36,157 kidney, 12,609 liver, 4532 heart, and 2656 lung transplant candidates were added to the waitlist, but only 22,817 kidney, 8906 liver, 3658 heart, and 2539 lung transplants were performed (http://optn.transplant.hrsa.gov).

Data for liver transplant (LiT) show that, in 2019, more than half of those who received a deceased-donor organ had to wait for more than a year, and 18%, that is of those listed, about 2580 patients, died or were too sick for transplant.[1] Regarding

Hofstra University at Northwell Health, 300 Community Drive, Manhasset, NY 11030, USA
* Corresponding author.
E-mail address: ckuntzen@northwell.edu

Clin Liver Dis 26 (2022) 291–312
https://doi.org/10.1016/j.cld.2022.01.012
1089-3261/22/© 2022 Elsevier Inc. All rights reserved.

liver.theclinics.com

kidney transplant, the wait time exceeds 5 years in most countries and in many areas of the United States,[2] and the waitlist mortality is around 3 per 100 patient-years.[3]

The predicament is similar worldwide. One strategy to increase the number of transplants is the expansion of the donor pool by inclusion of organs from increased-risk donors, including those infected with hepatitis C virus (HCV).

This article focuses on liver and kidney transplant. For review of heart and lung transplant, the authors refer the reader to the excellent articles by Aslam and colleagues and Weinfurtner and Reddy.[4,5]

Before new interferon (IFN) -free direct-acting antiviral (DAA) regimens became available starting November 2013, transplantation of HCV-positive livers into HCV-negative recipients led to poor outcomes and was rarely done.[6] Infection of an HCV-negative graft in an HCV-positive recipient or of an HCV-negative recipient after transplant of an HCV nucleic acid test (NAT) -positive liver is near universal, and the course of hepatitis in an immunocompromised host after transplant is accelerated, leading to cirrhosis within 5 years in about one-third of the cases.[6] Treatment with the first-generation protease inhibitors, boceprevir and telaprevir, which were Food and Drug Administration (FDA) approved in 2011, required use of IFN and ribavirin and generally yielded sustained virologic response rates 12 weeks after treatment (SVR12) of only 60% to 75%. Data in posttransplant patients were very limited: a study of 37 patients treated for recurrent hepatitis C after transplant found SVR12 rates of 20% with telaprevir-based regimens and 71% with boceprevir-based regimens.[7,8] Therefore, HCV-positive livers were reserved for HCV-positive recipients and were 3 times more likely to be discarded.[9]

Similarly, infection after an HCV donor-positive recipient-negative (D+/R−) kidney transplant is associated with increased mortality (relative risk, 1.85).[10] Hence, 4144 HCV antibody (Ab) -positive kidneys were discarded in the 10 years until 2014, although most were of good quality.[2]

With the introduction of effective DAA agents with SVR12 rates between 92% and 98% in noncirrhotic patients, the possibility of hepatitis C treatment after solid organ transplant of HCV-positive grafts into HCV-negative recipients has gained attraction, and an increasing number of studies has shown excellent results for kidney, liver, heart, and lung transplant.[4,11,12]

In addition, the opioid epidemic in the United States has led to a surge of hepatitis C infections and drug-related deaths. More HCV-positive organs are available, which are often from much younger donors than the average and promise greater longevity if the infection can be treated. Indeed, the median age of HCV-positive liver donors decreased from 47 to 35 years between 2012 and 2016,[13] and the annual number of HCV donor-positive to recipient-negative liver transplants (HCV D+/R− LiT) has increased 35-fold between 2016 and 2019, from 8 to 280.[14] Although the discard rate of hepatitis C–positive livers has decreased from almost 30% in 2008 to a rate of less than 10% since 2016,[1] that is, equal to that of HCV-negative organs, most livers are still used for HCV-positive recipients (84% of NAT+ and 73% of Ab+/NAT− livers), and utilization for HCV-negative recipients still varies widely among transplant centers in the United States.[6,15,16]

Increased use of HCV-positive livers for HCV-negative patients will be especially helpful for patients with long wait times, such as those with hepatocellular cancer in regions with high median end-stage liver disease (MELD) scores at transplant.[14]

In patients listed for kidney transplant, significantly shorter wait times, 16 versus 60 months, were observed in those who accepted HCV+ organs in a study in Long Island, New York by Jandovitz and colleagues.[17] In contrast to HCV-positive livers, HCV-positive kidneys were still twice more likely to be discarded than HCV-negative organs between 2015 and 2018.[18]

Several factors need to be considered when hepatitis C–positive organs are used for transplant in HCV-negative recipients, including acceptance by the patient, who needs to consent beforehand, the insurance approval process, timing and duration of treatment, possible inability to swallow pills owing to postoperative complications, and medication interactions. In addition, the risk of immunologic complications, such as fibrosing cholestatic hepatitis (FCH) and acute cellular rejection (ACR), is still unclear. Inflammatory changes typical of hepatitis C infection have been detected in graft livers after successful LiT and subsequent treatment of hepatitis C with DAAs, the clinical significance of which is still uncertain.[19,20] Further, HCV-positive donors may be hepatitis B–positive, as illustrated by one study of 32 HCV D+/R− LiT in which 60% of the donors were also HBV NAT-positive or HBcAb-positive.[21] HCV infection has been associated with acute or chronic glomerulonephritis,[22] but is overall rare, and the frequency after HCV D+/R− transplant is not clear yet.[23]

The goal of this article is to summarize and discuss existing evidence for the use of HCV-positive organs in liver and kidney transplantation, the role of different DAA agents, and effective strategies in adopting this practice.

EVALUATION OF HEPATITIS C IN THE DONOR

The presence of hepatitis C in the donor organ is evaluated by anti-HCV Ab and NAT. The latter include RT-PCR with use of reverse transcriptase and DNA polymerase chain reaction, transcription-mediated amplification, which uses reverse transcriptase and RNA polymerase at a single temperature, or branched DNA technology, in which specific RNA is not amplified, but hybridized to a synthetic, branched DNA molecule labeled with multiple molecules of an enzyme, the activity of which is measured.[24] Detectable anti-HCV Ab develop between 28 and 72 days after exposure and remain positive lifelong. Sensitivities are 95% to 99%, and false-positive results occur in up to 8% (specificity, 92%–100%).[25] On the other hand, NAT usually detect viremia, that is, active infection within 5 to 7 days after exposure, significantly reducing the "window period" between infection and a positive test result. The sensitivities of NAT are 98% to 99%.[25]

Infection of the donor can occur after transplant of HCV NAT+ or Ab+/NAT− organs. The latter situation includes cases of patients that had cleared hepatitis C and got reinfected within a week before their death, false negative NAT, and possibly reactivation of hepatitis C owing to immunosuppression.[26–28] In the United States, NAT, in addition to HCV Ab testing, was mandated by United Network for Organ Sharing (UNOS) in 2015.[9]

VIRAL TRANSMISSION AFTER HEPATITIS C VIRUS DONOR-POSITIVE RECIPIENT-NEGATIVE LIVER OR KIDNEY TRANSPLANT

Transplant of HCV Ab+/NAT− livers into HCV-negative recipients led to hepatitis C viremia in 11% (9 of 80 patients) in 2 prospective trials. In all cases, viremia developed within 3 months after transplant.[29,30] Transplant of an HCV NAT+ liver leads to infection in almost all patients[31] (**Table 1**).

Transplant of an NAT D+/R− kidney leads to viremia in 227 of 233 recipients (97.4%) (**Table 2**).

VIRAL ERADICATION AFTER LIVER TRANSPLANT

Excellent outcomes of hepatitis C treatment after HCV D+/R− LiT have been found. Fifteen reports show SVR12 in 99.5% of the patients who were treated with DAAs in

Table 1
Studies of HCV D+/R− Liver Transplant: O

Study Design	Number, Status of Donors	Viremia	D+/R− Patients Started on Treatment	SVR12 Achieved/All who Completed Treatment and Had Sufficient Follow-Up	Treatment	Treatment Initiation, Median POD (IQR)	Treatment Duration (wk)	Mortality of Transplanted (%)	Donor Characteristics	Follow-up Time, Median (IQR)	Complications, n (%)	Comments
Bari et al,[29] 2018 Observational	26 Ab + NAT−	4	3 Ab+ NAT− (1 not started due to complicated course)	3/3 Ab + NAT−	LED/SOF 1 SOF/VEL 1 LED/SOF/ Riba 1	NR	NR	1/4 complicated course	NR	NR	ACR: 0 FCH: 0 GN: 0	NR
Luckett et al,[30] 2019 Observational	55 Ab+ NAT−	5	4/5 Ab+ NAT− 1/5 died POD 253	4/4 Ab + NAT−	NR	NR	NR	0/4	NR	NR	ACR: 0 FCH: 0 GN: 0	NR
Kwong et al,[12] 2019 Retrospective	10 NAT+	10	10	10/10 DNAT+	SOF/VEL 6 SOV/LED 3 SOF/DAC 1 Riba in 40%	43 (20–59)	12 (7 pt) 24 (3 pt)	0	Donor biopsies: steatosis 3/9 5%–10%, no fibrosis	380 (263–434)	ACR: 3 (1 before DAA, 2 during/after) FCH: 0 GN: 0	
Ting et al,[41] 2020 Retrospective	26 20 NAT+ 6 Ab+ NAT−	22 20 DNAT+ 2 Ab + NAT−	21 19/20 (1 died) 2/2	12/12 11/11 DNAT+ 1/1 Ab + NAT−	GLE/PIB 19 LED/SOF 1 SOF/VEL then LED/ SOF 1	within 12 wk	12 (20 pt) 24 (1 pt)	1 DNAT+ died within 1 wk of surgical complication	18/20 DNAT+ biopsied 1/26 NRH 5 moderate fibrosis (1 with rare bridging) 4 mild/minimal fibrosis 7 moderate steatosis≥20% 5 ≤10% steatosis	8 mo	ACR: 4 FCH: 0 GN: 0 2 ACR before tx 1 ascites due to preexisting NRH of donor	Many donors had significant liver disease
Anwar et al,[21] 2020 Prospective matched cohort	32 NAT+ (7 SLK) (1 died)	30/31 (1 died)	30	19/19	GLE/PIB 27/30 (90%) SOF/VEL 3/30 (10%)	47 (18–140)	12	2 (1 on POD 7 surgical complications before EOT, 1 on POD 180, likely before SVR12 assessed)	25/32 (78%) PHS increased risk 5/32 (16) HBV NAT+	259 d (41–582)	ACR: 2/32 (6%) FCH: 0 GN: 0 Comparator group: ACR: 1/29 (3%) matched comparator (P = 0.49)	Comparator group: 32 HCV− LT SVR12 in intention-to-treat analysis 63% 50% HBcAb+

Study	Cohort	NAT+	Transplanted	SVR	DAA regimen			Complications/deaths	Donor histology	Follow-up	ACR / FCH / GN	Notes
Crismale et al,[35] 2020 Prospective	19 (7 SLK) 13 NAT+ 6 Ab + NAT−	13 NAT+	13 1/13 died	12/12	SOV-based 7 GLE/PIB 6	42 (35–118)	NR	1 started on DAA, but died before wk 24	13/13 DBD: 6 steatosis 5 mild, 1 moderate) 10 fibrosis (4 stage 1, 1 stage 2)	16.4 mo (15.4–18.4)	ACR: 1[a] FCH: 0 GN: 0	1 stage 2 fibrosis
Kapila et al,[37] 2020 Prospective	6 NAT+ (2 SLK)	6/6	6 (2 SLK)	3/3	GLE/PIB	62 (25–90)	12	0	NR	NR	NR	Study included 64 kidney transplants
Bohorquez et al,[34] 2020 Retrospective	61 NAT+ (1 did not become viremic)	60/61	56/60 (4 not started: 1 complicated course, 3 died early)	50/51 (98%) 1 relapsed, then SVR12 after 2nd course	GLE/PIB 36 SOF/VEL 20 (1 relapsed, then SOF/VEL/VOX)	67 (36–69)	12	4 3 sepsis POD 7, 26, 76 1 recurrent cholangio-carcinoma POD 259 1-y survival 93% (vs 94% in DNAT− group)	All had biopsy ≤ Stage 2 fibrosis (Batts-Ludwig), ≤ stage 2 inflammation Steatosis 0%–20%	NR	ACR: 8/61 (13%) FCH: 0 GN: 0 Control group: NAT− LTs: ACR: 44/231 (19%, $P = 0.15$)	Request to treatment initiation: Median 21 (IQR 14; 26) Control group: NAT−transplants
Nair et al,[19] 2021 Retrospective	23 NAT+	23/23	23/23	23/23	GLE/PIB 13 SOF/VEL NR LED/SOF NR	118 (46–129)	NR	2 graft losses/ deaths in entire cohort, which included 10 NAT+ to NAT− LT	NR	1 y in 24 pt	ACR: 0 FCH: 0 GN: 0	Study included 10 D+R+ LiT
Aqel et al,[32] 2021 Prospective multicenter observational	20 NAT+ 14 Ab + NAT−	20/20 0/14	20/20	20/20	GLE/PIB 18 LED/SOF 2	27.5	12	2/20 1 MI on POD 610 1 sepsis	Donor fibrosis stage: 0: 12 (60%) 1: 5 (25%) 2: 3 (15%)	NR	ACR: 1 FCH: 0 GN: 1/20, AKI on POD 18, ESRD, died of sepsis	
Hudson et al,[36] 2021 Retrospective single center	18 NAT+	18/18	18	18/18	GLE/PIB 14 SOF/VEL 4	Entire cohort: average 46 ± 25	NR	0/18	NR	NR	ACR: 1 FCH: 0 GN: 0	Study total: 61 solid organ transplants, no FCH

(continued on next page)

Table 1
(continued)

Study Design	Number, Status of Donors	Viremia	D+/R− Patients Started on Treatment	SVR12 Achieved/All who Completed Treatment and Had Sufficient Follow-Up	Treatment	Treatment Initiation, Median POD (IQR)	Treatment Duration (wk)	Mortality of Transplanted (%)	Donor Characteristics	Follow-up Time, Median (IQR)	Complications, n (%)	Comments
Sobotka et al,[39] 2021 Retrospective single center	21 NAT+ 21 Ab + NAT−	20/21 NAT+ 2 Ab + NAT− (1/21 NAT+ did not become viremic)	20 NAT+ 2 Ab + NAT−	15/15	SOF/VEL 19 GLE/PIB 2 LED/SOF/ Riba 1	38		0/22	NR	NR	ACR: 1/21 NAT+ (5%, mild) FCH: 0 GN: 0 Control group: Ab + NAT−: ACR 4/21 (19%, 2 mild, 2 moderate)	Insurance approval 9 d if private insurance 17 d if government insurance
Early treatment:												
Bethea et al,[88] 2020 Prospective, single center, early treatment	9 NAT+	9/9	9/9	9/9	GLE/PIB	1.7 (mean) Maximum 5	12	0	NR	46 (20–76)	ACR: 1 (POD 50, resolved) FCH: 0 GN: 0	Crushed GLE/PIB used if required 2/9 did not receive insurance approval, which was generally difficult to get
Said et al,[38] 2021 Prospective, single center (VA), early treatment	8 NAT+	8/8	7/7 1/8 died after ETR	7/7	GLE/PIB 5 SOV/VEL 3	10 (range, 3–25)	12	1/8 after ETR			ACR: 1 FCH: 0 GN: 0	Crushed SOF/VEL in 3

Terrault et al,[42] 2021 Prospective, multicenter, Included kidney tx Early treatment	13	13 1/13 died before EOT	12/12	12/12	SOV/VEL	7 (6–12) per protocol	1/13 POD 152 due to GVHD	Minimal or no fibrosis	ACR: 0, but 1 AMR (POD 36) FCH: 0 GN: 0 1 GVHD POD 19, 1 intrahepatic biliary sclerosis POD 31, improved 1 idiopathic pericardial effusion, resolved	Also 11 kidney transplants 1 intraoperative Amiodarone, SOF/VEL started POD 25
Sum later treatment				189/190					ACR: 19 FCH: 0 GN: 1, ESRD, died	
Sum early treatment				28/28 NAT+					ACR: 2, AMR: 1 FCH: 0 GN: 0	
Total				181/182 NAT+ 217/218 all (both 99.5%)			Deaths within 1 wk: 3 (1.4%)		ACR: 21 (9.5%) FCH: 0 GN: 1 (0.5%)	

Numbers of duration of treatment given for entire study cohort.

Abbreviations: AMR, antibody-mediated rejection; DBD, donation after brain death; DNAT, donor nucleic acid test; IQR, interquartile range; MI, myocardial infarction; NR, not reported; Pt, patient.

[a] Noncompliance with immunosuppression.

Table 2
Studies of HCV D+/R- Kidney Transplant

Study	Number of NAT D+/R- Kidney Tranplants	Treatment Initiation (Median Day)	DAA Regimen	Treatment Duration (wk)	SVR12[a]	Complications, Comments
Goldberg et al,[82] 2017 (THINKER trial)	10	NR	ELB/GRZ	12	10/10	Delayed graft function: 1 De novo DSA: 1 FSGS: 1
Reese et al,[83] 2018	20	3	ELB/GRZ ELB/GRZ/Riba if NS5A resistance	12 16	20/20	Delayed graft function: 5 De novo DSA: 4 FSGS: 1
Friebus-Kardash et al,[84] 2019	7	7	LED-SOF SOV-VEL	8-12	7/7	No delayed graft function
Molnar et al,[60] 2019	53	76	GLE/PIB SOF/VEL SOF/LED	≥12	53/53	Delayed graft function: 3 De novo DSA: 16 FCH: 1 Acute rejection: 4
Crismale et al,[35] 2020	13	40	SOF-based GLE-PIB	NR	7/7	2 of 13 did not develop viremia
Kapila et al,[37] 2020	64	72	LED/SOF GLE/PIB SOV/VEL	NR	41/41	Death: 1 FCH: 2 3 of 64 did not develop viremia
Graham et al,[63] 2020	30	9	GLE/PIB SOF/VEL	12	30/30	Delayed graft function: 27% (8 patients) vs 60% in age-matched cohort Acute rejection: 2 (6.6%)
Terrault et al,[42] 2021	11	16.5	SOF/VEL SOF/VEL/VOX for failures	12	11/11	1 additional patient did not develop viremia

Study	No.	Timing	DAA regimen	Duration	SVR12	Outcomes
Jandovitz et al,[17] 2020	25	13	LED/SOF SOF/VEL GLE/PIB	NR	24/25	1 failure achieved SVR12 with SOV/VEL/VOX
	233				203/204	Delayed graft function: 17/233 (7%) De novo DSA: 21 (9%) FCH: 3 Acute rejection: 6 No transmission: 4
Preemptive treatment						
Sise et al,[45] 2020	30	3	GLE/PIB	8	30/30	ACR: 3 BK viremia: 3
Durand et al,[85] 2018	10	Before surgery	ELB/GRZ ELB/GRZ/Riba,[b] ELB/GRZ/SOF[c]	12 16 12	10/10	NR
Franco et al,[86] 2019	4	6 h before surgery	GLE/PIB	8	4/4	NR
Durand et al,[46] 2021	10	Before organ perfusion	GLE/PIB	4	10/10	1 graft failure due to thromboembolism
Gupta et al,[50] 2020	15 40	Before surgery	SOF/VEL	2 d 4 d	44/50	Transmission rate 6/50 (12%): 30% (2 d) and 7.5% (4 d). SVR12 after 2nd DAA course
Duerr et al,[87] 2021	3	Before surgery	DCL/SOF	12	3/3	None

Abbreviations: DSA, donor-specific antibodies; NR, none reported, Riba = ribavirin.
[a] Patients with available data on first course of DAA.
[b] If NS5A RAS.
[c] If GT2 or 3.

the first few months after HCV D+/R− transplant and had sufficient follow-up: 181 of 182 patients who received a NAT+ graft, and 217 of 218 in total (NAT+ or Ab+ NAT− graft)[12,19,21,29,30,32–41] (see **Table 1**).

In the largest study by Bohorquez and colleagues,[34] 98.3% of the patients became viremic within 2 weeks after transplant. Treatment was generally initiated once the patient had recovered from surgery in 12 of the 15 studies, with median starting times between postoperative day 28 and 67.[12,19,21,29,30,32–41] Of note, 2 patients who received an NAT-positive organ did not have viremia after transplant and were not treated.[34,39] It is not clear if these cases were due to false-positive NAT of the donor or true viral clearance.

Three of the studies treated early with the pan-genotypic regimen, with median start times between 1.7 and 10 days after transplant[33,38,42] because of concerns of possible complications, including increased rates of rejection, development of FCH, and glomerulonephritis.[23] Viral eradication was achieved in all 28 patients. In the study by Terrault and colleagues,[42] several unusual complications were observed among the 13 patients: 1 case each of intrahepatic biliary sclerosis, idiopathic pericardial effusion (transient), graft-versus-host disease (GVHD), and Ab-mediated rejection. Whether this is due to DAA treatment in the first days after transplant or incidental is uncertain.

Most of the patients in the above studies were treated with the pan-genotypic regimens sofosbuvir/velpatasvir (SOF/VEL) or glecaprevir/pibrentasvir (GLE/PIB; see **Table 1**). A minority was treated with other sofosbuvir-containing regimens, and none with elbasvir/grazoprevir (EBR/GZR). Whether ribavirin in addition to ledipasvir/ sofosbuvir after HCV D+/R− LiT is of benefit cannot be concluded from the available studies and requires further research. However, in a large study of 512 post-LiT patients with recurrent hepatitis C who were treated after a median time of 7 years, the addition of ribavirin to ledipasvir/sofosbuvir (179 patients) or sofosbuvir/daclatasvir (335 patients) did not show higher SVR12 rates.[43] Similarly, a smaller study of 162 post-LiT patients with hepatitis C observed high SVR12 rates of 100% and 96% after 8 and 12 weeks of treatment with sofosbuvir/ledipasvir without ribavirin.[44]

The treatment failure occurred in Bohorquez and colleagues[34] after treatment with SOF/VEL, and the patient then achieved SVR12 after treatment with sofosbuvir/velpatasvir/voxilaprevir (SOF/VEL/VOX) for 12 weeks (see **Table 1**).

None of the studies reported cessation of treatment because of suspected side effects. Deaths and serious adverse events that are typical complications after transplant, such as sepsis and hepatic artery thrombosis, were thought to be unrelated to DAA treatment. Survival after HCV D+/R− LiT was analyzed in patients in the UNOS database of transplants performed in the United States between January 2014 and December 2018 by Thuluvath and colleagues.[16] HCV-negative recipients of NAT-positive grafts had a trend toward lower graft and patient survival. However, NAT-negative recipients had higher MELD scores than NAT-positive recipients (22.8 vs 18.1; $P = 0.001$), and worse Child-Pugh class (63% vs 41% in Child C; $P = 0.001$), and after adjustment for recipient factors, no differences were found. For Ab+/NAT− transplants, no significant differences were found.

Larger studies would be needed to determine whether any of these outcomes occur at a different rate than in general after LiT. [editing: please move the paragraph Duration and timing of treatment in liver transplante here]

VIRAL ERADICATION AFTER HEPATITIS C virusD + /R− KIDNEY TRANSPLANT

In 9 studies that involved 204 HCV D+/R− kidney transplant recipients who had persistent viremia after transplant, an overall SVR12 rate of 99.5% was observed (see **Table 2**). Those 2 patients who relapsed were then successfully treated with a second course. Median start was up to 72 days after transplant.

DURATION AND TIMING OF TREATMENT IN KIDNEY TRANSPLANT

Treatment duration in these trials was most often 12 weeks, but 8-week treatment[45] with GLE/PIB was successful as well (see later discussion and Table 2). Preemptive treatment, in which the first dose of DAA is given just before transplant, and short courses of 4 or 8 weeks of DAA treatment after transplant of kidneys and other non-reservoir organs, such as heart and lung from HCV-viremic donors to HCV-negative recipients, have been used successfully in small studies, in which the first dose of DAAs was given just before surgery (see **Table 2**).[33,45–49]

Durand and colleagues began treatment with EBR/GZR just before surgery and performed genotyping in parallel with the transplant[85]. Genotyping results were available within 7 days. In case of infections with GT1a with resistance-associated substitutions (RAS), ribavirin was added, and in case of GT2 or 3 infection, sofosbuvir. Treatment was given for 12 to 16 weeks and was successful in all patients. Treatment for 8 or 4 weeks with GLE/PIB was successful in 2 small studies with 4 and 10 patients, respectively (see **Table 2**).

Gupta and colleagues[50] evaluated ultrashort treatment with 2 or 4 doses of daily pan-genotypic SOF/VEL, starting just before transplant. Several patients had transient viremia detected at day 3 and/or 7. Viremia beyond postoperative day (POD) 14 developed in only 12% of the 50 patients, and in 7.5% of the 40 patients in the 4-day treatment group (see **Table 2**). Of the 6 patients with viremia, SVR12 was achieved in 3 patients with a 12-week course. Two additional patients were then successfully treated with a second course.

Although the number of cases is still small, these results suggest that hepatitis C infection by transplantation of an infected kidney can be suppressed quickly and that treatment courses shorter than 12 weeks may be successful.

DURATION AND TIMING OF TREATMENT IN LIVER TRANSPLANT

After liver transplant, the duration of treatment was generally 12 weeks[12,19,21,29,30,32–41] (**Table 1**). Whether eight-week courses with glecaprevir/piprentasvir or ledipasvir/sofosbuvir can be used in certain situations as in non-transplant patients is currently unknown, but given the excellent results, this should be explored. Given the risk of hepatitis C–related complications after NAT D+R– LiT, including development of FCH, there has been interest in early treatment, within the first week after transplant.

Three studies involving 28 patients reported results of this approach. Bethea and colleagues[33] treated 9 recipients of an NAT+ liver with pan-genotypic DAA regimens before the development of viremia, once bilirubin was less than 10 mg/dL or less than 50% of the pretransplant value and the international normalized ratio (INR) was less than 1.4. Treatment was started between POD 0 and 5, on average after 1.7 days. All patients developed viremia but achieved SVR at 12 weeks after treatment. One of these patients developed ACR but was successfully treated with increased immunosuppression. The authors used GLE/PIB, as sofosbuvir had not been approved for all chronic kidney disease (CKD) stages at the time of the study, acknowledging that GLE/PIB is not recommended in hepatic dysfunction with hyperbilirubinemia, as excretion is hepatic. The pills were crushed and put in suspension and fed via naso-gastric or orogastric tube if required. No adverse effects of treatment or other complications were noted in this study. The investigators reported significant difficulties in obtaining insurance approval, which could not be obtained in 2 of the 9 cases.

Said and colleagues[38] treated 8 recipients of an NAT+ liver within the Veterans Affairs (VA) system, which does not require prior insurance approval. All patients became viremic within an average of 3 days, and DAA was initiated within a median time of 10 days posttransplant. Three patients had dysphagia and were treated with SOF/VEL in crushed and suspended form. The others received GLE/PIB. One patient died of operative complications after end of treatment (EOT), before SVR12 could be assessed. The remaining 7 patients achieved SVR12. One patient had an episode of ACR, which was successfully treated.

The third study by Terrault and colleagues[42] included 13 patients, who received an NAT+ liver. All had viremia within 3 days, and DAA treatment was initiated on POD 7 on average. All patients achieved SVR12. This study reported complications that were not reported by previous studies. One patient developed Ab-mediated rejection, which resolved after administration of immunoglobulin. Another patient, who began treatment 6 days after surgery, developed intrahepatic biliary sclerosis starting day 31. This patient was noted to have abnormal-appearing bile ducts on cholangiography and elevated alkaline phosphatase. A third patient developed GVHD which led to multiorgan failure. The patient achieved SVR but died with multiorgan failure after 152 days. GVHD is a rare complication of LiT, but not one limited to HCV-positive donors.[51] The incidence of GVHD has been rate reported as 0.5% to 2% in general LiT.[52]

The above studies (see **Table 1**) included 2 patients who did not develop viremia after transplant,[34,39] and 3 who died within 1 week after transplant.[21,34,41] No cases of FCH developed, but 1 case of HCV-associated glomerulonephritis developed on POD 18, which led to the need of dialysis and likely contributed to the death of the patient of sepsis.

In 3 patients in Bohorquez and colleagues,[34] treatment was begun after clinical signs of hepatitis C developed, between POD 30 and 70 (persistent transaminase elevation, ascites, histologic hepatitis C activity). Two patients with abnormal liver serologies in the study by Ting and colleagues[41] were found to have histologic findings of ACR together with hepatitis 2 and 4 weeks after transplant, which prompted initiation of DAA treatment together with adjustment of immunosuppression.

OTHER OUTCOMES
Fibrosing Cholestatic Hepatitis

FCH is a severe form of recurrent disease in the setting of immunosuppression, which typically leads to liver failure and graft loss within 1 to 2 years after transplantation in the pre-DAA era.[53]

It is thought to occur owing to a direct viral cytopathic effect and is characterized by prolonged cholestasis and histologic cholestatic changes with prominent ductular reaction, ballooning of hepatocytes, fibrosis, and the absence of lobular inflammation and lymphoid aggregates. Viral titers are typically high but have not been found to be an independent predictor. Occurrence at least 1 month after transplant has been used as a diagnostic criterium, and most cases develop within 6 months after transplant.[54]

The frequency after LiT of patients with hepatitis C–related cirrhosis was 3.1% (42 patients) in 5 studies involving 1347 patients.[55–59] The frequency after kidney or other solid organ transplant is less certain.

No case of FCH has been reported in 15 studies involving 218 patients after HCV D+/R− LiT (see **Table 1**).

After kidney transplant, 3 of 345 patients developed FCH (see **Table 2**). In the study by Kapila and colleagues,[37] 1 patient developed biopsy-proven FCH 11 weeks after transplant. He achieved SVR12 after 16 weeks of DAA therapy. The second patient was diagnosed with FCH 14 weeks after kidney transplant, based on elevated bilirubin and liver enzymes and a high viral load. By the end of the study, he had completed 12 weeks of GLE/PIB and had normal liver serologies and no detectable viral load. A third patient in the study by Molnar and colleagues[60] was reported to have been successfully treated with DAA as well.

DAAs have been used successfully in a study of 23 patients, who developed FCH after LiT for hepatitis C.[53] Viral clearance occurred more slowly than in the general population, and treatment was extended up to 48 weeks. SVR12 was achieved in all 15 patients (100%) treated with sofosbuvir/daclatasvir and in 7 of 8 patients (88%) treated with sofosbuvir/ribavirin. One patient with HIV relapsed after sofosbuvir/ribavirin treatment.

Although the degree of fibrosis formation before SVR is achieved and long-term outcomes are unknown, the results indicate that the prognosis of FCH is significantly better than in the pre-DAA era.

Acute Cellular Rejection

ACR after HCV D+/R– LiT occurred in 21 of 220 cases (9.5%) overall (see **Table 1**).[12,19,21,29,30,32–41] The 2 largest studies by Bohorquez and colleagues[34] and Anwar and colleagues[21] included comparison groups, in which ACR occurred more frequently (see **Table 1**).

The rate is lower than the rates of 16% and 27%, which were observed in a large registry of 45,423 patients who underwent LiT between 2005 and 2013, and in a cohort of 890 living-donor transplants, respectively.[61] Of note, hepatitis C was a risk factor with hazard ratios of 1.1 and 2.2, respectively.[61] Historically, the rate of ACR ranged from 24% to 80% in different centers before 1995,[62] but the incidence has likely improved because of the advances in immunosuppression. It is associated with increased risk for graft failure and death.

ACR after HCV D+/R– kidney transplant occurred in 2.6% (9 of 345 patients), which is lower than the rate of 8% in the general population.[63]

A case of glomerulonephritis after HCV NAT D+R– LiT has been reported by Wadei and colleagues[64] (see **Table 2**). The patient developed viremia with 25 million IU/mL 12 hours after transplant and then immune-complex–mediated membranous glomerulonephritis after the insurance initially denied treatment and he required dialysis on POD 22. He improved after GLE/PIB was started on POD 24, but required dialysis for 3 weeks and continued to have nephrotic syndrome.

Significantly shorter wait times have been observed in patients who accepted HCV-positive organs and are likely to result in improved long-term outcomes. In 1 study by Jandovitz and colleagues[17] in New York State, 25 recipients of HCV NAT-positive organs spent less time on the waitlist (1.3 vs 5.0 years; $P<.01$), and the donors were younger (35 vs 45 years old; $P = 0.02$) compared with recipients of NAT– organs. Similarly, several small studies in HCV-positive recipients showed shortened waiting times if HCV-positive kidneys were accepted in Sawinski and colleagues[65] and references therein at 1.3 years versus 2.6 years.

Currently, it appears that hepatitis C–related complications within the first month, namely hepatitis, FCH, and glomerulonephritis, are infrequent, and that the numbers of these are similar to those in which the infection resolves after transplant and to the number of deaths within the first week. Furthermore, it is unknown whether the complications observed by Terrault and colleagues[42] (see above) are related to hepatitis C treatment. Therefore, the optimal time of starting DAA treatment after LiT may be within the first month, but after the patient has stabilized. In New York State, insurance approval of hepatitis C after infection via a hepatitis C–positive kidney transplant is currently obtained within a median of 2 days from almost all insurances,[17] and New York State Medicaid removed prior authorization requirements for hepatitis C treatment in 2020. If approval can be counted on within a few days, it is reasonable to order treatment after the patient has developed viremia and has clinically stabilized.

The American Association for the Study of Liver Diseases (AASLD) and the Infectious Diseases Society of America recommend treatment within the first month, with preference to start within the first week after LiT with pan-genotypic DAA regimens, provided the patients are clinically stable.

In contrast to LiT, no significant problems owing to an early start of DAA treatment in kidney transplantation have been reported and early treatment, before the patient develops viremia, should be attempted to avoid hepatitis C–related complications.

CHOOSING THE TREATMENT REGIMEN

First-line DAA regimens for patients with hepatitis C without cirrhosis in the United States are GLE/PIB for 8 to 16 weeks depending on genotype and prior treatment failures; SOF/VEL for 12 weeks; ledipasvir/sofosbuvir (LDV/SOF) for 12 weeks, or 8 weeks if viral load is less than 6 million IU/mL; EBR/GZR for 12 weeks, and, after DAA failure, SOF/VEL/VOX for 12 weeks.

GLE/PIB, SOF/VEL, and SOF/VEL/VOX are pan-genotypic and have a high barrier to resistance. Often, the treatment regimen depends on insurance approval. However, there are special considerations for a subset of the population for whom a specific regime may be preferred.

Renal Impairment

Both acute kidney injury and chronic kidney injury are common in liver and kidney transplant recipients. GLE/PIB, EBR/GZR, and ledipasvir are hepatically excreted and are safe.[66] Although sofosbuvir is mainly renally excreted and renal insufficiency leads to higher concentration of its primary metabolite, GS-331007, there is no associated toxicity, and several trials found sofosbuvir/ledipasvir and other sofosbuvir-containing regimens safe and effective in advanced renal disease with eGFR less than 30 mL/kg/min, including in patients with dialysis.[67] Hence, the FDA included patients with CKD of any severity, including those on dialysis in 2019, and AASLD guidelines recommend sofosbuvir-containing regimens independent of the presence of chronic kidney disease.[67]

Medication Interactions

Sofosbuvir is transported by P-glycoprotein, and medications that are known inducers of it, such as phenytoin and rifampicin, should not be coadministered. Use of sofosbuvir in patients taking amiodarone is contraindicated owing to life-threatening arrhythmias.

Ledipasvir is transported by P-glycoprotein and breast cancer resistance protein (BCRP).

Interactions with Immunosuppressive Agents

Calcineurin inhibitors and inhibitors of mammalian target of rapamycin inhibitors (mTOR) can interact with DAA regimens. Some combinations require dose adjustment and close monitoring, whereas others are not recommended.

Cyclosporine and tacrolimus are metabolized by CYP3A4. Cyclosporine is also a substrate and inhibitor of P-glycoprotein and inhibits organic anion transporting polypeptide OATP1B1.

Everolimus and sirolimus have not been studied in combination with first-line DAAs. Everolimus is also metabolized by P-glycoprotein. Interactions with DAAs may need close monitoring (see **Table 3**).[68,69]

Treatment with GLE/PIB inhibits CYP3A4 and P-GP weakly and increases the concentration of tacrolimus. Tacrolimus levels must be monitored closely.[69]

GLE/PIB levels do not influence the levels of cyclosporine but are increased by it. GLE/PIB is not recommended for use in patients requiring stable cyclosporine doses greater than 100 mg per day.

SOF/VEL and ledipasvir/sofosbuvir do not have significant drug interactions with tacrolimus, cyclosporine, sirolimus, everolimus, or mycophenolate mofetil.

SOF/VEL/VOX use is safe to use with tacrolimus and mTOR inhibitors but is not recommended together with cyclosporine owing to OATP1B1 inhibition by cyclosporine, which leads to significantly increased concentrations of voxilaprevir.

Grazoprevir is a weak inducer of CYP3A4, and tacrolimus concentrations must be monitored. Grazoprevir concentrations can also be increased markedly by cyclosporin via OATP1B1 inhibition, and coadministration is not recommended (see **Table 2**).[68,69]

Neurologic Complication

The incidence of seizures has been reported between 3% and 36% after liver and kidney transplant.[70] Most seizures are single episodes and are associated with toxic levels of immunosuppressant drugs or with central nervous system infections. These improve with cessation of the immunosuppressive agent or with treatment of the underlying infections.[71] Abscesses, brain lesions, or brain infarction during surgical procedure may require prolonged treatment with antiepileptic drugs. Levetiracetam, gabapentin, pregabalin, and lacosamide are drugs of choice in posttransplant patients[71] and do not interact with the first-line DAA regimens listed above. In contrast, carbamazepine, phenytoin, phenobarbital, or oxcarbazepine should generally be avoided, as they can decrease concentrations of several DAA agents. Valproic acid and lamotrigine are primarily metabolized in the liver and need to be used with caution after LiT but can be safely used with DAAs.[59,68]

Cardiovascular Patients

Cardiovascular diseases are common among patients who undergo liver or kidney transplant, with a prevalence of coronary artery disease in patients with liver cirrhosis and patients on the kidney transplant list of around 30%.[72] Coadministration of statins with DAA can lead to an increase in statin concentration and the risk for toxicity, including myopathy. Generally, low doses of several statins are tolerated, but some combinations are not recommended (**Table 3**).[4] Because the duration of treatment with DAAs is limited to 3 months, temporary discontinuation of the statin can be considered.[73]

Coadministration of amiodarone with ledipasvir/sofosbuvir is contraindicated because of severe bradycardia and heart block. Because of the long half-life of amiodarone, an interaction for several months after discontinuation of amiodarone is possible. Delaying treatment with ledipasvir/sofosbuvir for 6 and 3 months is recommended by AASLD and EASL guidelines (European Association for the Study of Liver Diseases), respectively.[68,69]

Apixaban, dabigatran, and rivaroxaban are non–vitamin K oral anticoagulants (NOACs), which are substrates of CYP3A4, P-glycoprotein, and BCRP, which are inhibited by DAA. Coadministration may increase bleeding risk, but few data about safety are available.[74] If NOACs cannot be avoided, dose reduction or close

Table 3
Medication interactions

	ELB/GZR	GLE/PIP	LED/SOF	SOF/VEL	SOF/VEL/VOX
Tacrolimus	2	2	0	0	2
Cyclosporine	3	2	0	0	3
Sirolimus	2	2	0	0	2
Everolimus	2	2	2	2	2
Dexamethasone	2	2	0	0	2
Acyclovir, valaciclovir	0	0	0	0	0
Ganciclovir	No data	No data	No data	No data	No data
Fluconazole	0	0	0	0	0
Omeprazole, es-omeprazole, panto-prazole, H2-RA	0	1	2	2	2
Atorvastatin	2	3	2	2	3
Rosuvastatin	2	2	3	2	3
Simvastatin	2	3	2	2	3
Pravastatin	0	2	2	0	2
Amiodarone	2	2	3	3	3
Diltiazem	0	2	2	2	2
Midazolam	2	0	0	0	0
Anticonvulsants: Phenobarbital, carbamazepine, phenytoin	3	3	3	3	3
Levetiracetam, gabapentin	0	0	0	0	0
Antihypertensives[a]: Diltiazem	0	2	2	2	2
Tenofovir, entecavir	0	0	0	0	0

0: no interaction, 1: potential weak interaction, 2: potential interaction, 3: do not coadminister

Ranking of clinical significance is based on www.hep-druginteractions.org (University of Liverpool). No interactions: basiliximab; mycophenolate; prednisone; methylprednisolone; antibiotics, including metronidazole, ciprofloxacin, meropenem, aztreonam, linezolid, trimethoprim/sulfamethoxazole, atovaquone; loop diuretics, hydrochlorothiazide, spironolactone.

[a]For individual interactions with calcium channel blockers, ACE inhibitors, angiotensin receptor antagonists, and other interactions, refer to the product label for dosing advice.

monitoring is recommended. Similarly, warfarin is metabolized by CYP enzymes, and NOAC coadministration can increase its levels and bleeding risk. At this time, it is advised to monitor INR and adjust as necessary. Heparin is not a substate of CYP enzymes, and thus far, no drug-drug interactions have been reported.[74]

Stress-Ulcer Prophylaxis

For critically ill patients in the intensive care unit, proton-pump inhibitors (PPI) or H2-receptor blockers are commonly used for prophylaxis against stress ulcers. Both ledipasvir and velpatasvir are best absorbed at a low pH. Use of PPI or H2 antagonists with these DAAs have been shown to decrease concentration of DAA agents. Therefore, PPIs should generally be avoided in these agents.[66] If PPIs are needed, use of omeprazole 20 mg 4 hours after administration of DAA is recommended. EBR/GZR and GLE/PIB can be used with PPI.[4]

Nasogastric/Percutaneous Endoscopic Gastrostomy Tube

SOF/VEL is the only pan-genotypic DAA regimen shown to have efficacy through the nasogastric tube and percutaneous endoscopic gastrostomy tube.[75,76] Other DAAs that can be used via feeding tubes include EBR/GZR and LDV/SOF.[77,78] GLE/PIB has been shown to yield favorable drug levels in healthy persons.[79] SOF/VEL, SOF/VEL/VOX, and LDV/SOF are not enteric-coated and can be dissolved in water with gentle spoon pressure. However, the pharmacokinetics of these drugs when dissolved, crushed, or split has not been studied.[4]

COST-EFFECTIVITY ANALYSIS

Patients who receive HCV-viremic livers have added cost to their transplant process. Recent model simulation by Bethea and colleagues[80] based on published data demonstrated that for HCV-negative patients with a model for MELD score ≥22, using HCV-viremic organ for LiT was more cost-effective and improved health care outcomes than remaining on waitlist. In kidney transplant, an analysis by Kadatz and colleagues[81] suggested that using an HCV-viremic organ in a HCV-negative recipient is cost-effective compared with remaining on the waitlist for an additional 2 years and receiving a hepatitis C–negative organ.

SUMMARY

Review of the published literature shows that DAAs are highly effective in hepatitis C transmitted by transplant of an HCV-positive liver or kidney into an HCV-negative recipient, with an overall SVR12 rate of 99.5 in 181 patients that received a NAT+ liver, and of 99.5% in 204 patients that received an NAT+ kidney. The rate of early complications after LiT may warrant treatment initiation within the first month after transplant, after the patient has stabilized. In kidney transplant, preemptive treatment initiated before the surgery appears safe and is likely the best approach, as shorter treatment courses of days to a few weeks may be effective. Whether treatment courses shorter than 12 weeks can be used after LiT remains to be determined. Further research is required to determine the necessary treatment duration in both cases.

Use of HCV-positive livers and kidneys in HCV-negative recipients is safe and should be offered to any patient who is willing to accept it.

CLINICS CARE POINTS

- Transplant of HCV-positive livers or kidneys is safe and may significantly shorten wait list times.
- SVR12 rates after liver or kidney transplant are nearly 100%.
- Pan-genotypic regiments can be used.
- Medication interactions need to be considered.

REFERENCES

1. Kwong AJ, Kim WR, Lake JR, et al. OPTN/SRTR 2019 annual data report: liver. Am J Transplant 2021;21(Suppl 2):208–315.

2. Reese PP, Abt PL, Blumberg EA, et al. Transplanting hepatitis C–positive kidneys. N Engl J Med 2015;373(4):303–5.

3. Homkrailas P, Bunnapradist S. Association between ethnicity and kidney transplant waitlist outcomes beyond estimated post-transplant survival score. Transpl Int 2021;34(10):1837–44. https://doi.org/10.1111/tri.13965.

4. Aslam S, Grossi P, Schlendorf KH, et al. Utilization of hepatitis C virus-infected organ donors in cardiothoracic transplantation: an ISHLT expert consensus statement. J Heart Lung Transplant 2020;39(5):418–32.

5. Weinfurtner K, Reddy KR. Hepatitis C viraemic organs in solid organ transplantation. J Hepatol 2021;74(3):716–33.

6. Cotter TG, Paul S, Sandıkçı B, et al. Increasing utilization and excellent initial outcomes following liver transplant of hepatitis C virus (HCV)-viremic donors into HCV-negative recipients: outcomes following liver transplant of HCV-viremic donors. Hepatology 2019;69(6):2381–95. https://doi.org/10.1002/hep.30540.

7. Charlton M, Dick T. Victory and defeat at Heraclea - treating hepatitis C infection following liver transplantation with telaprevir and boceprevir. J Hepatol 2014; 60(1):6–8.

8. Coilly A, Roche B, Dumortier J, et al. Safety and efficacy of protease inhibitors to treat hepatitis C after liver transplantation: a multicenter experience. J Hepatol 2014;60(1):78–86.

9. Bowring MG, Kucirka LM, Massie AB, et al. Changes in utilization and discard of hepatitis C-infected donor livers in the recent era. Am J Transpl 2017;17(2): 519–27.

10. Fabrizi F, Martin P, Dixit V, et al. Meta-analysis of observational studies: hepatitis C and survival after renal transplant. J Viral Hepat 2014;21(5):314–24.

11. Durand CM, Bowring MG, Thomas AG, et al. The drug overdose epidemic and deceased-donor transplantation in the United States: a national registry study. Ann Intern Med 2018;168(10):702–11.

12. Kwong AJ, Wall A, Melcher M, et al. Liver transplantation for hepatitis C virus (HCV) non-viremic recipients with HCV viremic donors. Am J Transpl 2019; 19(5):1380–7.

13. Gonzalez SA, Trotter JF. The rise of the opioid epidemic and hepatitis C–positive organs: a new era in liver transplantation. Hepatology 2018;67(4):1600–8. https://doi.org/10.1002/hep.29572.

14. Cotter TG, Aronsohn A, Reddy KG, et al. Liver transplantation of HCV-viremic donors into HCV-negative recipients in the United States: increasing frequency with profound geographic variation. Transplantation 2021;105(6):1285–90.

15. Da BL, Ezaz G, Kushner T, et al. Donor characteristics and regional differences in the utilization of HCV-positive donors in liver transplantation. JAMA Netw Open 2020;3(12):e2027551.

16. Thuluvath PJ, Yoo HY. Graft and patient survival after adult live donor liver transplantation compared to a matched cohort who received a deceased donor transplantation. Liver Transplant 2004;10(10):1263–8.

17. Jandovitz N, Nair V, Grodstein E, et al. Hepatitis C-positive donor to negative recipient kidney transplantation: a real-world experience. Transpl Infect Dis 2021;23(3):e13540.

18. Ariyamuthu VK, Sandikci B, AbdulRahim N, et al. Trends in utilization of deceased donor kidneys based on hepatitis C virus status and impact of public health service labeling on discard. Transpl Infect Dis 2020;22(1):e13204.

19. Nair SP, Marella HK, Maliakkal B, et al. Transplantation of liver from hepatitis C-infected donors to hepatitis C RNA-negative recipients: histological and virologic outcome. Clin Transplant 2021;35(5):e14281.

20. Whitcomb E, Choi WT, Jerome KR, et al. Biopsy specimens from allograft liver contain histologic features of hepatitis C virus infection after virus eradication. Clin Gastroenterol Hepatol 2017;15(8):1279–85.

21. Anwar N, Kaiser TE, Bari K, et al. Use of hepatitis C nucleic acid test–positive liver allografts in hepatitis C virus seronegative recipients. Liver Transplant 2020;26(5): 673–80.

22. Barsoum RS, William EA, Khalil SS. Hepatitis C and kidney disease: a narrative review. J Adv Res 2017;8(2):113–30.

23. Terrault NA, Feld JJ. Letter to the editor: safety first: favoring prophylactic/preemptive over delayed treatment in D+/R- transplants. Hepatology 2020; 72(2):787.

24. Gupta E, Bajpai M, Choudhary A. Hepatitis C virus: screening, diagnosis, and interpretation of laboratory assays. Asian J Transfus Sci 2014;8(1):19–25.

25. Colin C, Lanoir D, Touzet S, et al. Sensitivity and specificity of third-generation hepatitis C virus antibody detection assays: an analysis of the literature. J Viral Hepat 2001;8(2):87–95.

26. Castillo I, Rodríguez-Iñigo E, López-Alcorocho JM, et al. Hepatitis C virus replicates in the liver of patients who have a sustained response to antiviral treatment. Clin Infect Dis 2006;43(10):1277–83.

27. Lin A, Thadareddy A, Goldstein MJ, et al. Immune suppression leading to hepatitis C virus re-emergence after sustained virological response. J Med Virol 2008; 80(10):1720–2.

28. Vento S, Cainelli F, Longhi MS. Reactivation of replication of hepatitis B and C viruses after immunosuppressive therapy: an unresolved issue. Lancet Oncol 2002;3(6):333–40.

29. Bari K, Luckett K, Kaiser T, et al. Hepatitis C transmission from seropositive, nonviremic donors to non-hepatitis C liver transplant recipients. Hepatology 2018; 67(5):1673–82.

30. Luckett K, Kaiser TE, Bari K, et al. Use of hepatitis C virus antibody-positive donor livers in hepatitis C nonviremic liver transplant recipients. J Am Coll Surg 2019; 228(4):560–7.

31. Bunchorntavakul C, Reddy KR. Treat chronic hepatitis C virus infection in decompensated cirrhosis - pre- or post-liver transplantation? the ironic conundrum in the era of effective and well-tolerated therapy. J Viral Hepat 2016;23(6):408–18.

32. Aqel B, Wijarnpreecha K, Pungpapong S, et al. Outcomes following liver transplantation from HCV-seropositive donors to HCV-seronegative recipients. J Hepatol 2021;74(4):873–80.

33. Bethea ED, Gaj K, Gustafson JL, et al. Pre-emptive pangenotypic direct acting antiviral therapy in donor HCV-positive to recipient HCV-negative heart transplantation: an open-label study. Lancet Gastroenterol Hepatol 2019;4(10):771–80.

34. Bohorquez H, Bugeaud E, Bzowej N, et al. Liver transplantation using hepatitis C virus-viremic donors into hepatitis C virus-aviremic recipients as standard of care. Liver Transpl 2021;27(4):548–57.

35. Crismale JF, Khalid M, Bhansali A, et al. Liver, simultaneous liver-kidney, and kidney transplantation from hepatitis C-positive donors in hepatitis C-negative recipients: a single-center study. Clin Transplant 2020;34(1):e13761.

36. Hudson MR, Webb AR, Logan AT, et al. Outcomes of hepatitis C virus nucleic acid testing positive donors in aviremic recipients with delayed direct-acting

antiviral initiation. Clin Transplant 2021;35(8):e14386. https://doi.org/10.1111/ctr.14386.

37. Kapila N, Menon KVN, Al-Khalloufi K, et al. Hepatitis C virus NAT-positive solid organ allografts transplanted into hepatitis C virus-negative recipients: a real-world experience. Hepatology 2020;72(1):32–41.

38. Said A, Weiss M, Varhelyi A, et al. Utilization of hepatitis C viremic donors for liver transplant recipients without hepatitis C. A Veterans Transplant Center Report. Transpl Infect Dis 2021;23(2):e13466. https://doi.org/10.1111/tid.13466.

39. Sobotka LA, Mumtaz K, Wellner MR, et al. Outcomes of hepatitis C virus seropositive donors to hepatitis C virus seronegative liver recipients: a large single center analysis. Ann Hepatol 2021;24:100318.

40. Terrault NA, Berenguer M, Strasser SI, et al. International Liver Transplantation Society consensus statement on hepatitis C management in liver transplant recipients. Transplantation 2017;101(5):956–67.

41. Ting PS, Hamilton JP, Gurakar A, et al. Hepatitis C-positive donor liver transplantation for hepatitis C seronegative recipients. Transpl Infect Dis 2019;21(6):e13194.

42. Terrault NA, Burton J, Ghobrial M, et al. Prospective multicenter study of early antiviral therapy in liver and kidney transplant recipients of HCV-viremic donors. Hepatology 2021;73(6):2110–23.

43. Houssel-Debry P, Coilly A, Fougerou-Leurent C, et al. 12 Weeks of a ribavirin-free sofosbuvir and nonstructural protein 5A inhibitor regimen is enough to treat recurrence of hepatitis C after liver transplantation. Hepatology 2018;68(4):1277–87.

44. Kwok RM, Ahn J, Schiano TD, et al. Sofosbuvir plus ledispasvir for recurrent hepatitis C in liver transplant recipients. Liver Transpl 2016;22(11):1536–43.

45. Sise ME, Goldberg DS, Kort JJ, et al. Multicenter study to transplant hepatitis C-infected kidneys (MYTHIC): an open-label study of combined glecaprevir and pibrentasvir to treat recipients of transplanted kidneys from deceased donors with hepatitis C virus infection. J Am Soc Nephrol 2020;31(11):2678–87.

46. Durand CM, Barnaba B, Yu S, et al. Four-week direct-acting antiviral prophylaxis for kidney transplantation from hepatitis C-viremic donors to hepatitis C-negative recipients: an open-label nonrandomized study. Ann Intern Med 2021;174(1):137–8.

47. Reyentovich A, Gidea CG, Smith D, et al. Outcomes of the treatment with glecaprevir/pibrentasvir following heart transplantation utilizing hepatitis C viremic donors. Clin Transplant 2020;34(9):e13989.

48. Smith DE, Chen S, Fargnoli A, et al. Impact of early initiation of direct-acting antiviral therapy in thoracic organ transplantation from hepatitis C virus positive donors. Semin Thorac Cardiovasc Surg 2021;33(2):407–15.

49. Woolley AE, Singh SK, Goldberg HJ, et al. Heart and lung transplants from HCV-infected donors to uninfected recipients. N Engl J Med 2019;380(17):1606–17.

50. Gupta G, Yakubu I, Bhati CS, et al. Ultra-short duration direct acting antiviral prophylaxis to prevent virus transmission from hepatitis C viremic donors to hepatitis C negative kidney transplant recipients. Am J Transplant 2020;20(3):739–51.

51. Murali AR, Chandra S, Stewart Z, et al. Graft versus host disease after liver transplantation in adults: a case series, review of literature, and an approach to management. Transplantation 2016;100(12):2661–70.

52. Chan EY, Larson AM, Gernsheimer TB, et al. Recipient and donor factors influence the incidence of graft-vs.-host disease in liver transplant patients. Liver Transpl 2007;13(4):516–22.

53. Narang TK, Ahrens W, Russo MW. Post–liver transplant cholestatic hepatitis C: a systematic review of clinical and pathological findings and application of consensus criteria. Liver Transplant 2010;16(11):1228–35. https://doi.org/10.1002/lt.22175.
54. Verna EC, Abdelmessih R, Salomao MA, et al. Cholestatic hepatitis C following liver transplantation: an outcome-based histological definition, clinical predictors, and prognosis. Liver Transpl 2013;19(1):78–88.
55. Doughty AL, Spencer JD, Cossart YE, et al. Cholestatic hepatitis after liver transplantation is associated with persistently high serum hepatitis C virus RNA levels. Liver Transpl Surg 1998;4(1):15–21.
56. Gane E. The natural history and outcome of liver transplantation in hepatitis C virus-infected recipients. Liver Transplant 2003;9(11):S28–34.
57. Satapathy SK, Sclair S, Fiel MI, et al. Clinical characterization of patients developing histologically-proven fibrosing cholestatic hepatitis C post-liver transplantation. Hepatol Res 2011;41(4):328–39.
58. Schluger LK, Sheiner PA, Thung SN, et al. Severe recurrent cholestatic hepatitis C following orthotopic liver transplantation. Hepatology 1996;23(5):971–6.
59. Shuhart MC, Bronner MP, Gretch DR, et al. Histological and clinical outcome after liver transplantation for hepatitis C. Hepatology 1997;26(6):1646–52.
60. Molnar MZ, Nair S, Cseprekal O, et al. Transplantation of kidneys from hepatitis C-infected donors to hepatitis C-negative recipients: single center experience. Am J Transpl 2019;19(11):3046–57.
61. Levitsky J, Goldberg D, Smith AR, et al. Acute rejection increases risk of graft failure and death in recent liver transplant recipients. Clin Gastroenterol Hepatol 2017;15(4):584–593 e2.
62. Fisher LR, Henley KS, Lucey MR. Acute cellular rejection after liver transplantation: variability, morbidity, and mortality. Liver Transpl Surg 1995;1(1):10–5.
63. Graham JA, Torabi J, Ajaimy M, et al. Transplantation of viral-positive hepatitis C-positive kidneys into uninfected recipients offers an opportunity to increase organ access. Clin Transplant 2020;34(4):e13833.
64. Wadei HM, Pungpapong S, Cortese C, et al. Transplantation of HCV-infected organs into uninfected recipients: advance with caution. Am J Transpl 2019;19(3):960–1.
65. Sawinski D, Patel N, Appolo B, et al. Use of HCV+ donors does not affect HCV clearance with directly acting antiviral therapy but shortens the wait time to kidney transplantation. Transplantation 2017;101(5):968–73.
66. Smolders EJ, Jansen AME, Ter Horst PGJ, et al. Viral hepatitis C therapy: pharmacokinetic and pharmacodynamic considerations: a 2019 update. Clin Pharm 2019;58(10):1237–63.
67. AASLD-IDSA. Patients with renal impairment. Available at: https://www.hcvguidelines.org/unique-populations/renal-impairment. Accessed September 5 2021.
68. AASLD-IDSA. Recommendations for testing, managing, and treating hepatitis C. Available at: https://www.hcvguidelines.org/. Accessed September 5, 2021.
69. EASL. EASL recommendations on treatment of hepatitis C: final update of the series(✰). J Hepatol 2020;73(5):1170–218.
70. Bronster DJ, Emre S, Boccagni P, et al. Central nervous system complications in liver transplant recipients–incidence, timing, and long-term follow-up. Clin Transplant 2000;14(1):1–7.
71. Shepard PW, St Louis EK. Seizure treatment in transplant patients. Curr Treat Options Neurol 2012;14(4):332–47.

72. An J, Shim JH, Kim SO, et al. Prevalence and prediction of coronary artery disease in patients with liver cirrhosis: a registry-based matched case-control study. Circulation 2014;130(16):1353–62.
73. EASL recommendations on treatment of hepatitis C 2018. J Hepatol 2018;69(2): 461–511.
74. Smolders EJ, Ter Horst PJG, Wolters S, et al. Cardiovascular risk management and hepatitis C: combining drugs. Clin Pharm 2019;58(5):565–92.
75. van Seyen M, Samson AD, Cullen L, et al. Crushed application of sofosbuvir and velpatasvir in a patient with swallowing disorder. Int J Antimicrob Agents 2020; 55(6):105934.
76. Cáceres-Velasco C, Gómez-Sayago L, Marín-Ventura L, et al. 5PSQ-029 Safe administration of sofosbuvir/velpatasvir in a patient with percutaneous endoscopic gastrostomy. British Medical Journal Publishing Group; 2020.
77. Yap J, Jaiswal P, Ton L, et al. Successful treatment of chronic hepatitis C infection with crushed elbasvir/grazoprevir administered via a percutaneous endoscopic gastrostomy tube. J Clin Pharm Ther 2018;43(5):730–2.
78. Jindracek L, Stark J. Treatment of chronic hepatitis C virus infection with crushed ledipasvir/sofosbuvir administered via a percutaneous endoscopic gastrostomy tube. J Pharm Pract 2018;31(5):522–4.
79. Oberoi RK, Zhao W, Sidhu DS, et al. A phase 1 study to evaluate the effect of crushing, cutting into half, or grinding of glecaprevir/pibrentasvir tablets on exposures in healthy subjects. J Pharm Sci 2018;107(6):1724–30.
80. Bethea ED, Samur S, Kanwal F, et al. Cost effectiveness of transplanting HCV-infected livers into uninfected recipients with preemptive antiviral therapy. Clin Gastroenterol Hepatol 2019;17(4):739–47. e8.
81. Kadatz M, Klarenbach S, Gill J, et al. Cost-effectiveness of using kidneys from hepatitis C nucleic acid test-positive donors for transplantation in hepatitis C-negative recipients. Am J Transplant 2018;18(10):2457–64.
82. Goldberg DS, Abt PL, Blumberg EA, et al. Trial of transplantation of HCV-infected kidneys into uninfected recipients. N Engl J Med 2017;376(24):2394–5.
83. Reese PP, Abt PL, Blumberg EA, et al. Twelve-month outcomes after transplant of hepatitis C–infected kidneys into uninfected recipients: a single-group trial. Ann Intern Med 2018;169(5):273–81.
84. Friebus-Kardash J, Gäckler A, Kribben A, et al. Successful early sofosbuvir-based antiviral treatment after transplantation of kidneys from HCV-viremic donors into HCV-negative recipients. Transpl Infect Dis 2019;21(5):e13146.
85. Durand CM, Bowring MG, Brown DM, et al. Direct-acting antiviral prophylaxis in kidney transplantation from hepatitis C virus–infected donors to noninfected recipients: an open-label nonrandomized trial. Ann Intern Med 2018;168(8):533–40.
86. Franco A, Moreso F, Merino E, et al. Renal transplantation from seropositive hepatitis C virus donors to seronegative recipients in Spain: a prospective study. Transpl Int 2019;32(7):710–6.
87. Duerr M, Liefeldt L, Friedersdorff F, et al. Pan-genotype pre-exposure prophylaxis (PrEP) allows transplantation of HCV-positive donor kidneys to negative transplant recipients. J Clin Med 2021;10(1):89.
88. Bethea E, Arvind A, Gustafson J, et al. Immediate administration of antiviral therapy after transplantation of hepatitis C-infected livers into uninfected recipients: implications for therapeutic planning. Am J Transplant 2020;20(6):1619–28.

Simultaneous Liver–Kidney Transplantation

Gayatri Nair, MD, Vinay Nair, DO*

KEYWORDS

- End-stage kidney disease • Liver transplantation • Liver–kidney transplantation
- end-stage liver disease

KEY POINTS

- After the introduction of the model of end-stage liver disease (MELD) score the number of simultaneous liver–kidney (SLK) transplants has risen greater than 300%.
- Liver transplant recipients who develop end-stage kidney disease (ESKD) have significantly greater mortality than those who do not.
- Evaluation for SLK transplantation should include a thorough evaluation for chronic kidney disease (CKD).
- Recent changes in OPTN policy have created strict criteria for SLK listing and a safety net for patients with liver transplant alone (LTA) who develop ESKD within 1-year posttransplant.
- Patients with CKD and prolonged acute kidney injury (AKI) (including dialysis) greater than 6 weeks are at risk for developing ESKD after LTA and are candidates for SLK transplantation.
- Studies are underway to understand if the policy can decrease kidney utilization while maintaining current liver transplant outcomes.

INTRODUCTION

End-stage kidney disease (ESKD) after liver transplantation is associated with high morbidity and mortality. This increase in mortality can be offset by performing a kidney transplant at the time of the liver transplant in select cases. Accordingly, Margreiter and colleagues performed the first simultaneous liver–kidney (SLK) transplant in 1983.[1] The number of SLK transplants has increased by more than 300% since then (**Fig. 1**). In 1990%, 1.7% of all liver transplants in the United States were SLK transplants which increased to 9.9% by 2016.[2–4] This steep increase was likely due to the implementation of the model of end-stage liver disease (MELD) scoring system in 2002, which is heavily weighted by serum creatinine.[5–7]

Division of Kidney Disease and Hypertension, Donald and Barbara Zucker School of Medicine at Hofstra/Northwell, Hempstead, 400 Community Drive, Manhasset, NY 11030, USA
* Corresponding author.
E-mail address: vnair5@northwell.edu

Clin Liver Dis 26 (2022) 313–322
https://doi.org/10.1016/j.cld.2022.01.011
1089-3261/22/© 2022 Elsevier Inc. All rights reserved.
liver.theclinics.com

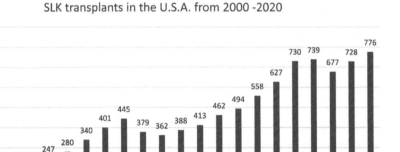

Fig. 1. SLK transplants in the United States from 2000 to 2020. (*Data Obtained from* Organ Procurement & Transplantation Network. Multiple Organ Transplants (Liver-Kidney) in the U.S. by Region from 2000-2020, www.//optn.transplant.hrsa.gov/data/view-data-reports/national-data/# ,accessed 8/25/2021.)

Since the inception of MELD, there have been several consensus conferences organized by the American Society of Transplant Surgeons (ASTS), American Society of Transplant (AST), United Network of Organ Sharing (UNOS), and American Society of Nephrology (ASN) to address the evaluation of kidney disease and candidacy for SLK transplantation in liver transplant candidates. However, it is only recently that the organ procurement and transplant network (OPTN) standardized rules for SLK listing in the United States.

There has been a historical variation in the way that SLK transplantation is practiced among liver transplant centers. This is concerning as SLK candidates are provided higher allocation priority than kidney alone candidates, raising questions regarding fair access to deceased donor organs, especially in kidney transplant alone (KTA) candidates that are highly sensitized, those with extended wait times, or are in the pediatric age group. In addition, the "best" kidneys, as determined by a low kidney donor profile index (KDPI) are often allocated to SLK transplants. KDPI is a score between 1% and 100%, which uses several predictive factors in the donor to determine kidney allograft longevity. High longevity kidneys with a KDPI of less than 35%, which are generally used in pediatric or younger KTA recipients, are historically used in almost 50% of SLK transplants.[8] To ensure fair and judicial use of such organs, the OPTN implemented a new SLK allocation policy in August 2017, which established medical eligibility criteria based on chronic kidney disease (CKD), sustained acute kidney injury (AKI), and certain metabolic disorders. This new policy also created a "safety net" allocation priority for liver transplant recipients with new or worsening kidney function within the first year after transplant.

The main goals of the new SLK allocation policy were to establish clear rules to provide:

- Fair access to transplants to improve patient and kidney allograft survival post-SLK transplant
- Blunt the rise of SLK transplantation without affecting postliver transplant survival
- Increase organ availability for KTA.

In this chapter, we will discuss the prevalence of CKD in end-stage liver disease (ESLD), challenges in accurately assessing CKD in liver transplant candidates, outcomes in SLK transplantation versus liver transplant alone (LTA), and candidate selection for SLK candidates including the 2017 OPTN policy, and the subsequent effect of the policy.

Prevalence of Chronic kidney Disease in Liver Transplant Candidates and Recipients

The true prevalence of kidney disease among patients with liver disease is unknown. In a retrospective study by Chen and colleagues, of 2862 liver transplants performed in Taiwan, 214 developed AKI in the postliver transplant period.[9] The patients that developed AKI postliver transplant were older, had a higher risk of preoperative hypertension (26.64% vs 19.98%, P = .0150), and were more likely to have a history of cerebrovascular events in the preoperative period (6.07% vs 2.76%, P = .006).[9] In another analysis of the OPTN from February 27, 2002, to September 30, 2012, among a total of 2280 adult patients with acute liver failure listed as status 1 or 1A, 56% had kidney dysfunction defined as an estimated glomerular filtration rate (eGFR) < 60 mL/min/1.73 m2 at the time of listing.[10] A higher prevalence of kidney dysfunction was noted in white patients and those who were on life support, and severe kidney dysfunction was associated with significantly increased mortality.[10]

Etiology of Kidney Failure in Patients with Liver Disease

Kidney dysfunction in patients with liver disease is usually multifactorial. AKI can occur due to intravascular volume depletion either caused by gastrointestinal bleeding, excessive diuretic use, or diarrhea from lactulose use.

AKI can also result from the use of nephrotoxic agents such as nonsteroidal antiinflammatory drugs or aminoglycoside antibiotics. Acute tubular necrosis (ATN) secondary to septic shock caused by bacterial infections is a common occurrence.

Patients with liver disease may also have parenchymal kidney diseases including IgA nephropathy and other immune complex-mediated glomerulonephritis associated with Hepatitis C and B. Hepatorenal syndrome (HRS) is a type of kidney failure seen in patients with severe liver cirrhosis. The criteria to diagnose HRS include:

- Cirrhosis with ascites
- Serum Creatinine greater than 1.5 mg/dL
- No improvement in serum creatinine after 2 days of diuretic withdrawal and volume expansion with albumin (1 g/kg)
- Absence of shock
- No current or recent treatment with nephrotoxic drugs
- Absence of parenchymal kidney disease.

The pathophysiology of HRS is mainly related to hypoperfusion of the kidneys secondary to a decrease in effective circulatory volume caused by splanchnic vasodilation that occurs in advanced liver disease. HRS has been divided into type 1 and type 2. In type 2 HRS, kidney dysfunction has a more insidious onset, while HRS type 1 is characterized by a rapidly progressive decline in kidney function which is frequently associated with severe bacterial infections, mainly spontaneous bacterial peritonitis.

Causes of worsening of kidney function after liver transplant are mainly due to:

- Perioperative ATN in the setting of hemodynamic instability
- Preexisting kidney disease

- Calcineurin inhibitor-induced nephrotoxicity
- Comorbid conditions sucha as diabetes mellitus and hypertension.

Evaluation of the Simultaneous Liver–Kidney Transplant Candidate

National Kidney Foundation Guidelines and the AKI Network and Acute Dialysis Quality Initiative Group definitions of AKI and CKD should be used while assessing the candidate's kidney function and category of CKD[11]. The most critical factors include determining AKI versus CKD and the duration of kidney dysfunction. Evaluation for CKD should include the history of comorbid conditions that cause CKD, the trend of GFR over time, kidney ultrasonography, and urinary studies. Comorbid conditions such as diabetes are often associated with CKD, and a higher incidence is seen in patients with microvascular damage such as retinopathy and neuropathy. Trending kidney function over time is extremely important as irreversible CKD requires at least 3 months of reduced kidney function. Kidney ultrasonography often shows small and echogenic kidneys in CKD. Proteinuria on urine analysis is a sign of CKD, while bland urine in the setting of low urine sodium (<20meq/dl) is often a sign of hemodynamic AKI, such as HRS. Recently cystatin C has been identified as a potentially more accurate assessment of kidney function in patients with cirrhosis.[12] Cystatin C is a protein produced by all nucleated cells which are easily filtered in the glomerulus and fully catabolized in the proximal renal tubule, thereby not returned to blood. Unlike serum creatinine, the concentration of serum cystatin C is not affected by gender, age, race, protein intake, and muscle mass which makes it valuable in assessing GFR. However, this method has not been universally accepted. Certain specific characteristics place patients at higher risk for ESKD after a liver transplant. Patients with ESLD with kidney biopsies demonstrating intra-renal fibrosis of greater than 30% and glomerulosclerosis greater than 40% are at high risk for progression to ESKD.[13] Those with low GFR due to CKD are at risk for progression to ESKD after liver transplant, while patients with HRS usually recover kidney function unless there is a prolonged length of kidney injury.[14] However, analysis with radionuclide scans suggests greater than 50% of patients may recover some degree of native kidney function after SLK transplantation.[15] Even among a study of SLK listed patients who receive liver transplantation alone, one-third improved their kidney function to an eGFR greater than 60 mL/min, and less than 5% needed kidney transplantation[16] in the subsequent year.

Once the patient is listed for SLK transplantation, kidney function should be periodically assessed at regular time points to calculate the MELD status and assess the reversibility of kidney dysfunction.

Organ Procurement and Transplant Network Simultaneous Liver–Kidney Allocation Criteria

Once a patient who is listed for SLK transplantation receives a local liver transplant offer, the kidney follows the liver. In other words, a patient with a high MELD who receives a local liver offer will pull the donor kidney regardless of kidney function and time with kidney dysfunction. This has led to significant variation in SLK listing and transplantation throughout transplant centers in the US. In an attempt to decrease the variation between SLK transplantation, and ensure fair utilization, OPTN introduced formal criteria for SLK listing on August 10th, 2017.[17] According to this policy, liver transplant candidates who meet one of the following criteria are eligible for SLK allocation.

1. Diagnosis of CKD with a Measured or Calculated GFR of ≤60 mL/min for More than 90 Consecutive d	AND at Least One of the following at the Time of Waiting List Registration: • ESKD on Dialysis OR • Measured or Calculated Creatinine Clearance or GFR ≤30 mL/min
2. Sustained AKI demonstrated by GFR < 25 mL/min	AND at least one of the following for the last 6 wks • Dialysis at least once every 7 d OR • Measured or calculated creatinine clearance or GFR of ≤25 mL/min documented at least once every 7 d
3. Metabolic Disease with a diagnosis of at least one of the following	• Hyperoxaluria • Atypical hemolytic uremic syndrome from mutations in factor H or factor I • Familial nonneuropathic systemic amyloidosis • Methylmalonic aciduria

Pediatric SLK candidates are exempted from medical eligibility criteria and can be listed for both organs on the waiting list to receive SLK offers.

In addition, a "safety net" was created to help LTA candidates whose kidney function did not improve or those who developed advanced CKD shortly after liver transplant. These patients are given priority for kidneys with a KDPI greater than 20% if they met they met the following requirements:

- The candidate must be registered on the kidney waiting list between 60 and 365 days after liver transplantation.

AND.

- The candidate is either on chronic dialysis or has a measured or calculated creatinine clearance or GFR of ≤20 mL/min.

The priority scheme of safety net patients is as follows:

Sequence a KDPI ≤ 20%	Sequence a KDPI > 20% < 35%	Sequence a KDPI ≥ 35% ≤ 85%	Sequence a KDPI > 85%
Not applicable	Highly Sensitized 0 ABDR mm Prior living donor Local pediatrics *Local Safety Net* Local adults Regional pediatrics Regional adults National pediatrics National adults	Highly Sensitized 0 ABDR mm Prior living donor *Local Safety Net* Local Regional National	Highly Sensitized 0 ABDR mm *Local Safety Net* Local and regional National

KDPI, kidney donor profile index; 0 ABDR mm, 0 HLA A, B, DR antigen mismatch.

Blood Type and Human Leukocyte Antigen (HLA) Compatibility

In both liver and kidney transplantation, the donor blood type should be compatible with the recipient's blood type. However, as opposed to liver transplantation alone, kidney transplantation requires more attention to HLA and HLA antibody testing as the kidney allograft is susceptible to antibody-mediated rejection.

Standard kidney transplantation is avoided in patients with elevated titers of anti-HLA antibodies to their donors as determined by solid-phase or crossmatch testing.

Interestingly when performing an SLK transplant, the liver confers some degree of protection to the kidney from antibody-mediated rejection. Mechanisms are unclear but may be related to the large surface area of the liver absorbing these antibodies or even by possibly changing the gene expression in the kidney.[18] However, even with the liver's protection, some studies have found greater degrees of chronic rejection in kidney allografts as part of SLK transplantation when performed across HLA compatibility barriers.[19] Thus, the risk versus benefit ratio must be considered when performing an SLK transplant when some degree of HLA incompatibility exists.

Surgical Technique

The liver is transplanted first, followed by the kidney. This is based on the shorter preservation time of the liver and because the liver (almost always from the same donor) can clear preformed antibodies that could otherwise have a detrimental effect on the kidney. The native liver is removed and then replaced by the donor liver in the same anatomic position. A bilateral subcostal incision with a midline extension to the xiphoid process is routinely used, and a hepatectomy is undertaken by either the classic or piggyback approaches. In the classic approach, the recipient IVC is resected with the interruption of the venous return. This hemodynamic change usually requires the institution of venovenous bypass to deliver blood from the infrahepatic IVC and portal vein via a pump into the SVC (superior vena cava) and right atrium. In the piggyback technique, the native IVC is preserved, avoiding the need for a venovenous bypass. According to the approach used for the hepatectomy, the implantation will entail a cava replacement (classic approach) or piggyback implantation whereby the donor IVC is attached to the recipient IVC either side-to-side or to the opening of the suprahepatic veins. After IVC reconstruction by either technique, the portal vein of the donor is anastomosed to the portal vein stump of the recipient. This allows for the reperfusion of the transplanted liver. Once the liver is reperfused, the hepatic artery and biliary system are also reconstructed. The biliary anastomosis can be performed either in an end-to-end fashion (between the bile ducts of the donor and the recipient) or by using a Roux-en-Y hepaticojejunostomy (if the recipient's bile duct is diseased). Based on the surgeon's preference, a biliary stent/tube can be left in place. After skin closure, the kidney is transplanted through a separate incision in the right or left lower quadrant of the abdomen. The native kidneys are not removed. The graft is placed retro- and extraperitoneally in the iliac fossa, most commonly on the right side. The anastomosis is usually performed between the donor renal and the recipient's external iliac vessels. The kidney is reperfused with blood, and the ureter is subsequently anastomosed to the bladder (a ureteral stent may be used based on the surgeon's preference). In patients on dialysis with prolonged operative times, continuous venovenous hemodialysis may be performed intraoperatively to maintain the stability of fluid and electrolyte status.

In recent years, an alternative approach called the en bloc technique has been used in some centers, whereby the liver and kidney are procured together.[20] The renal vein remains attached to the inferior vena cava, while the donor renal artery is anastomosed to the donor splenic artery, resulting in simultaneous reperfusion of both organs after implantation. This technique maintains renal outflow via donor infrahepatic vena cava and inflow via anastomosis of donor renal artery to donor splenic artery.

Outcomes in Liver Transplant Alone Versus Simultaneous Liver–Kidney Transplantation

The main impetus for performing SLK transplants is to abrogate the poor graft and patient outcomes in liver transplant recipients with kidney dysfunction.[21–24]

It is known that kidney dysfunction in itself can affect mortality after liver transplantation, especially in patients who are already requiring hemodialysis.[25] Furthermore, both the pretransplant and posttransplant creatinine are predictors of mortality in liver transplantation. Therefore, it could be assumed that performing a simultaneous kidney transplant would improve outcomes in these liver transplant recipients.

Several studies suggest that patients with CKD and especially dialysis dependence have worse mortality if they receive an LTA. Such complex patients have superior outcomes when they undergo an SLK transplant.[26,27] The outcomes of patients who undergo SLK transplantation show equivalent graft survivals compared with patients without CKD or ESKD that undergo LTA.[26] In one study, patients with serum creatinine greater than 2.5 mg/dl or dependence on dialysis had lower mortality with SLK versus LTA. Even when removing patients who died within the first 48 hours, outcomes with SLK transplantation were superior.

However, certain patients may be too sick to undergo SLK transplantation. Patients with SLK transplants have a higher incidence of bacterial infections, increased transfusion requirements, more prolonged ICU, and hospital length of stay than LTA. Lunsford and colleagues[28] found that SLK transplant recipients that needed renal replacement therapy 3 months after transplant did exceptionally poorly. These recipients had greater MELD scores, length of hospitalization, intraoperative base deficit, higher incidence of female donors, kidney and liver donor risk indices, kidney cold ischemia, and inferior overall survival.

Challenges to Simultaneous Liver–Kidney Transplantation

The most pressing challenge to SLK transplantation is appropriately identifying the best candidates for receiving 2 very scarce organs. As previously mentioned, patients with liver failure have higher mortality if they develop ESKD either before or immediately after liver transplant. Many of the patients at risk for developing ESKD postliver transplant are predialysis at the time of listing, making decision-making difficult. Transplanting a patient who may have adequate or reversible kidney dysfunction postliver transplant may pose an ethical dilemma as the organ could have been used for a patient on the kidney transplant waitlist. In addition, an SLK recipient often receives a kidney from a deceased donor with a KDPI of less than 35%, which would have otherwise been prioritized to a pediatric kidney alone recipient. This potentially decreases the total life-years gained from the kidney transplant. Several studies suggest that a kidney allograft will last longer if placed into a kidney alone recipient rather than used as part of an SLK transplant. For example, Hart and colleagues found poor 1-year kidney graft survival in SLK recipients compared with KTA.[29] SLK recipient's 1-year graft survival was 83% versus 93% in kidney alone transplants. This inferior graft survival is mainly driven by patient death.[30–38] The previously mentioned article by Lunsford and colleagues evaluating futility in SLK transplantation may explain this finding. Therefore, SLK transplantation should be reserved for liver transplant candidates who are unlikely to have kidney recovery after liver transplantation but are not too sick, whereby SLK transplantation will be futile.

As the formal OPTN SLK transplantation policy took place, studies have begun critically evaluating the policy change. The most recent study comes from Wilk and colleagues who performed a 2-year review of the OPTN policy. Within the 2 years after implementation (2017–2019), SLK registrations stayed relatively stable, whereas SLK transplantation was rising until 2017. In 2018, SLK transplants decreased by 9% but then increased by 8% in 2019. Two years after implementation, the net change was that the number of SLK transplants was still 1.6% below 2017. In 2020 the absolute number of SLK transplants was the same as prepolicy, but the total percent SLK remained below prepolicy numbers (due to a higher number of total transplants). Eligible kidney after liver safety net registrations continued to increase after policy implementation. The number of kidneys after liver transplants increased from 0.2% to 0.6% of all deceased donor kidney transplants. Wait times for kidneys after liver transplants decreased after the implementation of the safety net. One-year posttransplant patient and graft survival for SLK transplants was unchanged postpolicy. LTA patient and graft survival were unchanged. Overall, the data suggest that the OPTN policy resulted in slightly fewer kidney transplants in liver transplant candidates without change in mortality or graft outcome.

CONCLUSIONS

Kidney dysfunction in the postliver transplant period results in inferior liver transplant patient and graft survival. Such patients may benefit from SLK transplantation.

Assessing reversibility in kidney dysfunction is challenging but of utmost importance when deciding which patient should be listed for SLK transplantation. An ideal candidate is one with a low likelihood of kidney recovery but at the same time healthy enough so that the SLK transplant will not be futile. To ensure fair and proper allocation of these vital organs, the OPTN created standardized SLK criteria and a "safety net" in 2017. Early analysis of policy change suggests some degree of success in curbing the rising number of SLK transplants while not hurting liver transplant outcomes. Though this is a step in the right direction, there is a need for continued refinement and consensus to determine the best patients to undergo SLK. Further single-center and national database analysis are paramount to improving the practice of SLK.

REFERENCES

1. Margreiter R, Kramar R, Huber C, et al. Combined liver and kidney transplantation. Lancet 1984;1(8385):1077–8.
2. Puri V, Eason J. Simultaneous liver-kidney transplantation. Curr Transpl Rep 2015; 2(4):297–302.
3. Kim WR, Lake JR, Smith JM, et al. Liver. Am J Transpl 2016;16(Suppl 2):69–98.
4. Lum EL, Cardenas A, Martin P, et al. Current status of simultaneous liver-kidney transplantation in the United States. Liver Transpl 2019;25(5):797–806.
5. Edwards EB, Harper AM. The impact of MELD on OPTN liver allocation: preliminary results. Clin Transpl 2002;21–8.
6. Eason JD, Gonwa TA, Davis CL, et al. Proceedings of consensus conference on simultaneous liver kidney transplantation (SLK). Am J Transpl 2008;8(11): 2243–51.
7. Nadim MK, Davis CL, Sung R, et al. Simultaneous liver-kidney transplantation: a survey of US transplant centers. Am J Transpl 2012;12(11):3119–27.
8. Formica RN, Aeder M, Boyle G, et al. Simultaneous liver-kidney allocation policy: a proposal to optimize appropriate utilization of scarce resources. Am J Transpl 2016;16(3):758–66.
9. Chen HP, Tsai YF, Lin JR, et al. Incidence and outcomes of acute renal failure following liver transplantation: a population-based cohort study. Medicine (Baltimore) 2015;94(52):e2320.

10. Urrunaga NH, Magder LS, Weir MR, et al. Prevalence, severity, and impact of renal dysfunction in acute liver failure on the US liver transplant waiting list. Dig Dis Sci 2016;61(1):309–16.

11. Brennan TV, Lunsford KE, Vagefi PA, et al. Renal outcomes of simultaneous liver-kidney transplantation compared to liver transplant alone for candidates with renal dysfunction. Clin Transpl 2015;29(1):34–43.

12. Davis CL, Feng S, Sung R, et al. Simultaneous liver-kidney transplantation: evaluation to decision making. Am J Transpl 2007;7(7):1702–9.

13. Levey AS, Coresh J, Balk E, et al. National Kidney Foundation practice guidelines for chronic kidney disease: evaluation, classification, and stratification. Ann Intern Med 2003;139(2):137–47.

14. Poge U, Gerhardt T, Stoffel-Wagner B, et al. Calculation of glomerular filtration rate based on cystatin C in cirrhotic patients. Nephrol Dial Transpl 2006;21(3):660–4.

15. Pichler RH, Huskey J, Kowalewska J, et al. Kidney biopsies may help predict renal function after liver transplantation. Transplantation 2016;100(10):2122–8.

16. Ruiz R, Jennings LW, Kim P, et al. Indications for combined liver and kidney transplantation: propositions after a 23-yr experience. Clin Transpl 2010;24(6):807–11.

17. Nair S, Verma S, Thuluvath PJ. Pretransplant renal function predicts survival in patients undergoing orthotopic liver transplantation. Hepatology 2002;35(5):1179–85.

18. Gonwa TA, Klintmalm GB, Levy M, et al. Impact of pretransplant renal function on survival after liver transplantation. Transplantation 1995;59(3):361–5.

19. Gonwa TA, McBride MA, Anderson K, et al. Continued influence of preoperative renal function on outcome of orthotopic liver transplant (OLTX) in the US: where will MELD lead us? Am J Transpl 2006;6(11):2651–9.

20. Ojo AO, Held PJ, Port FK, et al. Chronic renal failure after transplantation of a non-renal organ. N Engl J Med 2003;349(10):931–40.

21. Narayanan Menon KV, Nyberg SL, Harmsen WS, et al. MELD and other factors associated with survival after liver transplantation. Am J Transpl 2004;4(5):819–25.

22. Organ Procurement and Transplantation Network. Simultaneous liver kidney allocation policy. 2017.

23. Levitsky J, Baker T, Ahya SN, et al. Outcomes and native renal recovery following simultaneous liver-kidney transplantation. Am J Transpl 2012;12(11):2949–57.

24. Hmoud B, Kuo YF, Wiesner RH, et al. Outcomes of liver transplantation alone after listing for simultaneous kidney: comparison to simultaneous liver kidney transplantation. Transplantation 2015;99(4):823–8.

25. Taner T, Park WD, Stegall MD. Unique molecular changes in kidney allografts after simultaneous liver-kidney compared with solitary kidney transplantation. Kidney Int 2017;91(5):1193–202.

26. Sellarés J, Reeve J, Loupy A, et al. Molecular diagnosis of antibody-mediated rejection in human kidney transplants. Am J Transpl 2013;13(4):971–83.

27. Lunsford KE, Bodzin AS, Markovic D, et al. Avoiding futility in simultaneous liver-kidney transplantation: analysis of 331 consecutive patients listed for dual organ replacement. Ann Surg 2017;265(5):1016–24.

28. Hart A, Smith JM, Skeans MA, et al. Kidney. Am J Transpl 2016;16(Suppl 2):11–46.

29. Singal AK, Ong S, Satapathy SK, et al. Simultaneous liver kidney transplantation. Transpl Int 2019;32(4):343–52.

30. Sung RS, Wiseman AC. Simultaneous liver-kidney transplant: too many or just enough? Adv Chronic Kidney Dis 2015;22(5):399–403.

31. Francoz C, Durand F, Kahn JA, et al. Hepatorenal syndrome. Clin J Am Soc Nephrol 2019;14(5):774–81.

32. Cheng XS, Khush KK, Wiseman A, et al. To kidney or not to kidney: applying lessons learned from the simultaneous liver-kidney transplant policy to simultaneous heart-kidney transplantation. Clin Transpl 2020;34(6):e13878.

33. Cheng XS, Kim WR, Tan JC, et al. Comparing simultaneous liver-kidney transplant strategies: a modified cost-effectiveness analysis. Transplantation 2018;102(5): e219–28.

34. Goyes D, Nsubuga JP, Medina-Morales E, et al. New OPTN simultaneous liver-kidney transplant (SLKT) policy improves racial and ethnic disparities. J Clin Med 2020;9(12):3901.

35. Bari K, Sharma P. Optimizing the selection of patients for simultaneous liver-kidney transplant. Clin Liver Dis 2021;25(1):89–102.

36. Cullaro G, Hirose R, Lai JC. Changes in simultaneous liver-kidney transplant allocation policy may impact postliver transplant outcomes. Transplantation 2019; 103(5):959–64.

37. Formica RN Jr. Simultaneous liver kidney transplantation. Curr Opin Nephrol Hypertens 2016;25(6):577–82.

38. Lee TC, Cortez AR, Kassam AF, et al. Outcomes of en bloc simultaneous liver-kidney transplantation compared to the traditional technique. Am J Transpl 2020;20(4):1181–7.

Chronic Kidney Disease After Liver Transplantation

Ramon O. Minjares, MD[a],*, Paul Martin, MD[b], Andres F. Carrion, MD[b]

KEYWORDS

- Chronic kidney disease • Acute kidney injury • Liver transplantation
- Immunosuppressive regimen

KEY POINTS

- The prevalence of renal dysfunction in liver transplant (LT) recipients continues to rise, paralleling increased long-term survival of the population.
- Etiology of renal dysfunction in LT recipients is typically multifactorial, with calcineurin inhibitors (CNIs) and pretransplant renal dysfunction representing major risk factors.
- Systemic hypertension is evident typically early after initiation of CNI therapy. Posttransplant diabetes is associated with the long-term use of CNIs. These conditions further increase the risk of renal dysfunction in LT recipients.
- Criteria to select candidates for simultaneous liver-kidney transplantation have been established, highlighting that recovery of renal function may not be anticipated in selected patients.
- Both delayed introduction of CNIs and renal-sparing immunosuppressive regimens offer some benefit with regards to reducing the progression of renal dysfunction and are currently used on an individual basis by most transplant centers.

INTRODUCTION

Improved survival after liver transplantation (LT) has led to an aging cohort of recipients at risk of renal dysfunction. The etiology of renal dysfunction in LT recipients is typically multifactorial; chronic immunosuppression with calcineurin inhibitors (CNIs), pretransplant renal dysfunction, and perioperative acute kidney injury (AKI) are important risk factors.[1,2] In addition, common metabolic complications such as hypertension (HTN), diabetes mellitus (DM), hyperlipidemia, obesity, and metabolic-associated fatty liver disease (MAFLD) contribute to the development of renal

[a] Department of Internal Medicine, University of Miami Miller School of Medicine, 1611 NW 12th Avenue, Suite 600-D, Miami, FL 33136, USA; [b] Division of Digestive Health and Liver Diseases, Department of Medicine, University of Miami Miller School of Medicine, 1611 NW 12th Avenue, Suite 600-D, Miami, FL 33136, USA
* Corresponding author. Department of Internal Medicine, University of Miami Miller School of Medicine, Jackson Memorial Hospital, 1611 NW 12th Avenue, Suite 600-D, Miami, FL 33136.
E-mail address: rom25@miami.edu

Clin Liver Dis 26 (2022) 323–340
https://doi.org/10.1016/j.cld.2022.01.006
1089-3261/22/© 2022 Elsevier Inc. All rights reserved.

liver.theclinics.com

disease.[3] Hepatitis C virus (HCV) infection is also associated with renal disease; however, the use of direct-acting antiviral agents has mitigated this complication.[4] Most LT recipients who survive greater than 6 months will develop some degree of renal dysfunction resulting in chronic kidney disease (CKD).[1] Although the severity of CKD is highly variable, 5% to 8% of LT recipients develop end-stage renal disease (ESRD) requiring renal replacement therapy (RRT) during the first 10 years posttransplant.[5]

DEFINITIONS OF AKI AND CKD

AKI refers to an abrupt decrease in kidney function and encompasses a spectrum of severity, from minor changes in markers of renal function to a requirement for RRT. Several consensus definitions of AKI have been developed based on the serum creatinine (sCr) and urine output (UO) (**Table 1**).[6] Etiologies of AKI include specific kidney diseases (eg, acute interstitial nephritis, acute glomerulonephritis, vasculitis, etc), nonspecific conditions (eg, ischemia, toxic injury), as well as extrarenal pathology (eg, obstructive nephropathy). It is possible that several of these conditions may coexist in the same patient. Prompt recognition is important, as even mild, potentially reversible AKI has important clinical consequences, including an increased risk of death.[7]

AKI has been difficult to define in patients with liver disease as diminished muscle mass in cirrhosis leads to spuriously low sCr levels. In 2012, the Acute Dialysis Quality Initiative (ADQI) recommended adaptation of the Acute Kidney Injury Network (AKIN) criteria to define AKI in patients with cirrhosis instead of the traditional definition using a fixed sCr level greater than 1.5 mg/dL.[8] In 2015, an International Consensus Conference and the International Club of Ascites (ICA) defined AKI in cirrhosis based on the Kidney Disease Improving Global Outcomes (KDIGO) definition, which is an increase in sCr $\geq$ 0.3 mg/dL within 48 hours or a $\geq$50% increase in sCr from baseline that is known or presumed to have occurred within the prior 7 days. The organization defined the 3 stages of AKI (stages 1, 2, and 3). However, recent data have suggested that stage 1 AKI consists of a heterogeneous group of patients with different clinical outcomes depending on whether the final sCr level is greater than or less than 1.5 mg/dL.[9] For this reason, current guidelines from the European Association for the Study of the Liver (EASL) recommend that clinicians should separate these 2 groups of patients into AKI stages 1a or 1b to describe patients with an sCr level at diagnosis below or above 1.5 mg/dL, respectively.[10] **Table 2** highlights the new definition of AKI in cirrhosis and incorporates the modification of AKI stage 1.

CKD is a heterogeneous group of disorders characterized by alterations in kidney structure and function. It is defined by the presence of kidney damage or diminished kidney function (<60 mL/min/1.73 m^2) for $\geq$90 days and it is classified based on glomerular filtration rate (GFR) and degree of albuminuria. The etiology of CKD is also included in the KDIGO revised classification. The purpose of staging is to guide management and stratify risk for progression and complications. In practice, patients who have estimated glomerular filtration rate (eGFR) < 60 mL/min/1.73 m^2 have a significantly increased risk for all-cause and cardiovascular mortality. The classification and staging of CKD are described in **Table 3**.

HEPATORENAL SYNDROME

Hepatorenal syndrome (HRS) is defined as renal dysfunction in patients with cirrhosis in the absence of an alternative explanation. It results from pathophysiologic derangements typical of severe chronic liver disease which may also occur in acute liver

Table 1
Diagnostic criteria and classification of acute kidney injury based on severity

	KDIGO (2012)	AKIN (2007)	RIFLE (2004)
Diagnostic criteria	Increase in sCr by ≥ 0.3 mg/dL within 48 h; or increase in sCr ≥1.5x baseline, which is known or presumed to be within the prior 7 d; or urine output < 0.5 mL/kg/h for 6 h.	Increase in sCr by ≥ 0.3 mg/dL within 48 h; or increase in sCr ≥1.5x baseline within 48 h; or urine volume <0.5 mL/kg/h for 6 h	Increase in sCr to ≥1.5x baseline, within 7 d; or GFR decrease >25%; or urine volume <0.5 mL/kg/h for 6 h
Staging	Stage 1: • Increase in SCr by ≥ 0.3 mg/dL or to 1.5–1.9x baseline OR • Urine output < 0.5 mL/kg/h for 6–12 h Stage 2: • Increase in SCr to 2–2.9x baseline OR • Urine output of <0.5 mL/kg/h for 12–24 h Stage 3: • Increase in SCr to ≥3.0x baseline OR • Increase in SCr to ≥4.0 mg/dL OR • Urine output of <0.3 mL/kg/h for ≥24 h or anuria for ≥12 h OR • Initiation of RRT	Stage 1: • Increase in SCr by ≥ 0.3 mg/dL or to 150%–200% baseline OR • Urine output of <0.5 mL/kg/h for 6–12 h Stage 2: • Increase in SCr to 200%–300% baseline OR • Urine output of <0.5 mL/kg/h for 12–24 h Stage 3: • Increase in SCr to >300% baseline OR • Increase in SCr by > 0.5 mg/dL to ≥4.0 mg/dL OR • Urine output of <0.3 mL/kg/h for >24 h or anuria for >12 h OR • Initiation of RRT	Risk: • Increase in SCr to 1.5x baseline OR • Urine output of <0.5 mL/kg/h for 6–12 h Injury: • Increase in SCr to 2x baseline OR • Urine output of <0.5 mL/kg/h for 12–24 h Failure: • Increase in SCr to 3x baseline OR • Increase in SCr by > 0.5 mg/dL to >4.0 mg/dL OR • Urine output of <0.3 mL/kg/h for >24 h or anuria for >12 h OR • Initiation of RRT Loss • Need for RRT for >4 wk End-stage renal disease: • Need for RRT for >3 mo

Abbreviations: AKIN, Acute Kidney Injury Network; GFR, glomerular filtration rate; KDIGO, Kidney Disease Improving Global Outcome; RIFLE, risk, injury, failure, loss, end-stage renal disease; RRT, renal replacement therapy; SCr, serum creatinine.

Table 2
International Club of Ascites (ICA-AKI) new definitions for the diagnosis and management of AKI in patients with cirrhosis

Subject	Definition
Baseline sCr	• A value of sCr obtained in the previous 3 mo, when available, can be used as baseline sCr. In patients with more than one value within the previous 3 mo, the value closest to the admission time to the hospital should be used. • In patients without a previous sCr value, the sCr on admission should be used as baseline.
Definition of AKI	• An absolute increase in sCr ≥0.3 mg/dL within 48 h; or, • A percentage increase sCr ≥50% from baseline which is known, or presumed, to have occurred within the prior 7 d.
Staging of AKI	Stage 1a[a]: Increase of 0.3 mg/dL from baseline in 48 h, 1.5–2 × baseline sCr. Absolute value of sCr < 1.5 mg/dL Stage 1b[a]: Increase of 0.3 mg/dL from baseline in 48 h, 1.5–2 × baseline sCr. Absolute value of sCr > 1.5 mg/dL. Stage 2: Increase of 2–3 × baseline Stage 3: >3 × baseline sCr, sCr ≥4 mg/dL with an increase ≥0.3 mg/dL, or initiation of RRT
Progression of AKI	• Progression: progression of AKI to a higher stage and/or need for RRT. • Regression: regression of AKI to a lower stage.
Response to treatment	• No response: No regression of AKI. • Partial response: Regression of AKI stage with a reduction of sCr to ≥0.3 mg/dL above the baseline value. • Full response: return of sCr to a value within 0.3 mg/dL of the baseline value

Abbreviations: AKI, acute kidney injury; RRT, renal replacement therapy; sCr, serum creatinine.
[a] Modified by the European Association for the Study of the Liver.

failure.[11] Importantly, HRS is a diagnosis of exclusion and may be particularly difficult to differentiate from acute tubular necrosis. Recent changes in the nomenclature of HRS need to be highlighted: Type 1 HRS, now renamed HRS-AKI, occurs in an acute setting and is a rapidly progressive decline in renal function associated with high

Table 3
Chronic kidney disease classification according to KDIGO and K/DOQI guidelines

GFR Stage	GFR (ml/min/1.73 m^2)	Terms
G1	≥90	Normal or high
G2	60–89	Mildly decreased
G3		
• G3a	45–59	Mildly to moderately decreased
• G3b	30–44	Moderately to severely decreased
G4	15–29	Severely decreased
G5	<15 (or dialysis)	Kidney failure

Albuminuria	Albumin Excretion Rate (mg/d)	Terms
A1	<30	Normal to mildly increased
A2	30–300	Moderately increased
A3	>300	Severely increased

mortality. Type 2 HRS, renamed HRS–non-AKI (HRS-NAKI), follows a more protracted clinical course evolving over weeks to months but is also associated with poor median survival (6 months).[12] The most recent diagnostic criteria and definitions for HRS are summarized in **Table 4**.

The pathogenesis of HRS includes both hemodynamic and inflammatory changes. Portal HTN triggers arterial vasodilation in the splanchnic circulation, which appears to play a central role in hemodynamic changes and decline in kidney function. The putative mechanism is increased production or activity of vasodilators in the splanchnic circulation (mainly mediated by nitric oxide). As the liver disease becomes more severe, there is an increase in cardiac output and a fall in systemic resistance despite activation of the renin-angiotensin-aldosterone system (RAAS) and sympathetic nervous system. The decline in kidney perfusion in this setting is associated with reductions in GFR and a fall in mean arterial pressure, despite intense renal vasoconstriction.[10,13]

Systemic inflammation may also have a role in the development of HRS. A synergic interplay of inflammation and microvascular dysfunction is responsible for the amplification of the signal that pathogen-associated molecular patterns and damage-associated molecular patterns exert on proximal epithelial tubular cells. Recognition of this signal and its subsequent spread to other proximal tubular epithelial cells may cause mitochondria-mediated metabolic downregulation. The sacrificed functions include the reabsorption of sodium and chloride. This consequently increases the delivery of sodium chloride to the macula densa, further activating the RAAS and thus lowering GFR. Furthermore, advanced cirrhosis is now considered a proinflammatory state. Patients with advanced liver disease have significantly higher levels of proinflammatory cytokines (ie, interleukin [IL]-6, tumor necrosis factor [TNF]-alpha, IL-7, IL-5, IL-12) and chemoattractants, including monocyte chemoattractant protein-1.[14,15] Cirrhosis is also associated with bacterial translocation from the intestinal

Table 4	
Current definition of hepatorenal syndrome	
Criteria to confirm HRS vs. other etiology of renal dysfunction	Diagnosis of cirrhosis with ascites
	Diagnosis of AKI according to ICA-AKI criteria
	Absence of shock
	No sustained improvement of renal function (sCr <1.5 mg/dL) following at least 2 d of diuretic withdrawal, and volume expansion with albumin at 1 g/kg/d up to a maximum of 100 g/d
	No current or recent exposure to nephrotoxic agents
	Absence of parenchymal renal disease as defined by:
	• proteinuria <0.5 g/d
	• no microhematuria (>50 RBCs/high-power field)
	• normal findings on renal ultrasonography
Definition of HRS-AKI	Patients who meet the criteria above and have a diagnosis of AKI according to International Club of Ascites – Acute Kidney Injury (2015 criteria).
Definition of HRS-CKD	Patients who meet the criteria for HRS and the rise of serum creatinine and changes in urine output are all progressive. eGFR <60 ml/min per 1.73 m² for ≥3 months.

Abbreviations: AKI, acute kidney injury; ICA, International Club of Ascites; RBCs, red blood cells; sCr, serum creatinine; eGFR, estimated glomerular filtration rate; HRS, hepatorenal syndrome; CKD, chronic kidney disease.

lumen, resulting in systemic endotoxemia; however, a clinically overt bacterial infection (eg, spontaneous bacterial peritonitis [SBP] or urinary tract infection) is often the main trigger for the development of HRS in this population.[16] All these findings suggest that the pathophysiology of AKI, and particularly of HRS-AKI, in patients with decompensated cirrhosis is more complex than previously hypothesized, supporting the concept that HRS-AKI is not purely functional in nature.

ASSESSING RENAL FUNCTION

Serum levels of some endogenous filtration markers (such as creatinine) are commonly used to estimate the GFR, as this is difficult to measure directly. However, sCr as a measure of renal function has important limitations in patients with chronic liver disease.[17] Diminished muscle mass and increased tubular secretion of creatinine result in spuriously low sCr levels, potentially overestimating renal function. As in the general population, sCr levels are lower in women than men and higher in non-Hispanic black people than non-Hispanic white people.[18] Furthermore, hyperbilirubinemia interferes with estimation of sCr levels when measured by some commercial assays. Commonly used formulas to estimate the GFR, such as the Modification of Diet in Renal Disease (MDRD), CKD-Epidemiology Collaboration (CKD-EPI), and Cockcroft–Gault include sCr and consequently frequently overestimate renal function in specific populations. Although accurate markers of GFR do exist (ie, inulin, iothalamate, iohexol, cystatin C, symmetric dimethylarginine, beta-trace protein, beta-2 microglobulin), their applicability in routine clinical practice is limited.[5]

Biomarkers of tubular injury such as urinary neutrophil gelatinase-associated lipocalin (uNGAL) have utility in differentiating the etiology of renal dysfunction in patients with cirrhosis: acute tubular necrosis (higher uNGAL levels) versus prerenal azotemia due to volume depletion, CKD, and HRS. Furthermore, uNGAL may also provide predictive information with respect to short-term inpatient mortality in patients with cirrhosis. Other biomarkers studied in patients with cirrhosis and renal dysfunction include IL-18, kidney injury molecule-1 (KIM-1), and liver-type fatty acid-binding protein (L-FABP).[19,20]

The use of UO as a criterion for AKI in patients with cirrhosis is somewhat controversial. Limitations of its use in this population include avid sodium and water retention due to splanchnic hemodynamic variations, frequent use of diuretics, and difficulties estimating the actual body weight. However, UO appears to be useful in stratifying the severity of AKI in patients with cirrhosis without elevation of sCr. A recent study in critically ill patients with chronic liver disease has demonstrated a significant increase in mortality in patients who met UO criteria for AKI.[21]

RENAL DYSFUNCTION IN LT CANDIDATES

Advanced liver disease can impact renal function because of several mechanisms, including acute bleeding with hypovolemia, glomerular diseases such as cryoglobulinemia in HCV infection and IgA nephropathy in alcohol-related cirrhosis, as well as a variety of other insults including nephrotoxic medications and intravenous contrast. Pre-existing renal dysfunction in patients with cirrhosis is an independent predictor of poor outcomes post-LT reflected in prolonged length of intensive care stay and need for RRT.[22] Renal dysfunction's prognostic significance is reflected by inclusion of sCr in the Model for End-Stage Liver Disease (MELD). Since the implementation of the MELD score-based allocation system, there has been a sharp rise in the number of transplant candidates with impaired renal function.[23] This may also be related in part to the increasing prevalence of metabolic risk factors such as obesity, HTN, DM, and

MAFLD. Although prolonged RRT (>6 weeks) has been clearly identified as a risk factor for mortality post-LT and is used as a criterion to qualify for simultaneous liver and kidney transplantation (SLKT), short-term (<4 weeks) need for RRT before LT has no impact on 1-year mortality posttransplant.[22]

MAFLD is independently associated with increased incidence of CKD.[24] Nonalcoholic steatohepatitis (NASH) is the second leading cause of liver disease in patients awaiting LT in the United States.[25] The severity of MAFLD correlates with stage of CKD[26] and compared with other etiologies of cirrhosis, LT candidates with MAFLD have the lowest GFR.[27] NASH is the fastest rising indication for SLKT in the United States, increasing from 6.3% of SLKT in 2002 to 19.2% in 2011.[28] Molnar and colleagues compared pre-LT eGFR and post-LT renal recovery in 4088 NASH LT recipients from the United Network for Organ Sharing (UNOS) database. Over a median follow-up of 5 years, NASH patients with preserved renal function had a lower risk of death than those with eGFR less than 30 mL/min/1.73 m^2; however, similar rates of death and graft loss were seen for NASH patients who had undergone SLKT and those with reduced renal function (<30 mL/min/1.73 m^2) at the time of LT and/or received dialysis within 2 weeks preceding LT. It is suggested that this mortality may have been driven by persistent kidney dysfunction post-LT and increased risk of cardiovascular mortality.[29]

Alcohol, hepatitis B virus (HBV) infection, and HCV infection are other leading worldwide indications for LT that can be associated with CKD. There is a strong association between infection with HBV or HCV and glomerulopathies. Membranous nephropathy, membranoproliferative glomerulonephritis, and polyarteritis nodosa are associated with HBV infection. Less commonly, this virus has also been implicated in other renal diseases such as mesangial proliferative glomerulonephritis, immunoglobulin A (IgA) nephropathy, focal segmental glomerulosclerosis, minimal change disease, and amyloidosis.[30] Although HCV infection has been suggested as a possible cause of membranous nephropathy, it remains unclear if there is a definitive association. In contrast to HBV infection, complement levels are usually normal in individuals with HCV infection and membranous nephropathy, and neither cryoglobulins nor rheumatoid factor are present. Membranoproliferative glomerulonephritis is characterized by the deposition of circulating antigen-antibody complexes in the mesangium and subendothelial space. Although HBV infection is a rare cause of membranoproliferative glomerulonephritis, cryoglobulinemia associated with HCV infection is a well-established cause of this glomerulopathy.[4] Renal dysfunction may occur because of immune complex deposition along the glomerular capillary walls and the mesangium. Moreover, alcohol-related cirrhosis is associated with alterations of IgA metabolism and increased risk of deposition in the glomerular mesangium that can lead to clinically overt IgA nephropathy, which can progress to CKD and adversely affect prognosis. IgA nephropathy may present with microscopic or gross hematuria and proteinuria ranging from mild to nephrotic range.[31]

RENAL DYSFUNCTION IN LT RECIPIENTS

AKI after LT has been reported in 17% to 95% of patients with the wide range mainly reflecting the lack of a standardized definition of AKI.[32] It has been estimated that up to 15% of LT recipients will require transient RRT.[25] Posttransplant AKI is typically due to a combination of factors which include ischemic renal insults, pre-existing renal dysfunction, intraoperative events, and drug-induced nephrotoxicity. Patients with decompensated cirrhosis are more susceptible to perioperative renal ischemia and are prone to develop AKI in the perioperative period. This is likely due to renal vasoconstriction induced by the activation of endogenous vasoactive systems during and after LT.[11]

Renal hypoperfusion with potential ischemic injury occurs during the anhepatic phase of LT as a result of cross-clamping of the portal vein and inferior vena cava. Reperfusion after unclamping the portal vein also frequently causes hemodynamic instability.[33] Prolonged hypotension defines the postreperfusion syndrome, which is characterized by decreased systemic vascular resistance, increased pulmonary resistance, and impaired cardiac output leading to ischemia.[33] This ischemia-reperfusion leads to the release of proinflammatory cytokines (eg, IL-6, TNF-alpha) which will trigger an inflammatory response and subsequent cellular damages (especially renal tubular injury), further increasing the risk of AKI. Vena cava–sparring techniques directed to maintain venous return, such as the cava-preserving piggyback (partial cava clamping during anhepatic phase), have not been shown to improve renal function or reduce renal complications post-LT.[34] If surgical portocaval shunt is not feasible, extracorporeal venovenous bypass can be used in patients with portal HTN to lessen hemodynamic instability. Although venovenous bypass improves hemodynamic parameters during this phase, it has not been consistently shown to reduce the incidence of postoperative AKI.[35] In contrast, improvements in surgical technique have markedly shortened the anhepatic phase and reduced intraoperative bleeding, with consequential lower incidence of postoperative AKI.

CNIs such as tacrolimus and cyclosporine remain the mainstay of immunosuppression post-LT. However, these agents are also the leading cause of renal dysfunction in LT recipients.[1,2] The nephrotoxic potential of CNIs is largely attributed to their vasoconstrictive effect on the afferent and efferent glomerular arterioles, with reduction of renal blood flow, ultrafiltration coefficient, and GFR. Although the precise mechanisms by which these agents cause renal vasoconstriction remains unclear, an imbalance of vasoactive substances such as nitric oxide, prostaglandins, endothelin, thromboxane, and angiotensin II has been described. Renal hypoxia from chronic vasoconstriction leads to the formation of reactive oxygen species that cause renal cellular injury and promote apoptosis. Intricate signaling pathways promote renal fibrosis through stimulation of synthesis and inhibition of degradation of extracellular matrix. Furthermore, chronic CNI nephrotoxicity leads to irreversible structural glomerular damage, characterized histologically by obliterative arteriolopathy, glomerular ischemic collapse, tubular vacuolization, and focal areas of tubular atrophy.[36]

Acute CNI nephrotoxicity is largely reversible following dose reduction or interruption of therapy and is primarily related to vasoconstriction of the afferent and efferent glomerular arterioles, resulting in diminished glomerular perfusion, typically manifesting as acute elevations in sCr levels. In contrast, chronic CNI nephrotoxicity is typically irreversible and characterized by progressive renal dysfunction due to glomerulopathy, vascular disease, tubular dysfunction, and chronic systemic HTN. Long-term use of CNIs resulted in eGFR $\leq$ 29 mL/min/1.73 m^2 in up to 18% of nonrenal solid organ transplant recipients (including liver, heart, and lung) during a mean follow-up of 36 months, and approximately one-third of these patients eventually progress to ESRD and require RRT.[1,19] Although some conflicting data exist, in general, CNI nephrotoxicity occurs with equivalent frequency with cyclosporine and tacrolimus.[1,37] Hence, substituting one agent for the other for the sole purpose of attenuating renal dysfunction is not recommended. There is a well-established relationship between CNI dose/plasma levels and nephrotoxicity.[38] Importantly, drug interactions leading to increased plasma levels may augment the nephrotoxic potential of CNIs. Preexisting intrinsic renal disease, as well as concomitant use of other potentially nephrotoxic agents or conditions associated with hypotension or volume depletion, may also increase the risk of CNI nephrotoxicity.

Systemic HTN is evident typically early after initiation of CNI therapy in LT recipients. Calcium channel blockade is the preferred approach. Posttransplant DM associated with long-term use of CNIs also increases the risk of future renal dysfunction. Optimal glycemic control is crucial to prevent microvascular complications, including renal disease. Renal tubular acidosis, magnesium wasting, and impaired potassium secretion resulting in hyperkalemia, hypophosphatemia, and hypomagnesemia are typically transient and rarely require dose adjustments. Hyperuricemia is also common but infrequently causes symptomatic gout.[39]

Although the inhibitors of the mammalian target of rapamycin (mTOR) appear to have no intrinsic nephrotoxic potential when used without concomitant CNIs, data from renal transplant recipients suggest that sirolimus inhibits renal tubular cell proliferation, resulting in impaired recovery from delayed graft function.[40] Furthermore, sirolimus has been implicated as a cause of cast nephropathy, proteinuria, and collapsing focal segmental glomerulosclerosis.[41] Although data about everolimus nephrotoxicity are limited, concurrent use of this agent with a CNI does result in increased sCr and proteinuria.[42,43]

The quality of the donor liver graft is also an important factor in the outcome of kidney injury. Donor variables associated with severe ischemia-reperfusion injury include advanced age, steatosis, prolonged cold, and warm ischemia time.[44,45] Early allograft dysfunction, which is more commonly seen with extended criteria donors, is associated with posttransplant AKI requiring RRT within the first month and long-term CKD.[46] Recipients of donation after circulatory death (DCD) liver grafts are at higher risk of developing renal dysfunction post-LT when compared with donation after brain death (DBD) or living donor liver transplantation.[47] A study published by the Birmingham group in 2012 showed that recipients of DCD liver grafts had higher rates of AKI and CKD within the first 3 years of transplantation.[48] Furthermore, AKI resulted in significantly lower 3- and 5-year survival rates. Conversely, a recent study reported no direct relation between the use of DCD or marginal DBD (donor age >70 years, donor BMI >35 kg/m^2, or cold ischemia time >12 hours) liver grafts and CKD post-LT. High MELD score and elevated sCr at transplant may also predict the need for post-LT RRT in DCD recipients, as reported by others.[47]

CKD AFTER LT

Most LT recipients recover from postoperative AKI, despite the frequent need for temporary RRT. However, a significant proportion of recipients develop CKD, resulting in ESRD requiring RRT or kidney transplantation years after LT. A 50% increase in sCr from baseline within 1 week post-LT has been associated with the development of CKD within 1 year.[49] In addition, even mild AKI was associated with reduced patient and graft survival.[49] A recently published large study using United Network for Organ Sharing and Organ Procurement and Transplantation Network (UNOS/OPTN) registry data (2002–2017) reported that patients with CKD at the time of transplant had an adjusted 16% increased risk of death post-LT—an effect that was independent of receiving an SLKT.[50]

In a large study published in 2014 from the Mayo Clinic, two-thirds of the recipients developed CKD 10 years post-LT.[51] However, there is a wide range between studies because of the different criteria used for CKD and variable follow-up. LT recipients seem to develop CKD after transplantation at higher rates compared with heart and lung transplant recipients, with a 5-year cumulative incidence of 22%.[32] The etiology of renal dysfunction was found to be attributable to one or more of the following etiologies: CNI toxicity (48%), hypertensive vascular changes (44%), membranoproliferative glomerulonephritis (17%), IgA nephropathy (9%), diabetic nephropathy (9%), proliferative glomerulonephritis with crescents (4%), and ATN (4%).[52]

PREVENTION AND MANAGEMENT OF RENAL DYSFUNCTION IN LT RECIPIENTS
Preoperative Prevention

Candidates for LT with cirrhosis and ascites are typically at high risk of developing AKI before and immediately after LT. Diuretics should be used with caution and be discontinued even in cases of a mild increase in sCr. Albumin should be administered in patients undergoing large-volume paracentesis or concomitantly with intravenous antibiotics for treatment of SBP.[53] However, there is no evidence that albumin in addition to antibiotics reduces the incidence of AKI in patients with bacterial infections other than SBP.[25] As bacterial infections are a frequent precipitant of AKI in cirrhosis, early antibiotic administration is essential in patients with confirmed or suspected infections.[54] It has been shown that primary prophylaxis of SBP in patients with low protein ascitic concentration delays HRS and improves survival.[25,55]

Nonsteroidal anti-inflammatory drugs should be avoided in LT candidates, as these may induce a variety of renal function, including hemodynamically mediated AKI through inhibition of prostaglandin synthesis.[56] Nephrotoxic antibiotics such as aminoglycosides should also be avoided, and contrast-enhanced imaging studies should be ordered judiciously to minimize the risk of contrast-induced nephropathy.

Posttransplant Renal Impairment

Diligent monitoring of renal function permits early identification of renal dysfunction and implementation of measures that may attenuate renal injury and minimize chronic sequelae. Therapeutic drug monitoring of plasma levels of CNIs and dose adjustments, implementation of renal-sparing protocols, and avoidance of nephrotoxic agents are fundamental interventions to prevent renal dysfunction post-LT. CNI dose reduction remains the most effective intervention to decrease the progression of renal dysfunction due to CNI nephrotoxicity. Although some data suggest that blockade of the RAAS with angiotensin-converting enzyme inhibitors or angiotensin receptor blockers may reduce renal fibrosis in animal models of CNI nephrotoxicity,[57] this benefit has not been confirmed in humans, with induction of hyperkalemia a possible consequence.

Delayed Introduction of CNIs

Delayed introduction of CNIs is a common strategy for patients with renal dysfunction at the time of LT. This can also be accomplished with the use of potent antibody-based induction therapy in addition to mycophenolate and/or steroids, which permits a 4- to 10-day delay in CNI introduction.[58] This approach improves renal function at 1- and 6-month posttransplantation without increasing the risk of acute rejection.[59,60] It should be noted that absorption of oral mycophenolate may be slow, so many units give mycophenolate intravenously for the first few days.

In a multicenter randomized controlled trial (DIAMOND study), immunosuppression with low-dose prolonged-release tacrolimus (0.15–0.175 mg/kg/d) immediately posttransplantation plus basiliximab and mycophenolate (without maintenance corticosteroids) was associated with significantly reduced incidence of impaired renal function and acute cellular rejection (ACR) when compared with higher first-dose of prolonged-release tacrolimus (0.2 mg/kg/d). Delayed higher-dose prolonged-release tacrolimus initiation significantly reduced renal dysfunction compared with immediate posttransplant administration, with comparable incidence of ACR. Delaying tacrolimus initiation for several days after transplantation to preserve kidney function is also supported by results from the ReSpECT trial.[61,62]

As reported by Verna and colleagues, basiliximab induction is effective in delaying CNI initiation and was associated with stability or return of renal function. The study group received basiliximab in addition to steroids and mycophenolate mofetil (MMF). CNIs initiation was achieved after significant improvement in renal function had occurred with a goal of starting the CNIs at lower doses.[58] Basiliximab induction resulted in 30-day and 1-year patient, graft, and renal outcomes comparable to those of a control group receiving standard CNI-based immunosuppression.

Addition of Other Drugs to CNIs

For those on long-term CNI regimens, combination therapy such as CNI, mycophenolate, and prednisolone or CNI and an mTOR inhibitor (sirolimus/everolimus) may allow use of lower doses of CNI. Most studies have demonstrated that use of mTOR inhibitors results in improvement in GFR.[42,43,63] Notably, the mTOR inhibitor containing arms did have higher adverse events such as infections, proteinuria, and dyslipidemia. The two main mTOR inhibitors studied have been sirolimus (SRL) and everolimus (EVR) with EVR demonstrating a better safety profile. A meta-analysis of randomized controlled trials of EVR with early withdrawal or CNI dose minimization reported improvement in GFR without increase in ACR, graft loss, or mortality.[64]

In a multicenter, open-label, randomized, prospective phase II study, LT recipients receiving standard-dose tacrolimus versus SRL and reduced-dose tacrolimus had an increased risk of sepsis, graft loss, and mortality at 24 months in the SRL arm. This led to early discontinuation of the study.[65] A higher rate of hepatic artery thrombosis and portal vein thrombosis was also observed in the SRL arm (8% vs 3%, $P = .065$). Increased rates of ACR and adverse events such as new-onset diabetes and cardiovascular events have also been reported in patients receiving SRL.[66,67]

Administration of short-term induction therapy with monoclonal or polyclonal antibodies with delayed introduction of CNIs in the immediate post-LT period as a renal protective strategy has also been studied.[68] Belatacept is a monoclonal fusion antibody that selectively inhibits T-cell activation through costimulation blockade. This molecule was also studied as a potential CNI reduction strategy. However, in a multicenter phase II trial, most belatacept-containing arms experienced higher rates of ACR, and the study was eventually halted because of higher rates of death in the belatacept-containing groups.[69]

Most data indicate that early nephroprotective strategies are more effective than late interventions. Introduction of mTOR inhibitors, both SRL and EVR, to replace CNIs beyond the first year of transplant has not shown to be substantially beneficial.[70,71] There are some data suggesting that reducing CNI doses with continued use of MMF may be beneficial in terms of improving renal function with no increase in ACR rates.[72] However, use of MMF alone with complete withdrawal of CNIs—while protective of the kidneys—is associated with increased rates of ACR and possible graft loss.

Withdrawal of CNIs

If necessary, patients can be switched to regimens such as SRL or EVR monotherapy, or prednisolone and mycophenolate, or azathioprine. There is little data to guide the timing of such withdrawal, but it is reasonable to consider this when the GFR falls below 50 mL/min/1.73 m^2. Most centers will start the recipient on the new regimen and, if well tolerated and target levels achieved, the CNI is gradually withdrawn. The use of EVR permits complete withdrawal of CNIs, with improvement in renal function and similar patient and graft outcomes after 5 years of follow-up. However, an increased risk of overall infections has been reported with the use of this agent.[64] SRL-based CNI-sparing regimens also improve renal function; however, rejection has been reported in 11% of patients, and proteinuria, hyperlipidemia, and oral ulcerations may be undesirable adverse events.[71] Conversion to SRL- or EVR-based regimens should not be considered if there is significant proteinuria. In those transplanted for hepatocellular carcinoma or who have developed some posttransplant de novo malignancies such as some skin cancers, earlier switching may be beneficial.[73] Neither mycophenolate nor mTOR inhibitors should be used in those who are planning pregnancy.

RENAL REPLACEMENT THERAPY

The optimal timing of RRT initiation remains a topic of much debate. Similar to non-transplant patients, the decision to initiate RRT should be made on clinical grounds, taking into account electrolyte and acid-base disturbances, oliguria, volume overload, and diuretic resistance. RRT should be considered as a bridge to LT in patients with HRS and not a definitive treatment option. Early RRT in non-ESLD patients with AKI has been suggested to confer mortality benefit; however, this finding has not been translated to ESLD patients. At the eighth International Consensus Conference of the ADQI group, it was recommended that RRT should be withheld in HRS-AKI unless there is an acute reversible component or a plan for LT.[8]

Intraoperative management of patients with cirrhosis and AKI during LT surgery remains challenging, particularly due to profound changes in intravascular volume status as well as acid-base and electrolyte disturbances. Data evaluating the use of intraoperative continuous RRT have been limited to case series and retrospective cohorts. Proponents of intraoperative RRT highlight the better control of temperature, electrolyte, and volume management during critical phases of LT surgery such as reperfusion. A recent pilot randomized-controlled trial suggests that intraoperative continuous RRT is feasible as an adjuvant measure, with no difference in complications, does not require anticoagulation, and offers promising 1-year survival (92%).[74] Nonetheless, intraoperative RRT carries risks and requires additional resources (eg, extracorporeal circuit, trained personnel, etc), and further studies are needed to corroborate its beneficial effect.[75]

SIMULTANEOUS LIVER AND KIDNEY TRANSPLANTATION

As discussed earlier, renal impairment is an important predictor of poor outcomes after LT; thus, it is important to identify candidates for SLKT during the evaluation process for LT. However, it is difficult to predict which patients will recover renal function after LT. A study published in 2015 comparing 3127 patients who underwent SLKT versus 422 patients listed for SLKT who underwent isolated LT showed that the latter group had higher mortality from cardiovascular events within 2 days of posttransplantation, as well as 1.2-fold and 2-fold higher odds of mortality and liver graft loss, respectively. In contrast, after excluding patients who received a kidney transplant within the first-year post-LT, 33% recovered renal function to a GFR greater than 60 mL/min/1.73 m^2 and only less than 5% needed renal transplantation.[76] Moreover, there are some differences in criteria for candidacy for SLKT (**Table 5**). In the latest guidelines from the UNOS/OPTN, eligibility criteria for SLKT are AKI requiring dialysis or having a GFR less than 25 mL/min/1.73 m^2 at least once every 7 days in the last

Table 5
Indications for simultaneous liver and kidney transplant in cirrhotic patients

United States (OPTN/UNOS)	European Association for the Study of Liver
• AKI and 6 wk of consecutive dialysis; or, AKI for 6 wk with an eGFR ≤ 25 mL/min; or, AKI and 6 wk of a combination of both • Patients with end-stage renal disease chronically administered dialysis • CKD stage 3 for >90 d with an eGFR of ≤30 mL/min • Presence of comorbid metabolic disease (eg, hyperoxaluria)	• AKI on RRT for ≥4 wk or AKI with eGFR ≤35 mL/min; or, measured GFR ≤25 mL/min ≥4 wk • CKD with eGFR ≤40 mL/min or measured GFR ≤30 mL/min • CKD with proteinuria ≥2 g a day • CKD with renal biopsy showing >30% global glomerulosclerosis or >30% interstitial fibrosis • Presence of inherited metabolic disease (eg, hyperoxaluria)

Abbreviations: AKI, acute kidney injury; CKD, chronic kidney disease; eGFR, estimated glomerular filtration rate; OPTN, Organ Procurement and Transplantation Network; UNOS, United Network for Organ Sharing.

6 weeks (or a combination of both).[77] In contrast, European guidelines recommend SLKT in patients with sustained AKI irrespective of its type, including HRS-AKI when refractory to drug therapy, with the following conditions: (1) AKI on RRT for ≥4 weeks or (2) eGFR ≤35 mL/min/1.73 m^2 or measured GFR ≤25 mL/min/1.73 m^2 for ≥4 weeks. Beyond these 2 conditions, the option of SLKT may be considered in the presence of risk factors for underlying undiagnosed CKD (diabetes, HTN, abnormal renal imaging, and proteinuria >2 g/d).[10]

SUMMARY

The prevalence of renal dysfunction in LT recipients continues to rise, paralleling increased long-term survival of the population. Its etiology is typically multifactorial, with CNI nephrotoxicity and pretransplant renal dysfunction being major risk factors. Eligibility criteria to select candidates for SLKT have been established, highlighting that recovery of renal function may not be anticipated in selected patients. Both delayed introduction of CNIs and renal-sparing immunosuppressive regimens offer some benefit with regards to reducing the progression of renal dysfunction and are currently used on an individual basis by most transplant centers.

CLINICS CARE POINTS

- Delayed introduction of CNIs with the use of induction therapy is a common strategy to prevent renal dysfunction after LT without increasing the risk of acute rejection.

- Therapeutic drug monitoring of plasma levels of CNI and implementation of renal-sparing protocols are fundamental interventions to prevent renal injury after LT.

- If CNI withdrawal is necessary, patients can be switched to regimens such as sirolimus or everolimus monotherapy, azathioprine or steroids and mycophenolate.

- The optimal timing of RRT initiation in the peri-transplant period is controversial, the decision should be made on clinical grounds.

- Since renal dysfunction is an important predictor of poor outcomes after LT, it is important to identify candidates for SKLT during the pretransplant evaluation process.

DISCLOSURE

The authors have nothing to disclose.

REFERENCES

1. Ojo AO, Held PJ, Port FK, et al. Chronic renal failure after transplantation of a non-renal organ. N Engl J Med 2003;349(10):931–40.
2. Bennett WM. Insights into chronic cyclosporine nephrotoxicity. Int J Clin Pharmacol Ther 1996;34(11):515–9.
3. Lucey MR, Terrault N, Ojo L, et al. Long-term management of the successful adult liver transplant: 2012 practice guideline by the American Association for the Study of Liver Diseases and the American Society of Transplantation. Liver Transpl 2013;19(1):3–26.
4. Baid S, Cosimi AB, Tolkoff-Rubin N, et al. Renal disease associated with hepatitis C infection after kidney and liver transplantation. Transplantation 2000;70(2): 255–61.
5. Carrion AF, Martin P. Care of the liver transplant recipient. Liver Transplant 2021;403–8.
6. Thomas ME, Blaine C, Dawnay A, et al. The definition of acute kidney injury and its use in practice. Kidney Int 2015;87(1):62–73.
7. Thakar CV, Christianson A, Freyberg R, et al. Incidence and outcomes of acute kidney injury in intensive care units: a veterans administration study. Crit Care Med 2009;37(9):2552–8.
8. Nadim MK, Kellum JA, Davenport A, et al. Hepatorenal syndrome: the 8th international consensus conference of the acute dialysis quality initiative (ADQI) group. Crit Care 2012;16(1):R23.
9. Piano S, Rosi S, Maresio G, et al. Evaluation of the acute kidney injury network criteria in hospitalized patients with cirrhosis and ascites. J Hepatol 2013;59(3): 482–9.
10. European Association for the Study of the Liver. Electronic address eee, European Association for the Study of the L. EASL Clinical Practice Guidelines for the management of patients with decompensated cirrhosis. J Hepatol 2018; 69(2):406–60.
11. Durand F, Graupera I, Gines P, et al. Pathogenesis of hepatorenal syndrome: implications for therapy. Am J Kidney Dis 2016;67(2):318–28.
12. Angeli P, Gines P, Wong F, et al. Diagnosis and management of acute kidney injury in patients with cirrhosis: revised consensus recommendations of the International Club of Ascites. J Hepatol 2015;62(4):968–74.
13. Adebayo D, Neong SF, Wong F. Ascites and hepatorenal syndrome. Clin Liver Dis 2019;23(4):659–82.
14. Dirchwolf M, Podhorzer A, Marino M, et al. Immune dysfunction in cirrhosis: distinct cytokines phenotypes according to cirrhosis severity. Cytokine 2016;77: 14–25.
15. Claria J, Stauber RE, Coenraad MJ, et al. Systemic inflammation in decompensated cirrhosis: characterization and role in acute-on-chronic liver failure. Hepatology 2016;64(4):1249–64.
16. Gines P, Sola E, Angeli P, et al. Author correction: hepatorenal syndrome. Nat Rev Dis Primers 2018;4(1):33.
17. Sherman DS, Fish DN, Teitelbaum I. Assessing renal function in cirrhotic patients: problems and pitfalls. Am J Kidney Dis 2003;41(2):269–78.

18. Jones CA, McQuillan GM, Kusek JW, et al. Serum creatinine levels in the US population: third national health and nutrition examination survey. Am J Kidney Dis 1998;32(6):992–9.

19. Carrion AF, Radhakrishnan R, Martin P. Diagnosis and management of renal dysfunction in patients with cirrhosis. Expert Rev Gastroenterol Hepatol 2020; 14(1):1–7.

20. Gupta K, Bhurwal A, Law C, et al. Acute kidney injury and hepatorenal syndrome in cirrhosis. World J Gastroenterol 2021;27(26):3984–4003.

21. Amathieu R, Al-Khafaji A, Sileanu FE, et al. Significance of oliguria in critically ill patients with chronic liver disease. Hepatology 2017;66(5):1592–600.

22. Horvatits T, Pischke S, Proske VM, et al. Outcome and natural course of renal dysfunction in liver transplant recipients with severely impaired kidney function prior to transplantation. United Eur Gastroenterol J 2018;6(1):104–11.

23. Gonwa TA, McBride MA, Anderson K, et al. Continued influence of preoperative renal function on outcome of orthotopic liver transplant (OLTX) in the US: where will MELD lead us? Am J Transplant 2006;6(11):2651–9.

24. Byrne CD, Targher G. NAFLD as a driver of chronic kidney disease. J Hepatol 2020;72(4):785–801.

25. Durand F, Francoz C, Asrani SK, et al. Acute kidney injury after liver transplantation. Transplantation 2018;102(10):1636–49.

26. Musso G, Gambino R, Tabibian JH, et al. Association of non-alcoholic fatty liver disease with chronic kidney disease: a systematic review and meta-analysis. PLoS Med 2014;11(7):e1001680.

27. Asrani SK, O'Leary JG. The changing liver transplant waitlist: an emerging liver purgatory? Gastroenterology 2015;148(3):493–6.

28. Singal AK, Hasanin M, Kaif M, et al. Nonalcoholic steatohepatitis is the most rapidly growing indication for simultaneous liver kidney transplantation in the United States. Transplantation 2016;100(3):607–12.

29. Molnar MZ, Joglekar K, Jiang Y, et al. Association of pretransplant renal function with liver graft and patient survival after liver transplantation in patients with nonalcoholic steatohepatitis. Liver Transpl 2019;25(3):399–410.

30. Fabrizi F, Martin P, Messa P. Hepatitis B and hepatitis C virus and chronic kidney disease. Acta Gastroenterol Belg 2010;73(4):465–71.

31. Morales JM, Pascual-Capdevila J, Campistol JM, et al. Membranous glomerulonephritis associated with hepatitis C virus infection in renal transplant patients. Transplantation 1997;63(11):1634–9.

32. Weber ML, Ibrahim HN, Lake JR. Renal dysfunction in liver transplant recipients: evaluation of the critical issues. Liver Transpl 2012;18(11):1290–301.

33. Aggarwal S, Kang Y, Freeman JA, et al. Postreperfusion syndrome: hypotension after reperfusion of the transplanted liver. J Crit Care 1993;8(3):154–60.

34. Widmer JD, Schlegel A, Ghazaly M, et al. Piggyback or cava replacement: which implantation technique protects liver recipients from acute kidney injury and complications? Liver Transpl 2018;24(12):1746–56.

35. Sun K, Hong F, Wang Y, et al. Venovenous bypass is associated with a lower incidence of acute kidney injury after liver transplantation in patients with compromised pretransplant renal function. Anesth Analg 2017;125(5):1463–70.

36. Charlton MR, Wall WJ, Ojo AO, et al. Report of the first international liver transplantation society expert panel consensus conference on renal insufficiency in liver transplantation. Liver Transpl 2009;15(11):S1–34.

37. English RF, Pophal SA, Bacanu SA, et al. Long-term comparison of tacrolimus-and cyclosporine-induced nephrotoxicity in pediatric heart-transplant recipients. Am J Transpl 2002;2(8):769–73.

38. Naesens M, Kuypers DR, Sarwal M. Calcineurin inhibitor nephrotoxicity. Clin J Am Soc Nephrol 2009;4(2):481–508.

39. Farouk SS, Rein JL. The many faces of calcineurin inhibitor toxicity-what the FK? Adv Chronic Kidney Dis 2020;27(1):56–66.

40. McTaggart RA, Gottlieb D, Brooks J, et al. Sirolimus prolongs recovery from delayed graft function after cadaveric renal transplantation. Am J Transpl 2003;3(4): 416–23.

41. Letavernier E, Bruneval P, Mandet C, et al. High sirolimus levels may induce focal segmental glomerulosclerosis de novo. Clin J Am Soc Nephrol 2007;2(2):326–33.

42. Fischer L, Klempnauer J, Beckebaum S, et al. A randomized, controlled study to assess the conversion from calcineurin-inhibitors to everolimus after liver transplantation–PROTECT. Am J Transpl 2012;12(7):1855–65.

43. Saliba F, De Simone P, Nevens F, et al. Renal function at two years in liver transplant patients receiving everolimus: results of a randomized, multicenter study. Am J Transpl 2013;13(7):1734–45.

44. Leithead JA, Rajoriya N, Gunson BK, et al. The evolving use of higher risk grafts is associated with an increased incidence of acute kidney injury after liver transplantation. J Hepatol 2014;60(6):1180–6.

45. Saidi RF, Kenari SK. Liver ischemia/reperfusion injury: an overview. J Invest Surg 2014;27(6):366–79.

46. Wadei HM, Gonwa TA, Taner CB. Simultaneous liver kidney transplant (SLK) allocation policy change proposal: is it really a smart move? Am J Transpl 2016;16(9): 2763–4.

47. Kollmann D, Neong SF, Rosales R, et al. Renal dysfunction after liver transplantation: effect of donor type. Liver Transpl 2020;26(6):799–810.

48. Leithead JA, Tariciotti L, Gunson B, et al. Donation after cardiac death liver transplant recipients have an increased frequency of acute kidney injury. Am J Transpl 2012;12(4):965–75.

49. Barri YM, Sanchez EQ, Jennings LW, et al. Acute kidney injury following liver transplantation: definition and outcome. Liver Transpl 2009;15(5):475–83.

50. Cullaro G, Verna EC, Lee BP, et al. Chronic kidney disease in liver transplant candidates: a rising burden impacting post-liver transplant outcomes. Liver Transpl 2020;26(4):498–506.

51. Allen AM, Kim WR, Therneau TM, et al. Chronic kidney disease and associated mortality after liver transplantation–a time-dependent analysis using measured glomerular filtration rate. J Hepatol 2014;61(2):286–92.

52. O'Riordan A, Dutt N, Cairns H, et al. Renal biopsy in liver transplant recipients. Nephrol Dial Transplant 2009;24(7):2276–82.

53. Sort P, Navasa M, Arroyo V, et al. Effect of intravenous albumin on renal impairment and mortality in patients with cirrhosis and spontaneous bacterial peritonitis. N Engl J Med 1999;341(6):403–9.

54. Fernandez J, Acevedo J, Wiest R, et al. Bacterial and fungal infections in acute-on-chronic liver failure: prevalence, characteristics and impact on prognosis. Gut 2018;67(10):1870–80.

55. Fernandez J, Navasa M, Planas R, et al. Primary prophylaxis of spontaneous bacterial peritonitis delays hepatorenal syndrome and improves survival in cirrhosis. Gastroenterology 2007;133(3):818–24.

56. Elia C, Graupera I, Barreto R, et al. Severe acute kidney injury associated with non-steroidal anti-inflammatory drugs in cirrhosis: a case-control study. J Hepatol 2015;63(3):593–600.

57. Mortensen LA, Bistrup C, Thiesson HC. Does mineralocorticoid receptor antagonism prevent calcineurin inhibitor-induced nephrotoxicity? Front Med (Lausanne) 2017;4:210.

58. Verna EC, Farrand ED, Elnaggar AS, et al. Basiliximab induction and delayed calcineurin inhibitor initiation in liver transplant recipients with renal insufficiency. Transplantation 2011;91(11):1254–60.

59. Yoshida EM, Marotta PJ, Greig PD, et al. Evaluation of renal function in liver transplant recipients receiving daclizumab (Zenapax), mycophenolate mofetil, and a delayed, low-dose tacrolimus regimen vs. a standard-dose tacrolimus and mycophenolate mofetil regimen: a multicenter randomized clinical trial. Liver Transpl 2005;11(9):1064–72.

60. Soliman T, Hetz H, Burghuber C, et al. Short-term induction therapy with antithymocyte globulin and delayed use of calcineurin inhibitors in orthotopic liver transplantation. Liver Transpl 2007;13(7):1039–44.

61. TruneCka P, Klempnauer J, Bechstein WO, et al. Renal function in de novo liver transplant recipients receiving different prolonged-release tacrolimus regimens-The DIAMOND Study. Am J Transpl 2015;15(7):1843–54.

62. Neuberger JM, Mamelok RD, Neuhaus P, et al. Delayed introduction of reduced-dose tacrolimus, and renal function in liver transplantation: the 'ReSpECT' study. Am J Transpl 2009;9(2):327–36.

63. Fischer L, Saliba F, Kaiser GM, et al. Three-year outcomes in de novo liver transplant patients receiving everolimus with reduced tacrolimus: follow-up results from a randomized, multicenter study. Transplantation 2015;99(7):1455–62.

64. Lin M, Mittal S, Sahebjam F, et al. Everolimus with early withdrawal or reduced-dose calcineurin inhibitors improves renal function in liver transplant recipients: a systematic review and meta-analysis. Clin Transplant 2017;31(2).

65. Asrani SK, Wiesner RH, Trotter JF, et al. De novo sirolimus and reduced-dose tacrolimus versus standard-dose tacrolimus after liver transplantation: the 2000-2003 phase II prospective randomized trial. Am J Transpl 2014;14(2):356–66.

66. Teperman L, Moonka D, Sebastian A, et al. Calcineurin inhibitor-free mycophenolate mofetil/sirolimus maintenance in liver transplantation: the randomized spare-the-nephron trial. Liver Transpl 2013;19(7):675–89.

67. Weir MR, Pearson TC, Patel A, et al. Long-term follow-up of kidney transplant recipients in the spare-the-nephron-trial. Transplantation 2017;101(1):157–65.

68. Calmus Y, Kamar N, Gugenheim J, et al. Assessing renal function with daclizumab induction and delayed tacrolimus introduction in liver transplant recipients. Transplantation 2010;89(12):1504–10.

69. Klintmalm GB, Feng S, Lake JR, et al. Belatacept-based immunosuppression in de novo liver transplant recipients: 1-year experience from a phase II randomized study. Am J Transpl 2014;14(8):1817–27.

70. Levitsky J, O'Leary JG, Asrani S, et al. Protecting the kidney in liver transplant recipients: practice-based recommendations from the American Society of transplantation liver and intestine community of practice. Am J Transpl 2016;16(9):2532–44.

71. Abdelmalek MF, Humar A, Stickel F, et al. Sirolimus conversion regimen versus continued calcineurin inhibitors in liver allograft recipients: a randomized trial. Am J Transpl 2012;12(3):694–705.

72. Goralczyk AD, Bari N, Abu-Ajaj W, et al. Calcineurin inhibitor sparing with myco-phenolate mofetil in liver transplantion: a systematic review of randomized controlled trials. Am J Transpl 2012;12(10):2601–7.

73. Duvoux C, Toso C. mTOR inhibitor therapy: does it prevent HCC recurrence after liver transplantation? Transpl Rev (Orlando) 2015;29(3):168–74.

74. Karvellas CJ, Taylor S, Bigam D, et al. Intraoperative continuous renal replace-ment therapy during liver transplantation: a pilot randomized-controlled trial (INCEPTION). Can J Anaesth 2019;66(10):1151–61.

75. Nanchal R, Subramanian R, Karvellas CJ, et al. Guidelines for the management of adult acute and acute-on-chronic liver failure in the ICU: cardiovascular, endo-crine, hematologic, pulmonary, and renal considerations. Crit Care Med 2020; 48(3):e173–91.

76. Hmoud B, Kuo YF, Wiesner RH, et al. Outcomes of liver transplantation alone after listing for simultaneous kidney: comparison to simultaneous liver kidney trans-plantation. Transplantation 2015;99(4):823–8.

77. Formica RN, Aeder M, Boyle G, et al. Simultaneous liver-kidney allocation policy: a proposal to optimize appropriate utilization of scarce resources. Am J Transpl 2016;16(3):758–66.

Moving?

Make sure your subscription moves with you!

To notify us of your new address, find your **Clinics Account Number** (located on your mailing label above your name), and contact customer service at:

Email: journalscustomerservice-usa@elsevier.com

800-654-2452 (subscribers in the U.S. & Canada)
314-447-8871 (subscribers outside of the U.S. & Canada)

Fax number: 314-447-8029

Elsevier Health Sciences Division
Subscription Customer Service
3251 Riverport Lane
Maryland Heights, MO 63043

*To ensure uninterrupted delivery of your subscription, please notify us at least 4 weeks in advance of move.

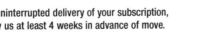

Printed and bound by CPI Group (UK) Ltd, Croydon, CR0 4YY

03/10/2024

01040474-0020